"From the moment I began an Integral Life Practice, it was as if my life was assigned a new trajectory and course setting from deep within the cockpit of my soul. 'Glory upon Glory' is the way my days are unfolding since I began to practice. An ILP is an incredible catalyst to growth in ways that I could never have imagined. See for yourself!"
— EDDIE KOWALCZYK, lead singer-songwriter of Live

"*Integral Life Practice* is an extraordinary achievement. Comprehensive, detailed, and powerfully rational, it inspires any and all of us to consider more deeply how profound is our embrace of the life we are living. The searing clarity of the integral perspective leaps off every page of this manual for personal evolution, clearly illuminating what it means to be fully alive!"
— ANDREW COHEN, spiritual teacher and founder of EnlightenNext

"Ken Wilber's Integral Theory has created a road map. Now Terry Patten, Adam Leonard, and Marco Morelli have added a GPS (Global *Practicing* System) with *Integral Life Practice*. Travelers on the spiritual path will find this book indispensable."
— BROTHER DAVID STEINDL-RAST, Benedictine monk, author of *Listening Heart: The Spirituality of Sacred Sensuousness* and *Gratefulness, The Heart of Prayer: An Approach to Life in Fullness* and cofounder of Gratefulness.org

"Once again, Ken Wilber and his colleagues have taken a big subject, swallowed the whole thing and the kitchen sink too, and then spent years working to understand it, digest it, metabolize it, and then translate it into clear prose and helpful practices. And the outcome? This wonderfully helpful manual for living: *Integral Life Practice*. A fantastic resource for a more peaceful, meaningful, intelligent, and exuberant life."
— ELIZABETH LESSER, author of *Broken Open: How Difficult Times Can Help Us Grow, The Seeker's Guide,* and cofounder of Omega Institute

"*Integral Life Practice* will help you build the healthy foundation from which you can wake up to your transcendent nature or Big Mind. Western aspirants have long needed a universal practice manual that wisely draws upon ancient traditions and modern science and psychology. Now we have it—an inspiring, straightforward guide for living a truly harmonious, awakened life."
— ZEN MASTER DENNIS GENPO MERZEL, author of *Big Mind, Big Heart: Finding Your Way*

"Ken Wilber and the authors of this clearly written, sensible, well-informed book are fellow explorers with George Leonard and me in the development of integral transformative practices. Such practices grow out of a philosophic vision dawning across the world that joins our aspiration for personal and social transformation with both science and the contemplative traditions. This book will advance this developing worldview and the disciplines needed to actualize it."
— MICHAEL MURPHY, author of *The Future of the Body* and *The Life We Are Given* and cofounder of Esalen Institute

"*Integral Life Practice* offers a finely honed distillation of some of the most effective and universal practices from the great wisdom traditions, at the same time presenting a context for practice that is both soaring and sensible. True to its title, it takes seriously the human need for fully balanced development, for depth as well as breadth, for psychological as well as spiritual development, for softness and toughness, for ethics and bold experimentation. Beautifully written, laid out in accessible modules, the book is truly an on-and-off-the-mat guide to 21st-century practice, arising from that place in us which stands in the best of tradition, yet rides the cutting edge."
— SWAMI SALLY KEMPTON, author of *The Heart of Meditation: Pathways to a Deeper Experience*

"This book spells out how to apply Integral philosophy to everyday life by working with body, mind, spirit, and the deeper psychological aspects of ourselves. *Integral Life Practice* presents a useful map of one's existential condition leading toward the attainment of the highest states of consciousness."
— TRALEG KYABGON RINPOCHE

"*Integral Life Practice* is a masterpiece guide of grounded, intelligent, self-transforming wisdom integrating the insights of all the great traditions of truth."
— CAROLINE MYSS, author of *Anatomy of the Spirit* and *Entering the Castle*

"*Integral Life Practice* brings the integral system from the mind to doable action in life. Here is a treasure of integral Upaya."
— RABBI ZALMAN SCHACHTER-SHALOMI, past holder of the World Wisdom Chair of Naropa University

"*Integral Life Practice* represents a particular milestone. It gives a lucid and easy to understand summary of the Integral thought-system, without dumbing it down—no mean feat. What's more, it describes in an engaging and practical way what to do in order to live from this elegant and inclusive worldview. If you want a clear and easy-to-follow map for waking up, read this book."
— BILL HARRIS, Director, Centerpointe Research Institute and creator of Holosync Meditation Technology

"Here we learn, through integral wisdom and disciplines, how to be freer and more fully authentic by ironing out the peaks of higher consciousness development into every nook and cranny of daily life. This is the secret of the integral life: transcending while including, and being there while getting there every single step of the way. Get ready to train your mind, open your heart, and awaken to your true universal Self."
— LAMA SURYA DAS, author of *Awakening the Buddha Within: Tibetan Wisdom for the Western World* and founder of the Dzogchen Meditation Centers

INTEGRAL LIFE PRACTICE

INTEGRAL LIFE PRACTICE

*A 21ˢᵗ-Century Blueprint for Physical
Health, Emotional Balance, Mental Clarity,
and Spiritual Awakening*

KEN WILBER, TERRY PATTEN,
ADAM LEONARD, and
MARCO MORELLI

INTEGRAL BOOKS
Boston & London
2008

INTEGRAL BOOKS
An imprint of Shambhala Publications, Inc.
Horticultural Hall
300 Massachusetts Avenue
Boston, Massachusetts 02115
www.shambhala.com

Cover images courtesy of iStockphoto.com, BigStockPhoto.com, Dreamstime.com, and Fotolia.com, and © of the respective artists. Also thanks to Wikipedia.org (Public Domain Portal) and Jenn Rensel (paints image, Flickr.com user "jenn_jenn," creative commons copyright).

9 8 7 6 5 4 3 2 1

FIRST EDITION
Printed in the United States of America

⊛ This edition is printed on acid-free paper that meets the American National Standards Institute Z39.48 Standard.
Distributed in the United States by Random House, Inc., and in Canada by Random House of Canada Ltd

Designed by Steve Dyer

Library of Congress Cataloging-in-Publication Data
Wilber, Ken
Integral life practice: a 21st-century blueprint for physical health, emotional balance, mental clarity, and spiritual awakening / Ken Wilber . . . [et al.].
p.   cm
Includes index.
ISBN 978-1-59030-467-9 (pbk.: alk. paper)
1. Self-actualization (Psychology)   I. Title.
BF637.S4W487 2008
158.1—dc22
2008015205

CONTENTS AT A GLANCE

CONTENTS

PREFACE

Welcome to the world of **Integral**! The fact that you have picked up this book means that you are ready to begin not just thinking about Integral but practicing and applying it as well. This is a truly momentous occasion, to judge from the developmental research itself.

Developmental models are in general agreement that human beings, from birth, go through a series of stages or waves of growth and development. The lower, earlier, junior stages are initial, partial, and fragmented views of the world, whereas the upper stages are integrated, comprehensive, and genuinely holistic. Because of this, the earlier stages are often called "first tier," and the higher stages are called "second tier."

The difference between the two tiers is truly profound. As pioneering developmental researcher Clare Graves put it, with second tier an individual "goes through a momentous leap of meaning." **That leap is what Integral is all about**—Integral Thinking and—yes—Integral Practice. At the Integral stages of development, the entire universe starts to make sense, to hang together, to actually appear as a **uni**-verse—a "one world"—a single, unified, integrated world that unites not only different philosophies and ideas about the world, but different practices for growth and development as well.

Integral Life Practice is just such an integrated practice, a practice that will help you grow and develop to your fullest capacities—to your ultimate Freedom and greatest Fullness in the world at large (in relationships, in work, in spirituality, in career, in play, in life itself). ILP is about developing your greatest FREEDOM from the world—freedom from your limitations, freedom from fragmentation, freedom from partialities—and your truest FULLNESS in the world—a fullness that includes and embraces all the seemingly partial aspects of yourself and your world into a seamless, whole, ultimately fulfilled life. Freedom and Fullness—to transcend all of life and to include all of life, unfolding and fulfilling your greatest capacities—is what Integral Life Practice is about.

As such, this "**transcending and including**" contains modules that address practices for the body, mind, spirit, and shadow dimensions of your own being. Because it is inclusive, this practice contains a distilled and condensed series of practices that are taken from premodern, modern, and postmodern approaches to growth and development. It is an "all-inclusive" practice in the sense that it takes the very best practices from all of them, and puts them together in a larger framework that uses—and makes sense of—all of them. **Premodern** practices include the world's great wisdom traditions and the meditation practices that drive them. **Modern** practices include scientific studies of human growth and ways to induce it. **Postmodern** practices include a pluralistic and multicultural composite map of the human territory—the territory of you—and ways to include (and not marginalize) all of the important dimensions of your own being (physical, emotional, mental, and spiritual—in self, culture, and nature).

Putting all of these together creates a "**cross training**" for human growth and spiritual awakening, a cross training that dramatically accelerates all of its dimensions—body, mind, spirit, and shadow—producing faster, more effective, more efficient practices than were ever possible prior to this time. It is the comprehensive, truly holistic, extraordinarily inclusive nature of Integral Life Practice that makes it the simplest practice you can do to truly wake up. Other approaches have part of the puzzle and therefore give you partial practices (and partial successes), whereas Integral Life Practice gives you a composite and comprehensive practice that covers all the essential bases, increasing the effectiveness and quickness of each, compared to when they are practiced alone. It is the dramatically increased speed and effectiveness of ILP that is one of its hallmarks.

ILP is practicing from the leading edge of evolution itself, from the In-

tegral stages and waves that are just beginning to evolutionarily unfold in
humanity at large. Being grounded in these Integral stages, ILP embodies, emerges, and attracts individuals to the same stages that produced it.
Put differently, Integral Life Practice is a second-tier practice—it comes
from second-tier, and it draws consciousness itself to second tier. Thus, it
trains both "altitude" and "aptitude"—altitude or vertical growth in consciousness, and aptitude or specific training in horizontal capacities. All
of this is included in the Integral Life Practice, which the following pages
will fully train you in. In short, ILP is a practice aimed at helping you discover your own "momentous leap of meaning," a leap that will radiantly
affect every aspect of your life.

So, once again, welcome to **Integral**. One of the advantages of this
particular book is the team of writers that created it. They have a broad
and fully qualified exposure to Integral Life Practice, both in its theory
and in its actual practice. The writing team is an integration of the richly
different backgrounds and perspectives of the co-authors. Although I did
not write any of these chapters myself, I fully participated in the writing
and its review, and oversaw the integration of the various perspectives and
experiences of the writers, reaching across generational and typological
differences. That's what Integral Life Practice is all about—integration—
and that is one of the many strengths of this book. The style turned out to
be accessible, transparent, and covering difficult topics with an easy-to-
understand clarity and humanity. I'm very happy with the results, and
proud to put my name on it.

Integral Life Practice is, as the name implies, the practice aspect of
Integral Theory. Integral Theory, in both its original form and critical
alterations of it, has had a profound impact on several million readers
around the world. If you want to just do Integral Theory and not also Integral Practice, that is fine. (Integral Theory is itself a mental praxis, and
it summarizes practices in all of the major dimensions—it is a composite Map of the world's most important methodologies.) But if we take
that composite Map and turn it into a composite Practice, the result is
Integral Life Practice, a practice that is therefore grounded in the very

best of Integral Theory itself. For this reason, ILP is a truly ground-breaking and leading-edge evolutionary practice for waking up.

Thank you for picking up this book and beginning your own "momentous leap of meaning." If you are ready, then let's get started!

Ken Wilber
Denver, Colorado, Winter 2008

ACKNOWLEDGMENTS

The book you are about to read has been thousands of years in the making. We have written it with conscious gratitude to the visionary pioneers of the past—those who endeavored to see further, feel deeper, love more fully, and live more mindfully than previously done—and those who left all endeavor behind in radical awakening. This extraordinary lineage—our ancient and modern brothers and sisters, teachers, and spiritual heroes—evolved "up from Eden" to create the fertile ground on which we've stood to birth what you now hold in your hands.

We would like to give special mention to the courageous founders of the human potential movement, which began in the 1960s and has been maturing ever since. These early practitioners experimented with new transformative techniques, methods, and syntheses—documenting both the powers and pitfalls of practice along the way. Especially significant were Michael Murphy and George Leonard, who joined Ken Wilber early on in calling for a more balanced or *Integral* approach to practice, which they described in their groundbreaking book *The Life We Are Given*.

We extend a huge thank you to the team of brilliant colleagues who helped us develop many of the ideas and practices presented in the following pages. They include Jeff Salzman, Huy Lam, Diane Hamilton, Bert Parlee, Willow Pearson, Rollie Stanich, Cindy Lou Golin, Sofia Diaz, Brett Thomas, Rob McNamara, and Shawn Phillips. These exceptional individuals have led numerous seminars, workshops, and practice groups, touching the lives of thousands of people, who, through their questions, feedback, and sincere application, also contributed to the evolution of ILP. Special appreciation goes to Genpo Roshi, who shared his Big Mind process through which seminar participants often glimpsed their "Original Face." (Indeed, the Big Mind process would have been included in this book, but it requires a full book or DVD—or better yet, a live workshop—to truly experience it. For more information on Big Mind, see BigMind.org.)

Others, too, like Nomali Perera, Clint Fuhs, Nicole Fegley, and Kelly Bearer made valuable contributions, as did Frank Marrero, Ted Phelps, and Marc Gafni (on whose work, along with that of Jonathan Gustin and Bill Plotkin, we've drawn in articulating our conception of "the Unique Self"). We also appreciate the editors and graphic designers who contributed their talents to this project. Our editors and readers include Liz Shaw, Kendra Crossen Burroughs, Annie McQuade, Deborah Boyar, Jordan Luftig, and Nick Hedlund. Joel Morrison, Kayla Morelli, and Paul Salamone created many of the elegant graphics that appear throughout the book. We also thank Jonathan Green, Sara Bercholz, and the entire Shambhala team, who have been helpful and professional throughout the process.

Our personal teachers—including S. N. Goenka, Richard Weaver, Adi Da Samraj, Rabbi Steven David Kane, Baba Muktananda, John Haught, Chögyam Trungpa Rinpoche, Byron Katie, Gangaji, Doc Childre, Rabbi Shaya Isenberg, Professor M. C. Dillon, Michael Scheisser, Adyashanti, Candice O'Denver, Genpo Roshi, Susanne Cook-Greuter, and too many others to name—inspired and awakened us to the insights we share in these pages. We've been further uplifted, informed, and clarified by our friends, colleagues, and teachers at Integral Spiritual Center, including Father Thomas Keating, Brother David Steindl-Rast, Rabbi Zalman Schacter-Shalomi, Roger Walsh, Saniel Bonder, Patrick Sweeney, Sally Kempton, and David Deida. Also thanks to Andrew Cohen for his penetrating advocacy in such forums as *What Is Enlightenment?* magazine.

We are perhaps most deeply grateful to our beloved partners, family members, and close friends, who have shared with us the day-to-day creative ordeal of producing this book, and without whose loving support and companionship it would have been far less pleasurable and fulfilling (if not impossible!).

This book would not have been even remotely possible without the monumental contributions of Ken Wilber. As the meta-author not only of this book, but of Integral Life Practice itself, he has literally defined the field in which these perspectives could arise. In his books and dialogues, he has outlined the Integral worldspace with clarity, compassion, erudition, and most graciously, a sense of humor. As our co-author, colleague, mentor, teacher, and friend, he has supported us from the beginning, with brilliance, eloquence, and generosity.

Finally, we would like to acknowledge you, our reader. The evolutionary spark that drew you to this book is the same impulse that motivated every pioneer who ever found him- or herself on the growing edge of consciousness. It's in your sincere use of what follows that Integral practice comes to life. We consider it a sacred privilege to share this embodiment of an Integral vision with you.

Terry Patten, Adam Leonard, and Marco Morelli
Summer 2008

INTEGRAL LIFE PRACTICE

THE GREAT EXPERIMENT

For thousands of years, in almost all parts of the globe, human beings have engaged in **practices** to transform and balance their lives. From the magical rituals of ancient shamans, to the contemplative science of the mystical traditions, to the latest scientific breakthroughs in health, nutrition, and physical exercise—we have always sought a way to connect with deeper truths, to achieve well-being and harmony, and to realize our highest potentials.

Now, in the information age, this incredible wealth of knowledge, teachings, and techniques—our evolutionary human legacy—is available to us like never before. The question is, how can we best use it? How can we put it all together? How can we make sense of the myriad approaches, from such diverse places and times, in a way that's relevant to our individual and collective lives?

Our answer to these questions amounts to an experiment in the deepest sense—an amazing and humbling and life-long adventure in consciousness itself, in humanity itself—a trek into the future of our own bodies, minds, and spirit. That's not to say this book presents an "experimental" or unproven approach—far from it. Rather, it means that in order to see the "data" (and taste the fruits) of practice, you must be willing to try the experiment yourself. This is, we believe, one of the most exciting and rewarding of all possible endeavors.

Integral Life Practice is a way of organizing the many practices handed down through the centuries—along with those developed at the cutting edge of psychology, consciousness studies, and other leading fields—using a framework optimized for life in the 21st century. It is, at once, ancient and modern, Eastern and Western, speculative and scientific, and yet also something beyond those dichotomies. Integral Life Practice (or ILP) is *Integral*—which means "comprehensive, whole, and balanced." It's a synthesis of the "best of the best" that our traditions have to offer, combined with the most state-of-the-art transformational techniques. ILP is a free and fearless exploration of the terrain of your own being and awareness.

The authors, along with a handful of other explorers, have been developing ILP for over thirty years, researching the most essential keys to human growth. We're proud to present the results in this book. To get started, all you need is the willingness to give it a try—to carry on the Great Experiment in your own life.

Whether you're a beginner or a more advanced practitioner seeking a more integrated approach to practice, we hope this book will be exceptionally useful to you. We look forward to helping you reach your highest aspirations, as we grow together toward a brighter here and now.

1

Why Practice?

Integral Life Practice starts where all practice starts—with inspiration, a yearning to grow, to become all that you can be.

Sometimes the choice to practice comes after you've been touched, opened, shaken, or maybe even awakened by something or someone profoundly *true*. Sometimes the decision to practice is triggered by the heartbreaking lessons of life—the experience of intense suffering, meaninglessness, or pain.

Maybe it's the inspiring example of someone living an uncompromised life or the reading of a book full of mind-blowing insights or the extraordinary presence of a wise teacher or saintly person. Maybe it's the death of a friend or loved one. Or maybe your conventional life is simply undone, because you suddenly see through your own game.

Somehow you get a glimpse of a freer, clearer, more authentic, loving, and true existence—and you want to live it.

People have been inspired like this for thousands of years. Those who got bit by the bug often became monks, nuns, shamans, or yogis—surrendering their lives to a mystical spiritual path. Others did it in alternative ways, becoming samurai or martial artists—giving themselves over with great intensity to a transformational discipline. Serious, traditional stuff, eh?

But it ain't necessarily so. Even though there's a lot of wisdom and beauty in the traditions, practice by nature is extremely *alive*. It continually reinvents itself. It breaks free of all bonds. It doesn't have to be a certain way—and certainly not *only* the way of the traditions. Though, of course, any tradition can be profoundly enlivened by the spirit of practice.

In truth, the traditions have always depended on innovation and improvisation. And so we continue the tradition of . . . breaking with tradition, while still drinking deeply from the wisdom of the past. Why? Because the world keeps changing. We keep changing. Human life has evolved—and so has practice. A personalized Integral Life Practice has many layers and dimensions. It goes as deep as you do, and flexes to fit your unique life. It can and will go through countless cycles and mutations. But the *essence* of ILP is simple, and it embodies the intention of authentic practice in every context, ancient or modern: to be *true, real,* and *whole*—to *wake up* in all directions and dimensions of your being.

Integral Life Practice means living for real. It's getting real with life—perhaps like never before. Or it's taking the real-ness you already have to a higher, more integrated level. ILP expresses your impulse to be as fully aware as possible—now and now and *now*—and to grow in that awareness over time.

It's also founded in deep care—care for ourselves, for others, and for this mysterious existence. This care inspires us to want to make a difference, to give more, to cut through the bullshit of narrow and fragmented views, and to magnify the freedom, love, openness, and depth in us, in others, and in this beautiful, terrible world.

And, from a certain perspective, practice is simply *what is*—it's a personal choice and a genuine lifestyle—not really something to make a big fuss about. . . .

Here are a few more possible reasons for engaging an ILP:

- Embracing and working with crisis, pain, or suffering
- Becoming a better person—on all levels, in all areas
- Living with integrity and excellence
- Getting over yourself
- Waking up!
- As a way to understand everything or make sense of it all
- Living according to your highest ideals
- Becoming more fully alive and creative
- Finding and/or living your deepest purpose
- Loving and caring for others more fully

- Making your highest contribution
- Communing with life, the universe, and Spirit
- Participating in the evolution of consciousness
- Because you're in love with the Mystery (or God)
- No specific reason — it's just what you're drawn to do

Many people come to ILP after an experience with a specific type of practice, which, at a certain point, no longer seems full or inclusive enough. ILP makes room for you to bring everything to the path:

- You may have experience training for physical excellence or competitive sports.
- Maybe you've disciplined your mind and emotions for peak performance in business.
- Perhaps you've practiced yoga or meditation, maybe even for decades.
- You may have done deep psychological exploration, facing your shadow and exploring your deep psyche.
- You might have come to practice out of your deeply felt devotion to God or a beloved teacher or guide.
- Maybe your interest in ILP comes through your scholarship, insight, and thirst for understanding.

Some radical teachers and teachings point out the limitations buried within many of our motivations for practice. Most of us at least begin practice as "spiritual materialists," seeking personal gain through spiritual pursuits, motivated to perfect or fulfill our separate-self sense. It's just a more refined form of egocentrism. But our exclusive commitment to self-centered motives tends to loosen and relax as we mature. The most fundamental paradox is that of *seeking*. Everyone begins the path as a seeker, and yet, the seeker must outgrow the notion that something's missing—and thus give up seeking—for the path to be fulfilled. So our motives do naturally evolve.

But none of those motives are necessarily wrong. We don't need to wait until our motives are perfectly pure. People find countless reasons for practice—and every motivation for practice is valid . . . and partial.

The beauty of practice is that it transforms us so that we outgrow our original intentions—and keep going! Our motivations for practicing evolve as we mature. They each contribute something to our path, even if we eventually leave them behind.

Ultimately, all our motivations and intentions converge in the present moment: What is our practice *right now?*

There's no single best or right way to practice, but there are plenty of less than optimal ways. ILP drops the baggage and cuts to the essentials, so you can easily find a practice that works for you, with a minimum of wasted time.

Shall we begin?

About the Practices in This Book

Peppered throughout this book are experiential practices. These are provided to help you convert theory into action. Some practices are explicitly "integral" and custom designed for ILP—these are called **Gold Star Practices**. Others are taken from different sources, but are adapted to an Integral context. Some Gold Star Practices also come in an ultra-condensed form called a **1-Minute Module**. You can use one of these any time as a virtually effortless way to bring practice into your daily life—instantly!

When we say "experiential," we mean this in the broadest sense. At a minimum, there are *bodily* experiences, *mental* experiences, and *spiritual* experiences. When you see a Gold Star Practice or a 1-Minute Module, try to open yourself to whatever form of experience is involved: bodily, mental, spiritual, or any combination of the above.

 1-MINUTE MODULE
What's Your Deepest Motivation?
It's important to connect with what practice means for you. Here's a way to check in with your motivation. You can try this now, but

really, it's a great thing to do regularly, at the beginning of any practice session—and it takes less than a minute!

Place both hands over your heart, and take a few deep breaths. Feel any activity in your mind, heart, and gut. Now, thoughtfully feel into your deepest motivation for practice. What is your real desire? What's behind the "pushes" or "pulls" that you're experiencing right now? What's arising in your self-awareness?

You might be seeking something extraordinary; you might just be curious about what will happen; or you might feel something that you can't really describe. Feel what motivates you most deeply in this moment and be aware of it.

Finally, feel or be aware of the Witness of your experience— the Witness being the part of your awareness that simply observes the content that is your experience. What is the experiencer behind this and every experience? What is it that's aware of, and therefore not, your motivations?

Breathe and relax into this awareness for a few moments. . . .

Then let it go, and move on.

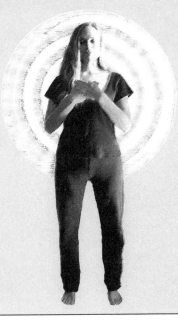

2

What Is Integral Life Practice?

Whatever your motivation, the intention to begin, renew, or deepen a practice is a wonderful first step. But once you've made that choice, how do you follow through with it? Thirty years of experience have shown us that your practice will turn to mush without a framework for organizing it. An *Integral* framework can help you make sense of the many options available to you, providing ultimate flexibility and inclusiveness, so you can most fully and deeply honor your intentions and fulfill your potentials.

A Radically Inclusive Approach

The Integral Life Practice framework allows for maximum flexibility. It's not a program you must follow uncritically, humorlessly, and perhaps even with a sense of superiority, until you're enlightened, more successful, better looking, and someday hopefully perfect. It gives you a set of tools for designing a unique and personalized practice, in whatever form works best for you right now, with the understanding that what works best will change over time.

The "Integral" part of ILP is that it is **radically inclusive**. To be this, it draws on a conceptual map called **AQAL** (which stands for "All Quadrants, All Levels"— we'll get deeper into this in a moment). AQAL (pronounced *ah-qwul*) is a *theory of everything*, a way of comprehending life and reality in very broad yet precise terms. AQAL is a map of consciousness, the Kosmos,

> **Kosmos** with a "K" is the word the ancient Greeks used to denote a universe that includes not just the physical reality of stars, planets, and black holes (which is what "Cosmos" usually means), but also the realms of mind, soul, society, art, Spirit—in other words, everything.

and human development, at every level and in every dimension that presents itself.

Technically speaking, AQAL is a map of maps, or a *meta-theory* that incorporates the core truths from hundreds of other theories. It organizes the profound insights of the spiritual traditions, philosophy, modern science, developmental psychology, and many other disciplines, into a coherent whole. AQAL accounts for the many perspectives that great thinkers, teachers, and researchers have brought to our understanding of self and world.

But it doesn't stop there, because AQAL is also intuitive—it describes the *terrain of your own awareness.* You don't need hi-tech equipment or an advanced degree to enjoy the benefits of an AQAL-informed perspective. All you need is to bring a new kind of awareness to your lived experience.

It's similar to learning a second language. At the beginning, it may feel a little awkward as you're memorizing new vocabulary and fumbling with new ways of expressing yourself. In time, however, you discover that the more you apply the new grammar to real life situations, the easier it becomes to remember and use it, even if you still instinctively think in your native language and translate to the second.

With practice, you begin to think in the new language with greater ease and mastery. Eventually, you even begin to dream in the new language. And you haven't lost your old language; you've only become bilingual. The more fluent you become, the more the language infuses your being and becomes a part of who you are. Soon the words effortlessly flow from you lips and you're able to communicate with different kinds of people in totally new ways. Your world has expanded to include new horizons that you may have never thought possible.

Integral Life Practice Is "Powered by AQAL"

Because AQAL attempts to map the Kosmos itself, ILP engages nearly every aspect of our lives. As you embark on an Integral Life Practice you will learn to hold more perspectives, and to do so more freely and flexibly, exercising every dimension of your being. It's not just a mental game, but a felt and lived embodied intelligence. Integral Life Practice is AQAL applied to life—a life of conscious evolution in all parts of your being.

In creating Integral Life Practice we asked some key questions:

- What are the most effective and essential practices of the ancient traditions?
- What new insights into practice are offered by the most current discoveries?
- How can we find the patterns that connect the most diverse insights and methodologies?
- How can we use this knowledge to promote a lifetime of growth and awakening?

We're not the first to attempt a synthesis of East and West, or to extract the spiritual wisdom from the religious traditions. It does seem though that AQAL provides some powerful missing keys to a truly universal approach to practice that is still capable of respecting—and even em-powering—the healthy differences between divergent paths.

As grand as this may sound, the basic principles are not particularly complex or difficult to grasp. Integral Life Practice is designed for and by people living within the pressurized schedules of the 21st century. You can't afford to waste your time any more than we can. That's why, if a practice isn't high-leverage, you won't find it here. ILP is perfectly com-patible with a fast-paced professional lifestyle. But we haven't cut corners either. If you want to go truly *deep* in your practice, ILP can help you do that quickly and directly.

How does ILP work? First, we suggest a **modular** approach to prac-tice. An ILP *module* is a category of practice that relates to a specific part of your being, such as body, mind, spirit, or shadow. Identifying your prac-tice modules will give you an overview of your practice life, allowing you to determine which areas you're exercising and which you're leaving out.

One of the benefits of a modular approach is that with just a handful of modules you can engage all the key areas of your life—while main-taining full choice of exactly *how* you do so. ILP does not dictate the specific practices you should do—and by "practices" we mean consciously and regularly performed activities such as yoga, weightlifting, journaling, acts of service, and so on. Rather, it suggests a few general areas—i.e., modules—that are essential, and others that are also important but optional, and then allows you to decide exactly how you want to engage those areas. This makes it easier to choose the practices that are right for you, while still covering all the bases.

Second, ILP is **scalable**, which means you can simplify and shorten your practice to accommodate your time frame. Do you often find yourself too busy for practice? You can do a basic form of Integral Life Prac-

Integral Life Practice is . . .

The Ultimate in Cross-Training,
working synergistically on body, mind, and spirit in self, culture, and nature.

Modular, allowing you to mix and match practices
in specific areas or "modules."

Scalable, adjusting to however much—or little—time you
have, down to the **1-Minute Modules**.

Customizable to your individual lifestyle—you design
a program that works for you, and adapt it on an as needed basis.

Distilled, boiling down the essence of traditional practices—
without the cultural or religious baggage—to provide a highly concentrated and effective form of practice for post-postmodern life.

Integral, based on **AQAL™ technology**, an "All Quadrants,
All Levels" framework for mapping the many capacities inherent in human beings.

tice in as little as ten minutes a day. Thus, *anyone*, no matter how busy, can have an Integral Life Practice.

Are you interested in deep and rapid transformation? You can also use the ILP principles to engage a committed life of practice at the deepest level—with the same intensity of a traditional monastic or an Olympic athlete. Your practices can stretch to several hours each day and may include attending retreats or living in a dedicated practice community.

Do you have a wide or very specific range of practice interests? ILP is **customizable**, letting you bring your unique interests, passions, and needs into play. It doesn't impose rigid structures on you, but rather creates a flexible, open space in which you can creatively engage the many dimensions of your being.

When we do suggest particular practices, such as the Gold Star Practices, these are **condensed** and **distilled**—keeping what's essential and discarding what isn't—in order to give you the "most bang for your buck." You can be sure you won't be wasting your time.

Finally, **ILP is Integral**, by which we specifically mean "powered by AQAL." AQAL is the most comprehensive map of consciousness available at this time, and Integral Life Practice puts it to use to create a cutting-edge form of practice for the 21st century. The AQAL structure of Integral Life Practice makes room not only for higher growth and self-actualization, but also and especially for awakening to, or recognizing, the Suchness or ever-present *is*-ness of this moment, and this one, and this . . .

The Universal (and Particular) Adventure of Waking Up

The adventure of awakening is among the most universal of human dramas. It takes every possible form, and thus it's an utterly creative, unpredictable, and unprogrammable process. The river's twists and whitewater sometime include passages such as the "dark night of the soul," or gates through which no one passes except on their knees. It can be experienced as an ordeal of transformation, a process of "blossoming," or as a romance with God.

The principles of ILP are remarkably clear and simple, putting practice within the reach of almost anyone. It provides an *organizing framework* for a lifetime of learning and transformation. By illuminating the big picture of consciousness, life, growth, and awakening, and distilling the essentials of practice, it helps you drop any unnecessary baggage and focus on the potent, juicy heart of the matter while giving you room to do so in your own style, in your own unique way.

Each traditional path paints a unique picture of what waking up looks like. Even modern scientific consciousness began with its own "enlightenment." ILP is not about rejecting any particular form of awakening in favor of the next new fad. It's about *understanding and supplementing* existing paths, enabling them to function even more deeply, in a way that adequately addresses life in the 21st century.

ILP presents a new, clear framework through which practitioners (of any path or religion, or no religion) can not only understand and upgrade their existing practice, but *communicate* deeply and meaningfully, across diverse paths, about the universal matter of practice.

That means that Christians, Jews, Muslims, Buddhists, Hindus, and any other religious, indigenous, and trans-traditional practitioners can all make use of this Integral approach and talk about their practices in a common language (which, incidentally, may provide new connections, highlighting how much they have in common — with each other and even with those that hold non-religious worldviews). Even atheists and agnostics can put ILP to work in their lives, since the AQAL framework is neutral with regard to "belief." It doesn't require (nor does it prohibit) any particular belief system.

This addresses a serious need. A Buddhist could easily discuss with a friend in the same tradition how to apply his or her spiritual practice to life challenges. But could a Buddhist do that with a Christian? Or a Muslim? The same holds true for spiritual aspirants outside of these traditions. We need to begin to engage a practice conversation across and beyond traditions. The growing international community of spiritual practice needs to establish a common vocabulary if we are to come together in service of the greater good.

Thus, this book begins a conversation about a new evolutionary direction in personal practice, one that will be continued by future explorers on the edges of human potential. Integral Life Practice is helping to define an emerging *field* of study, inquiry, and application.

Launch Pad: 4 Core Modules

Integral Life Practice has **4 Core Modules**:

- Body
- Mind
- Spirit
- Shadow

Additional important modules include:

- Integral Ethics
- Integral Sexual Yoga
- Work
- Transmuting Emotions
- Integral Parenting
- Integral Relationships
- Integral Communication

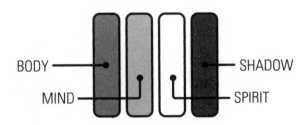

BODY ——— SHADOW
MIND ——— SPIRIT

Figure 2.1
*Start with the 4
Core Modules.*

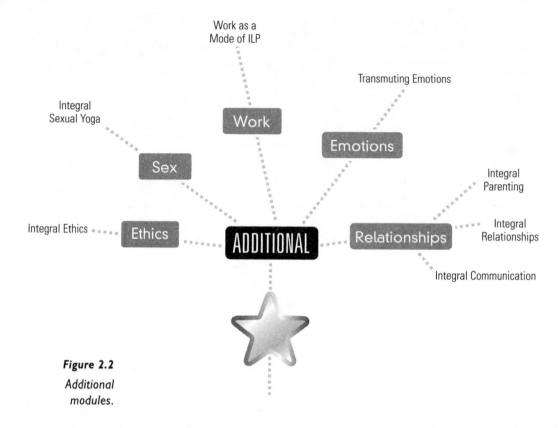

Work as a
Mode of ILP

Transmuting Emotions

Integral
Sexual Yoga

Work

Emotions

Integral
Parenting

Sex

Integral
Relationships

Integral Ethics

Ethics

ADDITIONAL

Relationships

Integral Communication

Figure 2.2
*Additional
modules.*

The universal starting point for ILP is the **4 Core Modules**. That's because they relate to four primary dimensions of your individual being: **body**, **mind**, **spirit**, and **shadow**. They don't require anything or anyone else but *you*. So you can, if you wish, work on them by yourself. If you consistently engage practices in each of these four areas, you'll empower and turbocharge your overall development. You will be better able to function inwardly and outwardly, through multiple perspectives, with greater clarity, presence, and vitality in practically any area of your life.

Traditional spiritual paths have usually emphasized only two or three of these modules—they almost never included the Shadow module. Modern and postmodern paths of self-development often do include shadow work, but some jettison the Mind module, and most usually lack the depth and rigor of the meditative traditions in the Spirit module.

If you only take on one practice in each of the 4 Core Modules, you'll be doing ILP. That's all it takes. And if you do it wisely, you'll avoid the common pitfalls that can otherwise hold back meaningful transformation.

Some people ask, "Well, what if I really need to focus on something else besides the 4 Core Modules?" Of course you do! You can bring awareness and care to all your key relationships and functions (career, intimacy, family, and more) in the additional modules. And *any* module could be your focus at any given time. *All* the modules—core and additional—are important. If you're in a phase where you're looking to align your career with your life's purpose or your heart's passion, then you probably want to focus on the **Work** module and on unfolding your **unique self**. If you've just fallen in love (or are looking for love), or are working on issues with your intimate partner, then you probably want to focus on the **Relationships** module. If you're starting a new family— well, then, you guessed it, the **Parenting** module.

The 4 Core Modules are a recommended foundation, not a rigid, dogmatic structure. The journey of your life will have many chapters, and the emphasis of your practice can shift accordingly. The ILP modules are just a way to account for the more central dimensions of your life. Moreover, you need not think of a module as a rigid, compartmentalized, abstract unit of your being—there's no need to relate to yourself in a detached and clunky way. Modules orient, balance, and integrate a life of practice. The exact terms are less important than the energy, clarity, sincerity, and intentionality with which you engage your practice.

Gold Star Practices

Each module contains any number of practices that you may choose from. For example, the **Body** module includes a broad range of practices, including weightlifting, aerobics, sports, swimming, yoga, qigong, diet, and nutrition. *Any* practice that focuses on the embodied aspect of your life can be considered a Body module practice. Likewise, practices such as prayer, meditation, and devotional worship belong to the **Spirit** module, because they relate to the spiritual dimension of your being.

We've developed a number of *recommended practices* in each of the 4 Core Modules. We call them **Gold Star Practices** and they're original, AQAL-based, and especially appropriate for 21st century life—integrating the best of traditional, modern, and postmodern approaches. Many Gold Star Practices are **distillations** of traditional practices—minus the religious and cultural baggage. In some cases, we invented a practice from scratch, to address a newly perceived need. All Gold Star Practices are streamlined and condensed, covering the most relevant aspects of practice.

Listed in figure 2.3 are some Gold Star Practices in the 4 Core Modules. All are described in more detail later in the book. The best way to find out if you like any of these practices, or if they really work for you, is to try them of course!

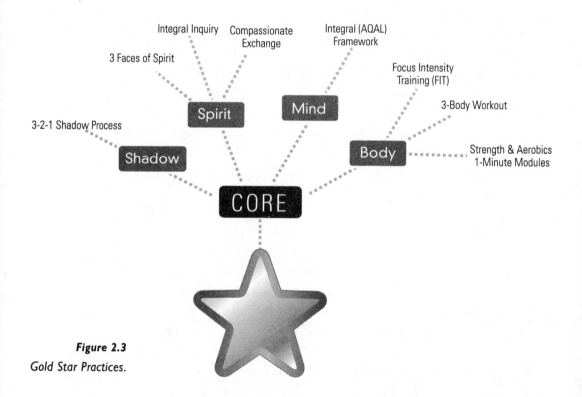

Figure 2.3
Gold Star Practices.

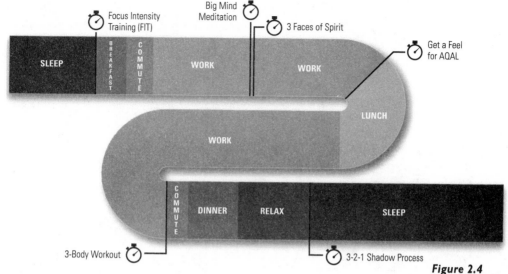

Figure 2.4

Sample ILP with 1-Minute Modules.

Pressed for Time? Try a 1-Minute Module.

Your ILP can be as rich and expansive as you want it to be. But for when you're in a hurry, we've created quick versions of the Gold Star Practices that are called **1-Minute Modules**. A 1-Minute Module is a Gold Star Practice condensed into a remarkably efficient and authentic exercise that takes very little time to complete. It's a Gold Star *mini*-practice, which you can do almost any time or anywhere—at work, on the subway, after lunch, between classes, just before bed . . . whenever.

The 1-Minute Modules are not a *replacement* for more intensive practices. Ideally, you might have an hour or two each day to deeply engage your practices; and sometimes, for example in an extended retreat, you would have even more. But when you don't have that much time, the 1-Minute Modules help you keep in touch with the *essence* of your practices, which is light years better then neglecting them completely.

By utilizing the 1-Minute Modules, you can do a full ILP, realistically, in about *ten minutes a day*. This makes it easy to maintain your practice even when you're busy—and it also eliminates the main excuse for not practicing! *Anyone* can make the time to practice ILP regularly.

The Integral Life Practice Matrix

Body	Mind	Spirit	Shadow	Ethics	Work	Relationships	Creativity	Soul
3-Body Workout ⭐	Reading & Study	Meditation	3-2-1 Process ⭐	Moral Inquiry	Right Livelihood	Conscious Commitment	Integral Artistry ⭐	Solitude
FIT (Strength Training) ⭐	Discussion & Debate	Prayer	Dream Work	Integral Ethics ⭐	Time Management	Weekly Check-Ins	Practicing, Playing & Writing Music	Nature Communion
Aerobic Exercise	Writing & Journaling	The 3 Faces of Spirit ⭐	Journaling	Volunteer Work	Professional Development	Intimacy Workshops	Creative Writing	Discovering/ Living Your Purpose
Balanced Diet & Conscious Eating	Looking At Your Meaning-Making	Integral Inquiry ⭐	Psychotherapy	Social Activism	Integral Communication ⭐	Integral Parenting	Dance & Drama	Depth Psychology
Yoga	Integral (AQAL) Framework ⭐	Spiritual Community	Family & Couples Therapy	Professional Ethics	Personal Productivity Systems	Being Vulnerable	Cooking & Interior Decorating	Resonance with Art, Music & Literature
Martial Arts	Pursuing a Degree	Worship, Song, & Chant	Transmuting Emotions	Philanthropy	Financial Intelligence	Integral Sexual Yoga ⭐	Creative Community	Vision Quest Journeys
Sports & Dance		Compassionate Exchange ⭐	Art, Music, & Dance Therapy	Heartfelt Service				

It's as simple as:

- Pick **one practice** from each of the **4 Core Modules**
- Add practices from the **Additional Modules** as you wish

(We particularly recommend the Gold Star Practices ⭐)

There is no end to practice. After years of dedication, experienced practitioners often work with the same modules in subtler, more nuanced ways. Once your whole life is practice, you tend to work more deeply with your states of mind and emotions. Your practice deepens in your relationships, work, and other additional modules. And, of course, you continue to return to Body, Mind, Spirit, and Shadow. Your practice should continually adapt, flex, and evolve as you move into each new phase of life and maturity.

The principles of ILP will help you to design and keep refining an overall practice that's effective, balanced, and high-leverage. You won't leave out any of the essentials, or neglect major dimensions of your development, even during periods when you concentrate on particular kinds of growth, such as an intensive phase of meditation practice or a period of focused training for an athletic event.

Practicing for 3 Kinds of Health

Regular practice changes us, in both dramatic and subtle ways. Looking at our **3 kinds of health** helps us to see this more clearly:

1. *Horizontal Health:* Our dynamic fulfillment of the possibilities for awareness, aliveness, and care available to us at our current stage of development
2. *Vertical Health:* Our continued growth into greater consciousness and complexity—thus outgrowing old ways of being, and moving into new stages of development
3. *Essential Health:* At any stage of development, our contact with, attunement to, and realization of Spirit—the Mystery, Suchness, or is-ness of this and every moment

ILP includes and integrates all three.

Even during phases of life in which practice apparently takes a back seat to work or family, you'll have tools so it can flex and morph appropriately. In fact, the way you engage the modules and practices of your Integral Life Practice can evolve over time: general guidelines can become firm commitments that can develop into a natural and inherent orientation to every moment of life. There's room not just for inhalation but also for exhalation — for all the qualities and phases of a healthy human life.

Principles of Practice

No Quick Fix

One reason we call it Integral *Life* Practice is because there's *no quick fix.* If there were, we'd be recommending it here. One of the primary hard-won lessons of the last half-century and the human potential movement is that weekend workshops wear off! The same is true for weeklong or monthlong intensives. A lasting, committed, daily practice is the only way to produce sustained transformation.

The quickest, shortest path to lasting change is a lifestyle that embraces some kind of ILP, including at least the 4 Core Modules. Although this might seem to require a lot of time (and sometimes even a minute seems like too much!), it pays huge dividends by unleashing our potentials, freeing up our energy and attention, and increasing our effectiveness and enjoyment in the rest of life. We've found that we don't have time *not* to engage in an ILP!

Integral Cross-Training

Typical cross-training is *flat.* You do some aerobics, some weightlifting, maybe some yoga — but it's all at the *physical* level. What if we applied the same cross-training principle — which holds that gains in one area will accelerate gains in others — across *all levels and dimensions of our being*? Well, that's the idea here. Preliminary research suggests, for instance, that a meditator who also lifts weights will progress faster in meditation than one who doesn't — and similarly, a weightlifter who meditates will progress faster in weightlifting. We can call this phenomenon *Integral cross-training synergy.* The 4 Core Modules simultaneously activate several powerful synergies, between body and mind, spirit and body, shadow (the unconscious) and spirit. Additional modules can further intensify these benefits.

Though some practices seem to focus on one module more than others, there's a ripple effect: by engaging a module in one area of life, you increase the effectiveness of every other module in every other area of life! That's the power of cross-training. The Shadow module, for instance, primarily addresses your interior, psychological dynamics. But realize how many aspects of life the shadow influences. Becoming aware of and owning your shadow material will bring greater intimacy and honesty to your relationships, free up repressed energy in your body, add clarity and effectiveness to your work, increase your capacity for authentic and ethical behavior, and may even help you improve your finances (if, for example, you have some unresolved, unconscious fears of money and power, and are able to face your fears and overcome them).

A Post-Metaphysical Approach

ILP is post-metaphysical. This principle is a bit more theoretical—but it's important. What "post-metaphysical" means here is that no perspective on reality is merely *given* to consciousness. Every perspective is *enacted*. In other words, you have to *do* something to *see* something. You have to look to know that it's raining. You have to use a microscope to observe an amoeba. You have to meditate to understand what Zen masters are really talking about.

Old-fashioned metaphysics assumes that reality is just given to awareness, unmediated by the contexts, actions, and perceptions of a person. A post-metaphysical, Integral approach claims that you must actually *do* an Integral practice to *experience* an Integral reality. Nothing presented in this book should be taken merely as a proclamation of truth. In all cases, you have to follow the practice injunction to determine for yourself whether or not what someone calls the "truth" is really true.

If you want to know if the moons of Jupiter really exist, you must actually learn some of the principles of astronomy and then look through a telescope. Likewise, if you want to know whether the Zen state of *satori*, or enlightenment, really exists, you must learn something about Zen and then meditate, looking into the nature of your mind. Instead of un-questioning belief or skeptical disbelief, a post-metaphysical approach requires an open, inquisitive attitude. In a sense, post-metaphysics is an expression of the scientific impulse — that is, of empirical experimenta-tion and experiential validation — but expanded to all levels and dimen-sions of our being, instead of only the material plane.

Awareness, Care, and Presence

At its core, Integral Life Practice is not limited to the performance of spe-cific practices. It's a sincere, inherent commitment to bring **awareness**, **care**, and **presence** to every moment of life — and thereby to *increase* one's awareness, care, and presence. An ILP practitioner naturally strives for a healthy body, a clear mind, an open heart, and a commitment to a higher purpose. This will then show up in how you breathe and feel as you go through your day, in how you do your job, how you treat your lover, how you respond to stress — it touches every aspect, every moment of life.

It's a profound thing to really be conscious, to really love — it means you're *seeing, feeling, being* in the moment — and yet you're not stuck in any one perspective, but free to flex and evolve with life itself.

Integral Life Practice is *paradoxical*. Your practices will progres-sively deepen over time, like in the classic "gradual paths" of some of the traditions, which can involve decades of diligent attention. But from the beginning, the path will often be punctuated by moments of sudden awakening and freedom. In these peak experiences, consciousness radi-cally reveals itself. The true nature of things is evident and obvious. But then soon, this vividness fades. Yet if peak states occur frequently enough, the spirit of free consciousness eventually seeps into the whole of life. So the universal path is *both gradual and sudden*.

It is also both specific and general. Although this book may seem like a "how to" manual, ILP is much more than a self-improvement program. It offers a distillation of the universal processes of awakening into higher states and stages of consciousness. Thus, in a way, you can "do it." But at a certain point, it begins to "do you."

The freedom into which human beings awaken has been present from the beginning. There was never a problem, never any need to transform ourselves. Paradoxically, transformation is also important, and we are profoundly grateful for it. At the moment of realization, our path is seen for what it was—a container for unconditional awakening. We practice for the goodness, truth, beauty, and joy of living our practice.

Your Integral Life Practice will keep evolving and deepening for the rest of your life, becoming more and more intimate and real. How do you practice with frustration, disappointment, and pain? How do you respond when someone attacks you? What do you do—what *can* you do—when someone you love dies? How do you face the stark reality of your own inevitable losses, aging, and death?

This is when practice matters most. If you can illuminate your shadow issues, if you can balance your body with proper exercise and nourishment, if you can see multiple perspectives, if your nervous system can release tension, if you can open into contact with more life and truth—all of these factors will determine your immediate experience, how present and loving you can be with whatever is arising, and whether—and how wisely—you can use it to grow.

But it's not just the hard stuff that practice can help with—it's the beautiful stuff too. Life is infinitely wonderful and awesome. Falling in love . . . the birth of a baby . . . having a brilliant new idea . . . serving a higher cause . . . starting a new business . . . traveling and experiencing another culture . . . having an insight into the nature of reality . . . creating or enjoying a beautiful work of art. . . . We're stretched by all of it, whether it's delicious or not.

Spirit's light can blind you like a billion suns. The beauty of a single teardrop can liquefy your heart. True love can crush you like a crumbling mountain.

Then your intimate partner says something that hurts or infuriates you, and you forget the beauty and the love.

And then you remember—or rediscover—it again. Balance. Freedom. Happiness. Sanity. Oneness. Ordinariness. And again. And that's what practice is for.

The Smart Way to Wake Up

The best thing is to just get started! Whether you're a beginner or a veteran practitioner, make use of this book to bring the most intelligent and useful practices to your own life.

Once you have the basics down, it's easy to begin your own ILP. Here is a summary of how simply and quickly you can do so:

- ILP has **4 Core Modules**: Body, Mind, Spirit, and Shadow. It works via the principle of *cross-training*.
- All you need to start an ILP is **one practice** in each of the core modules. See the **ILP Matrix** on page 20 for examples.
- **Design** your ILP and **scale** it to fit the realities (large or small) of your schedule, level of commitment, and state of inspiration.
- **Mix and match**. Include practices from additional modules as appropriate; focus on what's most relevant and needed in your life.
- **Gold Star Practices** are optimized for ILP—they're particularly distilled, concentrated, and effective, but not obligatory. Try a **1-Minute Module** if you're busy.
- **The hard part is the school of life itself**. But practice helps us be radically more present, alive, and capable of embracing both the difficulties and the pleasures of everyday life.

3

Get a Feel for Integral Awareness

"Integral" means comprehensive, balanced, and inclusive. Whenever we think, feel, or act in an Integral manner, it carries a sense of wholeness or completeness—like we're not leaving out anything important. Usually, this is an *intuitive* experience. It simply feels more right, more true, more in touch with reality.

There are also some very explicit ways that we can articulate an Integral sensibility. The AQAL Integral Framework is one such articulation. By using an Integral framework in our daily life, we can train our awareness to be more Integral more of the time. We can use AQAL to deepen our feeling-awareness, our intuition of wholeness, and our Integral Life Practice itself.

In chapter 2, we touched briefly on the AQAL Framework as a *theory* or *map of everything*. We said that Integral Life Practice is powered by AQAL—in fact, it's AQAL *applied to life*. AQAL is the **map** . . . and our being-in-the-world is the **territory**. AQAL functions as a kind of *reality-mapping technology* that shows how everything fits together and makes sense. Hence, we often say that AQAL "makes sense of everything." Yes, that's a tall order, so please check it out for yourself.

In this chapter, we're going to introduce and explore one of the most accessible aspects of the AQAL Framework: the **4 quadrants**. (This is the "all quadrant" part of AQAL.) These four facets of your own awareness are so close and self-evident they're easy to miss! Many conflicts or misunderstandings—personal, political, cultural, business-related, and even spiritual—result from neglecting to consider one or more of the quadrants. One of the first and best things we can do to get a feel for Integral awareness is to check in with the 4 quadrants of your own experience.

Four Dimensions of Being

The quadrants refer to four dimensions of your being-in-the-world: your **individual interior** (i.e., your thoughts, feelings, intentions and psychology), your **collective interior** (i.e., your relationships, culture, and shared meaning), your **individual exterior** (i.e., your physical body and behaviors), and your **collective exterior** (i.e., your environment and social structures and systems).

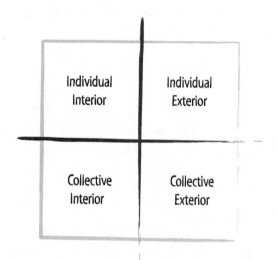

Figure 3.1

Taken together, the 4 quadrants are four aspects of your being-in-the-world.

They also refer to four corresponding perspectives in your present awareness: **I**, **We**, **It**, and **Its**.

Our Integral Life Practice is always arising in and as all 4 quadrants (this is part of the Integral-ness of it), but sometimes a practice will emphasize one quadrant more than another.

In the next four sections, we're going to present exercises that can be used to explore each of the 4 quadrants through the lens of their "I," "We," "It," and "Its" perspectives. That way, we'll begin to get a sense of the multiple dimensions in which all of our experiences arise—the terrain of our practice.

4 Quadrants = 360° of Life

Our lives, and our Integral Life Practice, arise 360°. Since our life arises in and as all 4 quadrants, we can engage it with more balance and intelligence by accounting for these four primordial perspectives. But Integral Life Practice doesn't break life into four, or four hundred, pieces. It's grounded in awakeness to life's wholeness and singleness, its "Integral-ness." While particular practices will often emphasize one quadrant more than the others, all 4 quadrants are still present in every practice occasion.

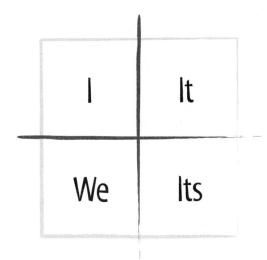

Figure 3.2
The 4 quadrants are four perspectives in your present awareness.

Get a Feel for "I"

Tune into your "I" space, your interior as a conscious individual, an intentional sentient being with a sense of "self." What's going on in there? What's arising within the landscape of your own consciousness? No one can fully answer this except you. Your behavior can provide clues, but your inward eye is best suited to answer these questions, because your interior, your "I" space is invisible to others.

An itch here, a tickle there. Pain in your lower back. Energy after an intense workout. Exhaustion after a long day. Tingling pleasure from the soft touch of a lover. Hunger for a midnight snack. Sore feet. The stickiness of dried sweat. What sensations do you feel in your "I" space?

Anger toward a world gone slightly mad. Compassion toward all of us doing the best we can. Apathy when you don't feel you can make a difference. Excitement when receiving a paycheck. Disappointment after opening it. Happiness walking in the moonlight. Boredom at work. Intense love blowing open your heart. Melancholy for no reason. Fear that you won't reach your potential. Gratitude for who you are right now. Envy that you're not there, doing that, with them. Joy waking up. What emotions do you feel in your "I" space?

Inner voices chime in constantly: the controller, the skeptic, the protector, the critic, the judge, the pusher, the wounded child. "You're not good enough." "That's not safe." "Push harder." "That's wrong." "Do this instead." "That's bullshit." And that traumatic memory keeps popping up. Abused as a child. Abandoned by your father. Betrayed by a friend. And the long shadow bag we drag behind us, stuffed with all those qualities we've disowned and project onto others. "I'm not angry, but she is." "I'm not jealous, but he is." Or the deadening numbness that comes from dissociating completely with a part of ourselves. What psychological dynamics occur in your "I" space?

Thoughts, ideas, opinions, intentions, motivations, purpose, vision, values, worldview, and life philosophy all exist within your personal interiors. All concepts from "I think she likes me" to "$E = MC^2$" arise in

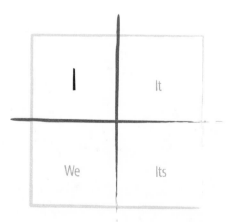

Figure 3.3

4 quadrants:
emphasis "I."

this "I" space. Dreams light up in interior display with subtle images doing the strangest things. Whether they're horrifying, sexual, or luminous and exhilarating, dreams open a subtle realm much different from our normal, waking state. And that's obviously just a taste of the phenomena that could arise in the "I" space, the individual interior of this and every moment.

By practicing introspection or focused "I" gazing, moments of grace may occur in which the moving waters of your interior become still. In place of the typical currents and rapids, an illuminated mirror mind appears, lucidly reflecting your face, your Original Face—usually elusive, yet so obviously ever-present. Radiant stillness opens the gateless gate of radical transparency all the way down to the ocean bottom of your own awareness. Witness the empty space holding the bubbly water that is your interior consciousness, your "I" space.

Get a Feel for "We"

Choose any relationship that you're in and imagine being together with this other person. Recollect the shared feelings and emotions present whenever you're with them. Although you may not always agree with them, you can relate to them in some way. They have become a "you" rather than an "it." A "We" space exists when there is mutual recognition, communication, and shared understanding. You and I experience shared feelings and visions and desires and conflicts, a vortex of love and dis-

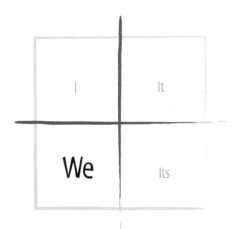

Figure 3.4

4 quadrants:
emphasis "We."

appointment, obligations and broken promises, the ups and downs of almost everything we call "important" in life. Right now you can feel the actual texture of those shared experiences, thoughts, insights, and emotions—this miracle called "we."

When **I** encounter **you**, and you and I communicate, **we** begin resonating, sharing, and understanding each other, at least enough to exchange some sense of meaning. Two "I's," become a "we." Think back to the last time you struck up an engaging conversation with a stranger. Recall how you felt before and after the interaction. When you first encountered the stranger he was an It, an object that you could see, but did not really know. Then you began talking with him, exchanging stories, picking up on each other's emotional state, witnessing the human experience expressed in each other's eyes. You could actually feel a new "we" coming into being. With each word, each head nod, each smile, each gesture of mutual understanding, each shared experience, the *we* grew stronger.

Consider the vast diversity of "We" spaces: the family we, the workplace we, the romantic we, the sports team we, the best friend we, the neighborhood community we, the meditation group we, the national we, the global we, and on and on. Notice that these shared spaces have actual felt textures, each unique. "We" spaces are so common that it's easy to forget what an incredible miracle it is that two or more people can understand each other. In order for communication to be possible, somehow you must be able to get into my mind, and I must be able to get into yours, enough so that we are in each other to the point that we both agree that we can see what the other sees. Amazing, isn't it?

Doesn't it feel wonderful to be on the same wavelength with another person who truly "gets" you? This magnificent "we" forms as you and I understand each other, and love each other, and hate each other, and in so many ways *feel* each other's existence as *part of our own being*, which indeed it is.

Get a Feel for "It"

In contrast to the mutual understanding of "We" space, "It" space is the perspective of looking at surfaces, objectifying things and people, and sensing behaviors. "It" space has a feeling of "thingness" because it's the realm of individual exteriors. You can see it, touch it, taste it, smell it, hear it, and point to it.

Turn your attention to the exterior dimension of your self, your "It" space. The physical or gross body is a truly astonishing vehicle (and work of art) allowing you to interact with the world. Many layers of complexity—from subatomic particles to atoms to molecules to cells to tissues to organs to organ systems—compose our physical body.

Take a look right now at just one square inch of skin on your arm. Consider that in this square inch there are 4 yards of nerve fibers, 1,300 nerve cells, 100 sweat glands, 3 million cells, and 3 yards of blood vessels. With a microscope and a lot of free time you could look at each of these. How strange to think that each of us spent about half an hour as a single cell, and today we have around 1,000 billion cells! And by the way, 50 million of those cells will have died and been replaced in the time it took you to read this sentence.

Our brain is perhaps the pinnacle of physical complexity. Nearly 45 miles of nerves run from the brain to all parts of the body, and information races across these nerve networks as electrical impulses at speeds topping 200 miles per hour—generating enough electricity to power a 10-watt light bulb (or perhaps a race of intelligent machines). The brain's 100 billion neurons allow virtually limitless possibilities for unique pathways.

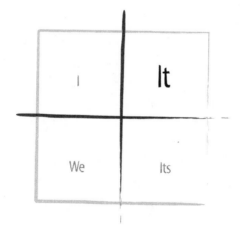

Figure 3.5
4 quadrants:
emphasis "It."

> ## Our Innards Are Actually Exteriors
>
> Though our brain, blood, and guts may be located inside our physical bodies, they're still in our "It" space because they're still exteriors of our being. You can see them as physical objects. You may have to cut the body open, but you can see every cell and every organ because they're all objects or exteriors.

Stop and feel the "It" space that is the thump . . . thump . . . thump of your physical heart. See the veins bulging from your arms filled with blood being circulated through the body about 1,000 times each day over 60,000 miles of blood vessels. Thump . . . thump . . . thump 40 million times per year.

What you do with your physical body—*your behavior*—is also an example of "It" space. How do you show up in the world? What do you do? It actually takes more facial muscles to frown (43) than it does to smile (17). Facial expressions occur in "It" space as do all body movements and behaviors. And speaking of body movements, the World Health Organization reports that approximately 100 million acts of sexual intercourse occur each day. The good news is you burn 26 calories in a one-minute kiss, let alone . . . well, never mind. All this covers only one of your bodies: your gross physical body. Your "It" space also contains a subtle body and causal body. More on all 3 bodies later.

Get a Feel for "Its"

Take a moment to look around at your immediate environment. Where are you reading this book? In your bed? In a library? On a train? In the lobby of your dentist's office? On a hammock in the Caribbean? Wherever you are, you're in relationship with local exterior surroundings such as other nearby organisms, buildings, and geographical landforms (such as mountains, rivers, forests).

Now take a look at your clothing. Where did it come from? Who made it? What material was used? What financial system allowed you to purchase it? How was it transported to a store near you? Or did you buy it over the phone or the Internet? What laws were in place to make sure you weren't cheated? What political system governs the laborers who manufactured the clothing? What pollution escaped into the ecosystem during its production? All these questions point to the many different systems in which we're enmeshed—and that's just tracing some of the systems surrounding the clothes on your back.

Try this visualization: zoom out from your immediate family system to your neighborhood to your city to your country to your planetary hemisphere to the whole Earth to the solar system to the Milky Way galaxy to the entire universe. Now reverse: start with the universe then zoom in to the Milky Way to the solar system to the Earth to your planetary hemisphere to your country to your city to your neighborhood to your family system. As you visualize the great web of life, feel your connection with the many physical ecosystems in your "Its" space.

A feeling of interconnectedness is natural once a person can comprehend his or her participation in the world's countless intertwining systems. Examples of shared exteriors include political systems, legal systems, and economic systems. Institutions (for example, educational, governmental), businesses (such as Google), and nonprofit organizations (like the Red Cross) mesh together to form society's infrastructure. The intersecting meshwork of social systems profoundly affects our lives and development in countless ways.

These intersections include, perhaps most interestingly, extensive

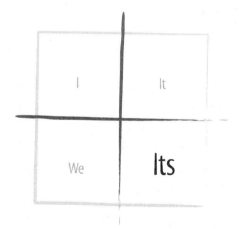

Figure 3.6
4 quadrants:
emphasis "Its."

The Big 3: I, We, and It

Sometimes, for convenience, the right-hand quadrants (It and Its) are combined, and the 4 quadrants are simplified into "The Big 3": I, We, and It.

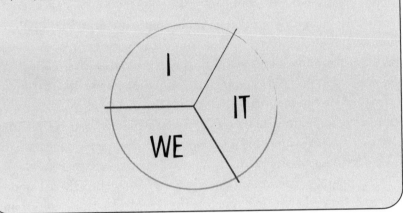

systems and *networks of communication* that link us all together. An increasingly wired society connects us through new ways of exchanging information. The exterior of communication refers to the distribution mechanisms through which information travels, such as mass media, book publishers, cell phone networks, direct TV satellite systems, and, of course, the Internet. Sound familiar?

Nature and society together form your "Its" space—the exterior contexts in which you exist.

All 4 Quadrants, All the Time . . .

You've probably noticed that although we've considered them one at a time these four dimensions of being are always *co-arising* (or, more precisely, *"tetra-arising,"* which means arising as four different aspects of the same occasion). None of these dimensions exists separately and independently from the others. And yet, when we talk or think about them, we tend to explore them one at a time.

Do you forget I and We when you explore It and Its? Do you forget We

and It when you explore the I dimension? Most people tend to privilege
one or two quadrants and ignore the others. At the extreme, we try to explain away or reduce the other dimensions of existence to the one we
want to focus on—and that's not Integral at all!

One essential skill for Integral awareness is the ability to hold *paradox*.
Integral theory has sometimes been described as "both/and" thinking,
rather than "either/or" thinking. While we can consciously choose to
focus on one or another quadrant, depending on the situation, we also
can implicitly recognize that *both* the I and It are important, both the We
and Its matter. All four simultaneously. Try to feel them all.

 1-MINUTE MODULE
Get a Feel for Integral Awareness—Right Now!
It's easier than you may think to go from theory to practice—and
you can do so at any moment. Here are five quick steps to bring a
more Integral awareness to your life right now, by getting in touch
with the 4 quadrants.

1. What are the 4 quadrants? They're a way of representing
the interiors (e.g., your thoughts and feelings) and exteriors (e.g.,
your body and behavior) of individuals (e.g., you) and collectives
(e.g., your culture and environment).

Individual Interior	Individual Exterior
Collective Interior	Collective Exterior

I	It
We	Its

2. Quickly expand your awareness. Take a moment to feel your "I-ness"—everything inside you that makes you *you*. Now, feel your "We-ness"—your relationships with others. Next, feel your "It-ness"—your physical body in all its complexity, including all the energies surrounding your objective presence in the world. Finally, feel your "Its-ness"—your membership and participation in the many systems in which your life is embedded. Just feel your awareness expand into these important dimensions of reality.

3. Notice where you tend to get stuck. According to Integral Theory, all of your 4 quadrants—I, We, It, and Its—are essential and irreducible. Yet, most people tend to focus on just one or two of these quadrants. For instance, they are only interested in *exterior* facts and ignore *interior* interpretations. Or, they are solely focused on *individual* experiences without acknowledging *collective* or communal issues. Which quadrant do you tend to focus your attention on when it comes to your job, your health, or your intimate relationship? Are you mostly concerned with *I, We, It,* or *Its?*

4. Use all 4 quadrants! All are important and real. At any moment, feel into the 4 quadrants of your existence, which are simply your *I, We, It, and Its* dimensions. Then notice where you tend to get stuck. Are you constantly looking outward (It and Its) and never within (I and We)? Or do you find yourself lost in relationship (We) and are unable to find your individual center (I)? Are you only concerned with your exterior bodily health (It), but out of touch with your emotional well-being (I)? Or do you actually need to get out of your head (I) and maybe clean up your living space (Its)? *All 4 quadrants are important, essential, real, and irreducible!*

Now take it to infinity: Notice that all 4 quadrants are arising *within* your awareness right now—an awareness that includes everything, so big that it's sometimes referred to as Big Mind. Feel your own pure awareness—where even your little I or ego arises, along with your We, It, and Its perspectives. Feel that open, pleasurable awareness, and go on about your day.

That's just a quick way to get a feel for Integral awareness in your life. (See chapter 5 for an expanded discussion of AQAL.) More advanced applications of the AQAL Framework use the 4 quadrants, along with other unique concepts, to unravel issues in medicine, ecology, business, spirituality, politics, and many other fields. The AQAL Framework is being used by scholars, professionals, leaders, and visionaries around the world to bring a more inclusive, balanced, and comprehensive approach to their work and personal lives—and it forms the theoretical basis of Integral Life Practice.

4

The Shadow Module

What Is the Shadow?

Everyone is familiar with the notion of "body, mind, and spirit," but ILP adds "shadow" as a core component of any truly Integral practice. Body, mind, spirit, *and shadow* are the minimum areas of focus required in practice—otherwise the transformative process tends not to stick, for reasons we'll explore. We present the Shadow module first because in other approaches to practice it is the most sorely neglected area.

The term "shadow" refers to the "dark side" of the psyche—those aspects of ourselves that we've split off, rejected, denied, hidden from ourselves, projected onto others, or otherwise disowned. In the language of psychotherapy, the shadow is referred to as the "repressed unconscious"—repressed because we've pushed or "pressed" it out of our awareness, and unconscious because we're not aware of it!

But the fact that we are not conscious or aware of the shadow does not mean that it has no effect: it just expresses itself through distorted and unhealthy means—or what are typically called "neuroses."

The purpose of shadow work, and of the Shadow module, is to undo this repression and *reintegrate* the shadow in order to improve our psychological health and clarity. The benefits of shadow work naturally extend to the other core modules (Body, Mind, and Spirit)—as well as to virtually every other area of life, from relationships and sex, to emotions and vitality, to work and personal finances.

One of the greatest benefits of shadow work is that it *frees up energy* that would otherwise be spent shadowboxing within ourselves. Maintaining our shadow is hard work! It takes a lot of energy to be constantly camouflaging undesirable aspects of ourselves from ourselves. Shadow work frees up that energy, which we can then use for growth and transformation.

Imagine that the energy you have available for transformation is represented by a bank account with $600 in it, and it takes $800 to move to your next stage of development. What if you had an extra $400 tied up in your repressed unconscious? If you could free up even $200 of that "energy-money," it would be enough to get you to the next stage. Not only does shadow work relieve the pain and suffering inherent to struggling with psychodynamic issues—it can make the difference between growth and stagnation.

Psychotherapy and shadow work are among the modern West's most important contributions to the endeavor of transformative practice. Profound as their understanding of spiritual development may be, the ancient spiritual traditions don't adequately address the psychodynamic shadow. In fact, one of the big mistakes the spiritual traditions make, which ILP shadow work attempts to correct, is to assume that practices such as meditation can transform the whole individual, whereas in fact they generally leave out some very important aspects of the self, including and especially the shadow. The result, all too often, is a realization of higher *states of consciousness,* without a correspondingly rigorous and conscious integration of the practitioner's "dark side."

Freud made some big mistakes, and while it's now fashionable to debunk him, his basic insight into the nature of the shadow remains indispensable: *unacceptable drives and feelings are repressed from conscious awareness, where they surreptitiously shape your life.*

Decades of shadow work by thousands of researchers and therapists around the world have demonstrated time and again this basic insight into the nature of the shadow.

To complicate matters, it's the nature of the shadow to remain hidden from awareness. At least in part, *you don't **want** to see your shadow.* That's why it takes a special kind of work to address it. But until it's seen, it will tend to subtly impose its obscuring nature on your choices and behavior, sometimes sabotaging your whole life.

Whether you like it or not, this is your choice:

Own your shadow. That is, work to become aware of your repressed unconscious drives, feelings, needs, and potentials, and to become able to make freer choices in life . . .

Or be owned by it. That is, let your disowned drives and feelings shape your life outcomes, entirely apart from your conscious choices.

There are many ways to do shadow work. For decades, most people who have tackled serious shadow work have sought the help of a trained psychotherapist. Although this usually takes the form of individual psychotherapy, it can also take place through intensive seminars or group therapy sessions.

The field of psychotherapy is remarkably diverse. Within it, you'll find numerous schools of psychoanalysis, other psychodynamic therapies, several general categories of cognitive therapy, a wide variety of therapies for sensing, integrating, and healing emotions, and numerous somatic or body-based approaches to therapy. And that just barely skims the surface of what's available.

The human psyche can get bruised and cramped and injured in many different ways at each stage of human development. And we also naturally contract and close in the face of existence itself. Each kind of wound or contraction results in a unique and distinct kind of shadow or neurosis. The emerging field of **Integral Psychotherapy** maps these different pathologies and identifies the therapeutic approaches that are best able to address them.

Other factors affect therapeutic choices too. Sometimes only brief therapy is possible or appropriate. Sometimes long-term therapy is absolutely necessary, given the depth and severity of the pathology. An integrally informed psychotherapist is able to make precise judgments about these important choices and has access to the widest range of treatment options.

Some unfortunate individuals suffer especially profound psychological disabilities. Those with psychoses like schizophrenia are currently getting best results with physiological approaches like psychopharmacology; for them, psychotherapy is often a secondary treatment. As a rule, however, an Integral treatment approach will take both interior and exterior methodologies into account and attempt to strike a judicious balance, even in extreme cases.

For the rest of us—people who function reasonably well, and who want to *enhance our lives* through "cleaning out the basement," so to speak—psychotherapy can be a highly desirable luxury. It is a way to get expert and compassionate help digging deeply into one's shadow material, expanding self-awareness, and opening up new options in our inner world.

But if you don't have the means, time, or inclination to seek out professional therapy now—and even if you do, but also want something effective you can do on your own—a distilled form of shadow work can be especially useful.

The **3-2-1 Process**, a Gold Star Practice, is a direct, economized, and highly efficient exercise for contacting and integrating the shadow. (Like every ILP Gold Star Practice, the 3-2-1 process is optional— shadow work itself, on the other hand, is definitely *not* optional if you are interested in an Integral life.) In the next section, we'll teach the 3-2-1 process. But first we'll set the stage by looking at the origins of shadow, along with some examples of how it shows up in life.

The 3-2-1 Shadow Process

The Origins of the Shadow

If a little child becomes angry with her mother, but that feeling of anger is a threat to her self-sense ("I depend completely on my bond of love with Mommy"), then she might dissociate or repress the anger.

But denying the anger doesn't get rid of it; it merely makes the angry feelings appear alien in her awareness: she might be feeling anger, but it cannot be *her own* anger. The angry feelings are put on the other side of the self-boundary and they appear as alien or foreign events in her awareness.

Repression and projection can be mapped in three phases as in the following example:

1. I'm furious at Mommy. But being angry with Mommy threatens my connection to warmth, food, comfort, love, security, and survival. I'm really mad!

2. But it's not okay! So I repress my fury. I might project the anger onto my inner image of "you," or "them," or worse, onto actual people whom I don't even know. The anger continues to arise, but since it cannot be me who is angry, it must be somebody else. All of a sudden, the world appears full of very angry people!

3. If I repress it fully enough, I no longer even acknowledge the anger. Anger has nothing to do with me. I'm scared and sad (which makes perfect sense living in this angry world). Through the repression of my anger, my primary actual (and thus "authentic") emotion ("mad") is now experienced only in the form of a secondary reaction and thus an "inauthentic" emotion ("scared and sad and depressed"). In other words, I've created an internal decoy—that's what we mean by *secondary, inauthentic* emotions (of sadness and fear, in this case) that further distance me from my unacceptable anger, which was my original, or primary and authentic, feeling. A secondary emotion may be very powerfully and sincerely experienced, but it is not the root cause and can't be effectively processed all by itself.

Shadow work is a core module because I'm never going to get over that sadness and fear without first recognizing the actual emotion at play—anger—and then *owning* it.

Whenever I disown and project my drives, feelings, and qualities, they appear "out there" where they frighten me, irritate me, depress me, or turn into an obsession. Much of the time, the things that most disturb, upset, fascinate, or compel me about others are actually my own shadow drives or qualities, which are now perceived not as originating in me but as existing "out there."

To me, the shadow seems "out there," but it informs my feelings and motivations. My shadow subconsciously and inadvertently shapes my behavior, creating patterns I don't seem to be able to escape. There is only one way out: through.

Let's look at the origin of the shadow in a little more detail.

1st-Person Identification: The split-off self was once a part of what the self knew as I or me. But, for whatever reasons or life conditions, this aspect posed a threat to my sense of self. If we were able to acknowledge and accept the primary emotion or drive: "I am angry (or scared or depressed or jealous) and that's okay," it would not have become dissociated and then displaced onto someone or something "out there."

2nd-Person Identification: When aspects of the self become unacceptable, we might push them out of awareness into the 2nd person. In other words, the disowned aspects of our self that we fear, are ashamed of, or disapprove of become part of what I see in you, not me. "*You* are stingy or impatient or lazy, not me."

You are angry.

You are grief-stricken.

You are _____. (Fill in the blank.)

But *I* am not. *I* am not angry. *I* am not grief-stricken . . . or whatever the rejected emotion may be.

3rd-Person Identification: Finally, when the threat of this emotion or situation is so great to the sense of self that it requires a total rejection, we move from owning it ourselves (1st person) to relating to it as something that belongs to others (2nd person) to finally banishing it totally as an It—an object that has nothing to do with me (3rd person). By making it an It, we push the rejected quality furthest from our awareness. "Anger? What are you talking about?"

The split-off quality becomes a dissociated "it" that remains unknown and dark to us—the shadow.

Here is another example of the shadow in action:

Harry wants to do his taxes so he goes up to his office to begin. But a strange thing happens as he sits down to go through the records. He cleans his desk. He sharpens his pencils. He reorganizes his files. He browses some websites on tips for saving money on taxes. He reads some other interesting websites. He leafs through some of his favorite magazines.

1st person = the one speaking (I)

2nd person = the one being spoken to (you)

3rd person = the one being spoken about (him/her/it)

He starts to have second thoughts. Maybe he should just hire a book-keeper and an accountant.

He doesn't leave the office, because his desire to do his taxes is still greater than his desire not to. But he is starting to forget his own drive, so he will start to alienate and project it.

In the back of his mind, Harry knows that *somebody* wants him to prepare his taxes. And that's precisely why he is still puttering around. But at this point, he's almost completely forgotten *who* wants him to do his damn taxes. He gradually becomes angry and annoyed with the whole project.

All he really needs to complete the projection — that is, to totally forget his *own* drive to do his taxes — is a likely candidate on whom he can "hang" his own projected drive.

Enter the unsuspecting victim:

Harry's wife gets home. She innocently asks, "How are the taxes going?"

Harry snaps, "Get off my back!" The projection is completed. Harry now feels that it is not he, but his *wife* that wants him to do the stupid taxes. She acts so sweet on the outside, but subtly, she's been pressuring him all along!

If Harry were really innocent of the drive, he probably would have answered that he hadn't really begun, and that he was reconsidering whether he really wanted to continue. But he did not, because in his gut he knew that *somebody* really wanted him to prepare those taxes today. Since it feels clear that it *wasn't him*, it must have been somebody else. As his wife, the likely candidate, appears, he throws his projected drive onto her.

After projecting his drive, Harry experienced it as an external drive, a demand coming from the outside. Another word for external drive is *pressure*. In fact, *any time* a person projects some sort of drive, he or she will feel pressure coming from the outside. Believe it or not, this is what *all* external pressure amounts to, in the end. External pressure can only be effective if it can hook your own projected drive!

What if his wife really *did* nag him to do the taxes, and what if she marched in and demanded that he get them done? Wouldn't that change the whole picture? Wouldn't Harry be feeling her pressure instead of his own?

No. This doesn't change the story at all. She'd be a better "hook" for the projection by displaying the same quality Harry's about to project onto her. She'd make it oh-so-inviting, but . . .

. . . what matters is still *his* projected drive.

His wife might indeed be pressuring him to do something—and she might even be annoying him for other reasons—but he won't actually *feel* pressure unless he *also* wants to do it.

So what is to be done?

Because the true nature of any particular shadow element is, by definition, hidden from our conscious awareness, we have to learn how to recognize the *symptoms* of shadow and "reverse engineer" a solution. This is where Integral Theory can help. The shadow begins as a 1st-person impulse, drive, or feeling, from where it's falsely displaced or projected onto a 2nd- and then 3rd-person object. Again, the genesis of shadow is a 1-2-3 process. It happens that fast! Our only recourse is to reverse the process: 3 to 2 to 1. Hence, the **3-2-1 Shadow Process**.

The 3-2-1 process uses shifts in perspective to identify disowned projections or shadow material and reintegrate them into conscious aware-

---

Potential Outcomes of Practicing the 3-2-1 Shadow Process

- A re-integration of split off parts of self.
- An energetic boundary is dissolved and energy is freed up.
- Compassion or empathy arises.
- Other insights may emerge such as identifying the original source of the projection.
- Creative strategies or actions come into awareness.
- The situation or person is no longer irritating, compelling, devastating, or distracting.

ness. This practice helps us confront our hidden aspects by restoring con-tact with them and fully experiencing them in a healthier manner.

As long as we have little renegade splinters of our personality running around in our unconscious, they appear not as integrated aspects of "me," but as alienated "others." The more fragmented "others" we have loose in our psyche, the harder it is to grow. *When aspects of the self are pushed out of awareness, healthy stage development is compromised.*

Also remember: The energy that it takes to animate and repress shadow elements and keep them out of awareness is the same energy that cannot be available for developing to the next stage of our potential.

Bringing the Light of Consciousness to the Shadow

As the aikido masters know in their bones, what we don't know can truly hurt us, whereas what we do know is always workable. To gain awareness of and recover the split-off aspects of the self, this 1-2-3 of dissociation, we must come back into association with that quarantined aspect of the self. In other words, we enter into relationship with that which was disowned.

We start with the "3" part of the process by taking what was made other as the "it" (3rd-person perspective) and face it by coming back into asso-ciation and making direct contact with it. We then take what was seen as "it" and restore that aspect of ourselves to partial awareness as "you" (2nd-person perspective). We talk to it, engage it, dialogue with it, relate to it. At the "2" part of the process, we approach that hook, but we don't yet identify with it. Then, lastly, in the "1" part of the process we take what was only partially illuminated as a "you" and fully claim it as "me" or "mine" by *being* it (1st-person awareness). Thus we have the 3-2-1 process: 3rd-person perspective to 2nd-person perspective to 1st-person perspective. What was "it" is restored to "you," which is ultimately re-stored to "me" as an aspect of my very self.

We *face it, talk to it,* and finally, *"be" it.* That's the essence of the 3-2-1 process, a very simple way to gain profound self-understanding in rela-tion to repressed dimensions of the psyche.

GOLD STAR PRACTICE
The 3-2-1 Shadow Process

First choose what you want to work with. It is usually easiest to begin with a "difficult person" to whom you are attracted or by whom you are repelled or disturbed (for example, a lover, boss, or parent.) Alternatively, pick a dream image or a body sensation that distracts you or otherwise causes you to fixate on it. Keep in mind that the disturbance may be a positive or negative one.

You can recognize the shadow in two ways. Shadow material either:

> Makes you negatively hypersensitive, easily triggered, reactive, irritated, angry, hurt, or upset. Or it may keep coming up as an emotional tone or mood that pervades your life.

OR

> Makes you positively hypersensitive, easily infatuated, possessive, obsessed, overly attracted, or perhaps it becomes an ongoing idealization that structures your motivations or mood.

Then follow the 3 steps of the process:

3 – Face It
Observe the disturbance very closely, and then, using a journal to write in or an empty chair to talk to, describe the person, situation, image, or sensation in vivid detail using 3rd-person pronouns such as "he," "him," "she," "her," "they," "their," "it," "its," etc. This is your opportunity to explore your experience of the disturbance fully, particularly what it is that bothers you about it. Don't minimize the disturbance—take the opportunity to describe it as fully and in as much detail as possible.

2 – Talk to It
Enter into a simulated dialogue with this object of awareness using 2nd-person pronouns ("you" and "yours"). This is your oppor-

tunity to enter into a relationship with the disturbance, so talk directly to the person, situation, image, or sensation in your awareness. You may start by asking questions such as, "Who/what are you? Where do you come from? What do you want from me? What do you need to tell me? What gift are you bringing me?" Then allow the disturbance to respond back to you. Imagine realistically what they would say and actually write it down or vocalize it. Allow yourself to be surprised by what emerges in the dialogue.

I – Be It

Now, writing or speaking in 1st person, using the pronouns "I," "me," and "mine," be the person, situation, image, or sensation that you have been exploring. See the world, including yourself, entirely from the perspective of that disturbance and allow yourself to discover not only your similarities, but how you *really* are one and the same. Finally, make a statement of identification: "I am _____" or "_____ is me." This, by its nature, will almost always feel *very* discordant or "wrong." (After all, it's exactly what your psyche has been busy denying!) But try it on for size, since it contains at least a kernel of truth.

This last step (the I of the 3-2-1) often has a second part, in which you complete the process of fully re-owning the shadow. Don't just see the world from that perspective momentarily, but actually *feel* this previously excluded feeling or drive until it resonates clearly as your own. Then you can engage it and integrate it.

To complete the process, let the previously excluded reality register not just abstractly but on multiple levels of your being. This engenders a shift in awareness, emotion, and subtle energy that frees up the energy and attention that was taken up by your denial. You'll know that the process has worked because you'll actually feel lighter, freer, more peaceful and open, and sometimes even high or giddy. It makes a new kind of participation in life possible.

Sample 1: Phil Visits His Childhood Friend

3 – FACE IT

I'm dreading going to visit my childhood best friend. The last time I visited, the whole scene with him and his wife and family really got on my nerves. He's such a wimp! His wife runs his life! He's got a super safe, secure, and dead-end job. He's not drinking from the cup of life and letting the juice run down his neck; he's never feeling the wind through his hair! If he'd just walk on the wild side once in a while, he'd be twice as alive. He's betraying himself. It makes me sick. It drives me nuts to be around him.

2 – TALK TO IT

Phil: Why do you let your wife make all the decisions?
Joe: I don't. But I respect her perspective.
Phil: Why are you satisfied with your grade B, dead-end job?
Joe: Hey, it's good honest work, and I enjoy it.
Phil: Why don't you consult or form your own company?
Joe: I prefer what I've got. It's more secure and takes less work. What's wrong with that?

Back and forth, Phil continues exploring—and what comes out is that Joe wants to be safe and secure and not have dramas in his life, whereas Phil believes in risk-taking and pushing the envelope and going for the max.

1 – BE IT

Phil becomes Joe. Phil says, "*I want safety and security and a smooth, predictable life.*"

Re-owning the Shadow

Phil realizes he's disowned his own needs for safety and security so much that he's easily triggered by Joe's qualities. He, like everyone, has needs for both sides: thrills, aliveness, risk, passion, intrigue, bigger rewards on one side, and safety, security, predictability, comfort on the other. Having disowned one side, he can become more whole and make conscious choices that take the whole spectrum of values into account.

This usually takes the form of both an insight and an energetic shift. Phil may go on to more deeply understand and reintegrate his need for safety and security and thus feel freer to make new choices in his life. He may feel a new kind of compassion and empathy for Joe. He may realize, for example, that his idealization of the swashbuckling father he lost when he was just 12 has cast a shadow over other important parts of his inner world. And he may even have new ways of coping with his life challenges; for example, he might realize that he can gratefully enjoy Joe and his family for a day and a half, and that he wants to stay in a hotel for the rest of his stay, so as to avoid an overdose. It might include all of these possibilities, and it might be nothing more specific than a relaxation of his previously triggered reactivity.

Sample 2: Kathy Gives Her Power to Bill

3 – FACE IT

I first met Bill through an online dating service where I specified that I was looking for a *very intelligent* man. I felt an instant pull toward Bill after reading his bio: professor at the University of Chicago with two PhDs, one in theoretical physics and the other in philosophy!

During our first couple dates, I hung on Bill's every word—totally enamored of his range of knowledge and insight. The more he talked about black holes and M-Theory, Kant and Kierkegaard, the more attracted I felt to him.

I've been seeing Bill for about three months now and am beginning to notice something that really bothers me. *I lose my voice when I'm around him.* He knows so much about so much that I don't know what I can contribute to the conversation. He's already so smart there's just not much he could learn from me.

I still love spending time with Bill because he's such a brilliant guy, but I'm not sure if he feels satisfied with our conversations.

2 – TALK TO IT

Kathy: Do you enjoy spending time with me?

Bill: Of course I enjoy spending time with you. That's why I've wanted to see you so much over the past few months.

Kathy: But don't our conversations bore you? You don't learn anything new from me.

Bill: On the contrary Kathy, I see you as one sharp lady. You've learned more than you think from starting your own business and building it from the ground up. It takes more than luck to run a company as successful as yours. I've certainly never done anything like that, and I learn a lot from listening to you talk about it.

Kathy: But don't you notice how timid and agreeable I am around you?

Bill: Just because I've spent over half my life in school, doesn't mean I'm right about everything! I invite you to challenge me, disagree with me, and speak your mind. I greatly value independent thinkers and unique perspectives and would love to hear more of your views—especially if they're different from my own!

1 – BE IT

Kathy becomes Bill. Kathy says, "I am intelligent. I have valuable perspectives to contribute."

Re-owning the Shadow

Somewhere in her past, Kathy learned that displaying her intelligence around men was not okay. So she disowned and hid her own intellectual capacity. In this case, Kathy's shadow was a positive quality: intelligence. She projected her intelligence onto Bill. Kathy felt such a strong initial attraction to Bill because she was "shadow hugging." Her infatuation was not just with Bill, but also with her disowned intelligence. Through the 3-2-1 process, Kathy reclaimed her own intelligence.

This occasioned a re-assessment of her whole self-image, a process she pursued by journaling actively for the next several days. As she came to terms with this insight, she felt more grounded and less prone to give away her power to others. After taking a short break from Bill, she decided to continue the relationship. But she no longer found herself idealizing Bill's intelligence as if she needed it to fill a void in herself. She felt much more self-respect. And on that basis, she could see his egotism and foibles, and appreciate him as a peer, a multi-dimensional human being.

Sample 3: Tony Meditates with a Monster

Shortly after his divorce, Tony begins to have horrible nightmares that recur many times each week. Every nightmare features the same grotesque monster with sharp teeth and cold, slimy skin who relentlessly stalks him through various dreamscapes. The vicious monster hates Tony and wants to kill him. Right when the monster is about to ensnare him, Tony wakes up sweating in the darkness, terror pulsing through his body.

Tony, a long time meditator, takes the issue to his meditation teacher, who advises him to meditate on the fear associated with the monster. Over the next several months, Tony follows his teacher's instruction, witnessing the fear, feeling into the fear, relaxing into the fear, so that it may uncoil and "self-liberate." The idea is that when Tony allows his mind to relax completely and "just be," the coiled up, contracted energy in his emotions can be released and thus liberated to be used more freely.

After four months of diligent practice, the nightmares remain the same and in some instances they intensify. For Tony, the monster is still scary as hell and still intent on killing him.

Tony decides to practice the 3-2-1 process in addition to his regular meditation. Here's an excerpt from one of his 3-2-1 process sessions:

3 – FACE IT

It's almost as though I'm inside a computer. Flashing lights and techno contraptions surround me. It feels like a harsh, foreign, and unnatural environment. I sense something is pursuing me, stalking me as if I were helpless prey. Glancing over my shoulder I catch a glimpse of a tall menacing figure, shrouded in darkness. I know this monster hates me and wants to kill me. Fear grips every muscle in my body. I awkwardly try to escape and stumble through this alien world. Yet despite all my efforts, the killer gains ground . . . closer . . . closer until it's almost on top of me. I scrunch my eyes shut as the fear completely paralyzes me.

2 – TALK TO IT

Tony: Why are you chasing me?
Monster: Because I hate you and want to kill you.
Tony: Why do you hate me and want to kill me?
Monster: Because I'm so damn angry with you.
Tony: Why are you angry with me?
Monster: Because you're hateful and contemptible and deserve to die!
Tony: How does that feel?
Monster: Like a roaring furnace of rage!

Tony and the monster continue to explore the monster's feelings and experience.

1 – BE IT

Tony becomes the monster. Tony says, "I'm freaking angry!" "I'm seething with rage and fury and I want to kill!"

Re-owning the Shadow

Through practicing the 3-2-1 process, Tony realized that a fierce anger lurked behind his fear. After his divorce, he had dissociated his anger into a split-off shadow element, which showed up in his nightmare as an angry monster. Only by re-owning his anger could Tony reclaim his shadow repression and free up the power of a more integrated self.

He realized he'd been subtly depressed for several years. Tony had felt depleted, since he had been continually depriving himself of the raw energy of the primary emotion he'd so totally denied. He started exercising more vigorously at the gym, especially enjoying a kick boxing class there. He also found a good therapist with whom he worked to recapture and channel the raw energy of his being.

Meditation alone couldn't do it. Tony did an exemplary job of witnessing his fear during his daily sittings. But the fear itself was an *inauthentic* emotion, a symptom of the primary emotion, anger. Tony could have witnessed his fear for twenty years (as many people do) and the primary repression—anger—would still be in place. Without owning this authentic emotion, Tony's anger would be projected to create monsters all around him, which would bring up fear in him (which is really fear of his own anger, not fear of the monsters), and while he would get in touch with that fear and think he was transmuting that fear—he would never contact or liberate the primary and authentic emotion, anger, the root cause of his nightmares and terror.

Failing to work with the actual mechanism of dissociation (1 to 2 to 3) and therapeutic ownership (3 to 2 to 1), meditation becomes a way to get in touch with your infinite Self, while reinforcing the inauthenticity in your everyday finite self, which has broken itself into fragments and projected some of them onto others. Here the disowned fragments hide,

Symptom	← manifests from	Original Shadow Form
Resentment of outside pressure	←	Drive
Rejection ("Nobody likes me")	←	Rejection ("I reject them")
Guilt ("You make me feel guilty")	←	Resentment (of another's demands)
Anxiety	←	Excitement
Self-consciousness	←	Outward focus (on others)
Sexual Dysfunction	←	"I wouldn't give him/her the satisfaction"
Fear ("They want to hurt me")	←	Hostility ("I'm angry and attacking without knowing it")
Sad	←	Mad
Withdrawn	←	Rejecting
I can't	←	"I won't, dammit!"
Obligation ("I have to")	←	Desire ("I want to")
Hatred	←	Self-hatred
Envy ("You're soooo great")	←	"I'm better than I realize." (A golden shadow form)

Figure 4.1

Secondary, inauthentic emotions and drives translated to their primary, authentic forms.

Often, you can translate a 3rd-person shadow symptom back into its original 1st-person form. Use the chart above as a handy reference guide. These are some of the more common examples of how shadow translates into symptom (and vice versa). As you continue to practice with the 3-2-1 Shadow Process, you'll gain more insight into your own individual shadow dynamics.

1-MINUTE MODULE
The 3-2-1 Shadow Process

You can do the 3-2-1 process any time you need it. Two particularly useful times are right when you wake up in the morning and
just before going to bed at night. Once you know 3-2-1, it only
takes a minute to do the process for anything that might be disturbing you.

Morning: First thing in the morning (before getting out of bed)
review your last dream and identify any person or object with an
emotional charge. *Face* that person or object by holding it in mind.
Then *talk* to that person or object (or resonate with it, just feeling
what it would be like to be face to face.) Finally, *be* that person or
object by taking its perspective. For the sake of this exercise, there
is no need to write anything out—you can go through the whole
process right in your own mind.

Evening: Last thing before going to bed, choose a person who
either disturbed or attracted you during the day. In your mind, *face*
him or her, *talk* to him or her, and then *be* him or her (as described
above).

Again, you can do the 3-2-1 process quietly by yourself, any
time you need it, day or night.

even from the sun of contemplation—shadow-mold in the basement that
will sabotage every move you make from here to eternity.

More Advanced Forms of Shadow Work

Lighter Shades of Shadow

Several distinct *types* of shadow exist. For most of this chapter we've
focused on one of the main types—the repressed unconscious shadow,
the drives, feelings, and needs that were so threatening to our conscious-

ness that we've repressed our awareness of them. This shadow material is the source of projections—both negative and positive. The work of shining light on it never ends.

Another kind of shadow is also worth mentioning. It's the shadow of our emergent capacities that we have not yet owned and inhabited. This is the shadow cast by *higher* parts of ourselves that want to come down and be lived by us. Often, our conditioned identity doesn't allow for aspects of our deep, unique calling and capacity. We keep these out of awareness, in shadow. Certain kinds of growth can't take place until this repression is relaxed, letting us know ourselves and show up fully as utterly unique individuals.

Put another way, sometimes our highest intelligence, intuition, and capacities don't fit our images of ourselves. In this type of situation, we function in ways consistent with old, fixed identities, unable to responsibly integrate and incarnate our highest potentials and awareness. We're stuck being a lower self than we're really supposed to be. It's important to recognize that sometimes the shadow can hold not just "low" or primitive aspects of the psyche, but also some of the "highest" evolved aspects. Be aware of this possibility. And when you recognize it operating in you, find the clarity and courage to choose to live your highest capacities. In the afterword, "The Unique Self," we will discuss this process of opening up to our own special dynamism and purpose. Both of these kinds of "golden shadows" represent a golden opportunity for growth.

For example, some people may have a high capacity for leadership, but they dislike that aspect of themselves that wants to be "in charge." It's too aggressive, masculine, self-assertive—and besides, who are they to tell other people what to do? Because they associate leadership with perceived negative qualities of control and domination, they've created a golden shadow in themselves. They may admire the leadership capacity *in others*, while resenting their own greater power. By exploring a 3-2-1 process, they might come to see their own desire to be a leader—which might also be the cutting edge of their own practice and growth: a "golden shadow," which, if re-owned, could be transformed into a gift of visionary light.

The Strange Logic of the Psyche

In doing shadow work, it's important to account for the sometimes strange logic of the psyche. The deep psyche often responds to the *opposite image* of our shadow parts in much the same way that it responds to the shadow parts themselves. We can become activated, agitated, frozen, disoriented, or withdrawn not just in response to the presence of the parts of ourselves we have denied, our shadow, but also in the presence of their mirror image, or emotional opposites.

In our first example above, Phil had disowned his needs for safety, and so his relatively timid childhood friend, Joe, triggered this shadow element in him. These same disowned needs might have been triggered again, albeit differently, if Phil was confronted by someone quite the opposite of Joe, say a different friend, Raul, an extreme daredevil. He might feel that his own courage, wildness, and intensity were dwarfed in comparison. If he then did a 3-2-1 process on Raul, this wild person, he might have ended by saying "Life is about intensity and aliveness or it is nothing; I care nothing for safety or security." And this would have touched an important psychological truth. But the inverse—the denial of safety needs at which Phil arrived in our original example—might have been even *more* deeply revealing.

Thus, at the completion of the 3-2-1 process, as you "try on" whatever originally triggered you, let your intuition notice whatever disowned parts of the self you can most deeply recognize. Sometimes they may show up in what seem to be the *opposite* of the feeling with which you began.

Transmuting Your Authentic Primary Emotions

Shadow work is important, but it's often just the first step in clarifying our emotional lives. Once you've done your shadow work, and you're no longer lost in secondary, inauthentic emotions, you have an opportunity to creatively reclaim and use the energy of that primary authentic emotion. (Technically speaking, this is not true "shadow work," but it is very often the next appropriate step in practicing with emotions.)

The raw energy of your authentic, primary emotion is an expression of the primordial energy of your being. All of it is essential and necessary to your wholeness. If your emotions are apparently "negative" ones, such as anger, fear, or grief, it may seem that they are only sabotaging your effectiveness or poisoning your mind and heart. It is common to think that such emotions need to be eliminated. However, this is not a realistic option. The effort to "get rid" of negative emotions only tends to drive them into the shadow. That was the problem in the first place! A more fruitful approach is to transmute these emotions into their pure and essential energy for expression and release.

This simple five-step approach conveys the essence of the traditional spiritual practice of transmuting negative emotions:

1. Notice what you are feeling and how this shows up in your body, both physically and energetically.
2. Relax the tendency to judge, suppress, or otherwise react to it, and just allow it to be what it is, embracing it with awareness.
3. If your emotion is about someone or something, relax your relationship to the object. Let the emotional energy be there. Notice that it is arising within you (rather than happening to you, as in "she makes me feel this way.") Relax into full responsibility for your emotional patterns and energies.
4. Feel the energy of your emotion and the situation or relationship in which it is arising. Breathe and allow the energy of the emotion to flow. Notice how that can take place constructively rather than destructively. Take several breaths and notice how the emotion changes as it is channeled and circulated.
5. Pay attention until you recognize the transitory nature of the emotion and allow its raw energy to self-liberate, like water boiling into steam, as a free, unobstructed, and positive expression.

The essence of this process is the *acceptance* and *allowance* of the emotion, which relaxes the tension and resistance surrounding it. Then you let the emotion show itself to you. You let it reveal the liberated, unobstructed, or awakened expression of its raw energies.

Consider, for example, the transmutation of anger. There is great energy behind anger. If it is liberated into its pure, authentic essence, what does it become? Often it reveals itself as the energy and commitment to discriminate and penetrate, to cut through confusion into clarity. Sometimes it is the energy and will to change what needs to be changed. Emotional energy such as anger need not disappear; in fact, it can be a valuable resource in service of compassion and freedom.

Ongoing Emotional Transmutation

Emotions are deeply habitual. After you have transmuted an emotion, you will sometimes find yourself falling back into the same old pattern. The newly revealed emotional energies need to find new ways to organize themselves. To transmute emotions successfully over time requires persistent practice. They will self-liberate, apparently completely, only to arise again at a later time, so that you'll have to work with them again. Lasting results require patience and persistence. With practice, over time, you may notice how quickly and powerfully your emotions respond to negative experiences, and you may be amazed to discover that, with conscious practice, even such visceral emotions will naturally self-liberate. As your practice becomes more natural, you'll have more energy, insight, and skill in working with challenging emotions and energies in your life.

How the transmutation of emotions fits together with shadow work:

- In the shadow work process, what was "it" or "you" is realized to be a disowned part of the "I."
- In the process of transmuting emotions, these dimensions of the "I" are witnessed by the "I AM."
- In the process they are released and no longer identified with. Instead of your emotions having you, you have them. Instead of shaping the "I" they become "mine."

In other words, inauthentic secondary emotion transforms into authentic primary emotion, which transmutes into awakened transcendental energy.

Since words cannot precisely capture the fluidity of emotions, no

Shadow Work with Transmuting Emotions

One of Sigmund Freud's famous summations of the psychothera-peutic process was, "Where It was, there I shall become." Like-wise, for shadow work and transmuting emotions:

What was "it"
becomes "I."

What was "I"
becomes "mine"

and is witnessed by I AM.

Thus, its energy is reclaimed and liberated.

categorical generalizations can be fully accurate. Nonetheless, the corre-spondences shown in figure 4.2 (see page 64) might be useful.

Evolving Your Relationship with Your Emotions

The process of transmuting emotions, together with shadow work, offers the opportunity for extra spaciousness in relationship to your emotional life. This spaciousness makes it possible to relax and experience your feel-ings directly. You can be curious and investigate them. You can trust that the process will be liberating, rather than just painful. Valuing the raw energy of your emotions, you can work with them, knowing they will eventually open from their contracted expressions into their authentic, free, and awakened expression. You can be confident that when this hap-pens you will be empowered. The tremendous energy they contain will become usable as additional vitality, awareness, and growth.

The 3-2-1 Shadow Process and Transmuting Emotions are inherently powerful and valuable practices. The benefits that follow from practicing them can change the whole climate of your inner experience, dramati-cally speeding up your growth and enriching your life. Most people are

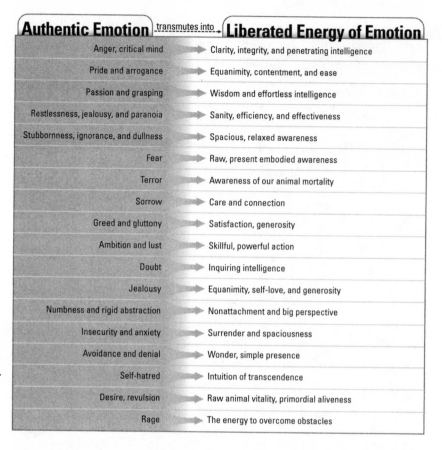

Authentic Emotion	transmutes into	Liberated Energy of Emotion
Anger, critical mind	→	Clarity, integrity, and penetrating intelligence
Pride and arrogance	→	Equanimity, contentment, and ease
Passion and grasping	→	Wisdom and effortless intelligence
Restlessness, jealousy, and paranoia	→	Sanity, efficiency, and effectiveness
Stubbornness, ignorance, and dullness	→	Spacious, relaxed awareness
Fear	→	Raw, present embodied awareness
Terror	→	Awareness of our animal mortality
Sorrow	→	Care and connection
Greed and gluttony	→	Satisfaction, generosity
Ambition and lust	→	Skillful, powerful action
Doubt	→	Inquiring intelligence
Jealousy	→	Equanimity, self-love, and generosity
Numbness and rigid abstraction	→	Nonattachment and big perspective
Insecurity and anxiety	→	Surrender and spaciousness
Avoidance and denial	→	Wonder, simple presence
Self-hatred	→	Intuition of transcendence
Desire, revulsion	→	Raw animal vitality, primordial aliveness
Rage	→	The energy to overcome obstacles

Figure 4.2

Authentic emotion translated to liberated energy of emotion.

very afraid to experience some of their own feelings. This fear holds them back from being fully present in life.

This can change when you become confident that "scary" feelings conceal an opportunity to become more alive and powerful. Successfully doing this work not only frees the energy that was previously bound up in shadow emotions, but it also provides a realistic basis for a rich, compassionate relationship with your own emotional life.

The fruits of these emotional practices can be seen in many forms:

- The willingness to allow and experience more of life directly, including what were formerly difficult feelings
- More aliveness and empowerment where you were formerly numb and afraid

- The ability to be fully present in emotionally charged situations
- Sincere openness and relaxed curiosity about shadow emotions
- An inner atmosphere of self-acceptance and self-compassion
- A lessening of the tendency to become emotionally hijacked, and thus the ability to see life more clearly

Integrating Light and Dark, Spirit and Shadow

We can now begin to draw some conclusions regarding the shadow, as well as make a couple of crucial connections between shadow work and other aspects of ILP—specifically, spiritual practice and meditation.

Face the Shadow, or It Will Find a Way to Trip You Up

Spiritual teachers have taught us many beautiful lessons. Hidden among them is a darker, inadvertent lesson: Even spending many hours in high meditative states won't necessarily turn the shadow into light. The reputations of many otherwise wonderful spiritual figures have been marred by scandals, involving sex, power, and money, engendered (sometimes subtly and paradoxically) by their unconscious *shadow* impulses.

You Can't See What You Can't See

If I meditate, and meditate very deeply, what can happen? I can watch my fear and sadness arise as objects in my awareness. I can relax my "identification" with them. I can even discover the timeless present in which fear and sadness don't really matter. **But unless I do shadow work in addition to meditating, I probably won't truly face my shadow.** This has become obvious after three decades of diligent sitting by Western students of Eastern paths. There is a big difference between advanced meditators who have meditated but neglected shadow work and those who've practiced both.

Working with the shadow, as in the 3-2-1 process, brings the relative self back into wholeness; it does not touch the infinite Self or Witness— which is untouched either way. Meditation helps us realize the Big Self, but it does not directly deal with the problems of the finite self. An Integral Life Practice does both: it heals the finite self by uniting it with its shadow, and discovers the infinite Self that has no self and no shadow, since it is unmanifest emptiness in all conditions.

Shadow Work Includes a Vast, Rich Territory

Aspects of shadow work pervade ILP.

Growth inherently requires us to tolerate discomfort. To see a more conscious choice, we must become aware of the unconsciousness of our previous habit or tendency. This involves at least a moment of unflattering self-awareness, which usually feels uncomfortable.

Immature people reflexively and persistently defend themselves against unflattering self-awareness. Practitioners develop a different response—that of relaxed curiosity and interest. New awareness of unconscious and unproductive patterns and tendencies is actually very good news. It means that new choices are possible—choices that can produce better results in our lives.

This core capacity—to face our limitations and learn from them, rather than responding with defensiveness and denial—is essential to every module of Integral Life Practice.

Shadow Work Is Forever

Shadow work is both necessary and never-ending. No matter how aware you become, there is no final perfecting of the psyche. In every new moment, the psyche can, yet again, slyly and invisibly, play hide-and-seek with itself. Thus, there's no end to the work of shining light into shadow.

But don't *wait* to become shadow-free. You can always go beyond yourself—right now, despite your shadows. It would be a mistake to get self-indulgently caught up in an endless "hall of mirrors" where all you see are warped reflections of the ego.

Still, doing the work matters. People who are working sincerely to re-own their projections become mature, self-responsible, and trustworthy. This is why shadow work is a core module. Psychotherapy sessions may end. But shadow work never ends. We become clearer and clearer—more capable of shining with the light of awareness—as our shadow work becomes more subtle and profound. But wherever there is a light, there is a shadow—and we want to integrate both.

5

The Mind Module

The Practice of Taking Perspectives

The Mind module of ILP has two primary dimensions:

1. The practice of increasing your capacity to take more nuanced, complex, and accurate perspectives
2. The practice of expanding the mental framework you use to organize those perspectives

Most of this chapter will concentrate on the AQAL Integral Framework. By learning and using this framework in your everyday life, you will radically increase your capacity to take perspectives, and those perspectives will *make more sense* within your expanded awareness. Indeed, we often call AQAL a "psychoactive" framework, because the very act of using it expands, intensifies, and illuminates our experience of the world and ourselves—we are able to make new connections, feel life more deeply, and intuit subtler dimensions of consciousness.

Increasing Your Capacity to Take Perspectives

In a classic experiment, Jean Piaget tested the ability of young children to take different points of view. A child was shown a cube with opposing sides of blue and yellow. When he held up the cube, he asked the child, "What color are you seeing?" And then he asked, "What color am I seeing?" Younger children who were shown the yellow surface assumed that he was seeing yellow too. But children of about age 5 consistently demonstrated a big transition. Even though the 5-year-old still saw yellow, he now understood that the researcher was seeing blue. The child could take the perspective of someone else, which allowed him to answer correctly.

Ideally, this perspective taking capacity keeps developing well into adulthood. Growth occurs through taking on wider and wider perspectives. Whereas previously we were embedded in a limited perspective, we become able to hold a more embracing view that goes beyond the limited truth of our previous way of seeing. Eventually, we learn to take perspectives on our own perspective-taking! And so proceeds the evolution of consciousness.

The simple intention to *see more perspectives* is a fundamental practice of the Mind module. Try to notice additional perspectives when possible, to continually wake up into new and larger perspectives—to take perspectives on your own perspective-taking. As a practitioner, hold the awareness that every perspective is both true and partial, *including your own*. Thus, try to be less defensive of your point of view and more curious about and open to new ways of seeing things.

Easy to say; hard to do. The practice of opening to new perspectives could take a million forms—from reading books, to talking to new people, to traveling, to experiencing art. The mind is truly infinite, and so are

The Mind Module and ILP

The Mind module *pervades* the whole of Integral Life Practice. In fact, we're doing a Mind module practice right now: *taking a perspective on practice itself.*

Successfully steering our way through our life practice requires all dimensions of self—including our mind. A developed mind allows us to take multiple perspectives and make better choices when designing our practice, dealing with challenges, and waking up to new realizations. A mature mental intelligence allows us to emerge not just as an expression of universal oneness, but distinctly, as who we each are—*the unique self.*

the perspectives available to you. That's what makes the AQAL Framework an indispensable tool. As a way *organizing* the many perspectives we can take, it actually creates room for more (and deeper) perspectives. Just as cleaning out a closet helps you fit more into it (and helps you find what you're looking for when you need it), using AQAL helps create "a place for everything in your life."

Elements of the Integral Framework

AQAL Integral Theory

AQAL is a power tool for mental integration. It identifies a handful of simple distinctions that can enable you to recognize, classify, and eventually transcend (and include) perspectives. Let's take a look at AQAL's key elements.

AQAL stands for "all **quadrants**, all **levels**, all **lines**, all **states**, and all **types**." This is the simplest set of distinctions that can account for the complexity of our evolving world and the depth and breadth of consciousness for which authentic practice strives.

We often say that AQAL "makes sense of everything." However, the AQAL Framework is not totalistic. In fact, it leaves most of the details out, to be filled in by new discoveries and individual experience. AQAL is a "theory of everything" because it *actively makes room for* and *consciously includes* as many *ways of knowing* as we're aware of—from phenomenology to systems science, cultural studies to empiricism, contemplation to developmental psychology, and more.* And it does so in a way that's based on millennia of wisdom, centuries of science, and decades of cross-cultural research. AQAL helps us realize that the Kosmos is a lot bigger than we might have previously imagined. It can thus serve as an expansive framework for virtually any human endeavor, including Integral Life Practice.

---

*Technically, this is called "Integral Methodological Pluralism." It's a way of honoring the truths and insights from a multitude of disciplines, by showing how their respective ways of knowing all fit together.

AQAL: All Quadrants, All Levels, All Lines, All States, All Types

Here is a brief overview of the elements of the AQAL Framework:

Quadrants combine two of the most fundamental distinctions in the Kosmos: interior/exterior and individual/collective. The four resulting intersections give us the *interior and exterior of the individual and collective* (I, We, It, Its).

Levels are higher-order structures that emerge as evolution breaks into new territory. These structures reflect altitudes of consciousness (such as egocentric, ethnocentric, worldcentric). Also sometimes called "stages" or "waves" of development.

Lines are specific areas in which growth and development can occur (for example, interpersonal, moral, musical, needs, cognitive). Also sometimes called "multiple intelligences" or "streams" of development.

States are temporary, changing, and sometimes heightened forms of awareness (for example, waking, dreaming, deep sleep, meditative states, "the zone," and peak experiences).

Types are horizontal differences (such as, masculine and feminine expressions, cultural differences, or personality types such as the Enneagram or Myers-Briggs).

A Place for Everything in Your Life

It's no secret that contemporary life can be overwhelming. The availability of so much information and so many varieties of experience is both a blessing and a curse. Information overload can feel smothering, demanding, intimidating, paralyzing, daunting, burdensome, and downright exhausting. Believe it or not, *an Integral framework simplifies the situation.* AQAL is aspirin for this information headache.

Information loses its usefulness without organization. Data amounts to nothing unless it relates to a bigger picture. Fragments of disconnected information lie around in idle, meaningless heaps, until we see the larger patterns that unite them. AQAL *helps turn heaps into wholes by identifying the most fundamental patterns that connect those heaps.* An Integral

But Is This Just a Head Trip?

Integrating mind with body and spirit is a critical task of any ILP. But that doesn't mean getting rid of the mind—after all, it's central to the equation! Many people view the mind as an obstacle to spiritual growth. We are urged to go beyond the mind, to let it go, to drop it. "Get out of your mind and into your body." Or, "stop being so heady and just be!" "If you're really spiritual, you should listen closely to the wisdom of your body and avoid intellectual distinctions."

When it comes to spirituality, there is a prejudice that the mind takes us out of our immediate experience—that the mind is "conceptual," while the body is "experiential." We want to feel some kind of unity or intimacy with Spirit, but the mind, with its divisions and distinctions, kills that feeling-experience. Not to mention the flood of thoughts and distractions (or "monkey mind") that comes up in meditation. And so the rule in popular spirituality has become, "Just be!"—in other words, don't get too intellectual.

It's definitely possible to get stuck in the head if you don't have a truly Integral practice. But ILP *includes* the mind and intellect; it doesn't leave them behind. It makes the mind a dimension of practice. Utilizing the AQAL Framework is itself a practice of body-mind-spirit (and shadow) integration.

Clear thinking is necessary for cultivating moral clarity, conscious choice, and even compassion; I have to be able to first *take your perspective* (a mental act) in order to *empathize* with you. It takes a healthy, developed mind to be truly spiritual.

vision reveals how seemingly unrelated aspects of our experience fit together, simplifying life's complexity without oversimplifying and offering a place for everything.

Quadrants

Sure, no map can include every detail, but it can *create space for them all*. For example, it would be impossible to fit every conceivable direction onto the face of a compass. Nevertheless, a compass makes room for every possible direction with two simple orientations: North/South and East/West.

Similarly, the 4 quadrants create a place for everything with two simple distinctions:

1. **Interiors** (including thoughts, feelings, meanings, and meditative experiences) and **Exteriors** (including atoms, brains, bodies, and behaviors)

and

2. **Individuals** (which have their own distinct forms and experience) and **Collectives** (which interact together in cultural groups and systems)

When we make these two distinctions, the same four dimensions or worldspaces emerge that we walked through in chapter 3: **I**, **We**, **It**, and **Its**.

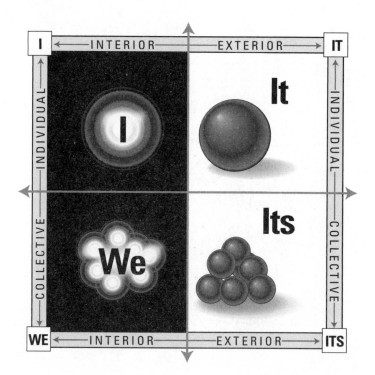

Figure 5.1
The 4 quadrants.

An Integral vision sees how realities in each of the 4 quadrants—from

consciousness and the shadow in the Upper-Left quadrant, to cultural values and relationships in the Lower-Left, to individual behaviors and physiological factors in the Upper-Right, to ecological and techno-economical systems in the Lower-Right—interpenetrate to give rise to each moment of life on this planet and in our own awareness.

Indeed, the four dimensions represented by the quadrants are present in every life situation. Visualize yourself walking into an office building in the morning. . . .

Upper-Left Quadrant, Interior-Individual "I" space: You feel excited and a little nervous about the big meeting today. Thoughts race through your head about how best to prepare.

Lower-Left Quadrant, Interior-Collective "We" space: You enter a familiar office culture of shared meaning, values, and expectations that are communicated, explicitly and implicitly, everyday.

Upper-Right Quadrant, Exterior-Individual "It" space: Your physical behaviors are obvious: walking, waving good morning, opening a

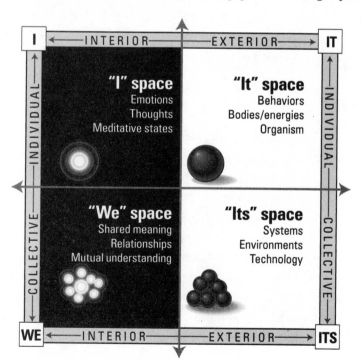

Figure 5.2

What's in the 4 quadrants?

door, sitting down at your desk, turning on the computer, and so on. Brain activity, heart rate, and perspiration all increase as the important meeting draws nearer.

Lower-Right Quadrant, Exterior-Collective "Its" space: Elevators, powered by electricity generated miles away, lift you to your floor. You easily navigate the familiar office environment, arrive at your desk, and log on to the company's intranet to check the latest sales numbers within the company's several international markets.

As you can see, phenomena arise in all four dimensions simultaneously. The 4 quadrants co-arise (or, more precisely, "tetra-arise") in the experience of every *now*. Moreover, *Integral Life Practice exercises aspects of your being in all 4 quadrants.* ILP is supported by noticing them all: your **Individual Interior "I,"** your **Individual Exterior "It,"** your **Collective Interior "We,"** and your **Collective Exterior "Its,"** which are always already present in every moment.

As you engage ILP and a life of practice, you may at some point notice yourself "forgetting" one or more of the quadrants of your life, focusing exclusively on certain parts of reality and leaving the rest out. As the Integral Framework becomes second nature, you'll more easily recognize all four dimensions of a situation.

Levels of Consciousness

This is the second basic element of the AQAL Framework. It maintains that there are indeed *higher and lower (or more and less evolved and aware) structures of consciousness,* and that we, as individuals and societies, can grow to higher levels in progressive *stages* or *waves* of development.

Many people find this idea difficult to swallow. They think if you talk about levels it means you're putting yourself above others; or they think the very notion of "higher consciousness" is somehow vague and new-agey. Unfortunately, they have a point: sometimes people do try to arrogantly elevate themselves above others—using their intellectual religion to imagine their false superiority. And yes, sometimes people *do* talk about "higher consciousness" in rather mushy, sloppy, or thoughtless

ways—which discredits the noble and profound matter of waking up in
the Kosmos.

But on the other hand, if we look at evolution, we see millions of tiny
incremental changes periodically give rise to *emergent properties*—and
something entirely new bursts forth into being (like living cells emerging from a primordial chemical soup, or art first emerging from early
humans). This demarks a whole new *stage, or level, or wave of development*. It happens in all four quadrants—in physical and biological evolution (It), in socioeconomic (Its) and cultural evolution (We), and in
the evolution of individual consciousness (I). And those stages *do* unfold
in a discernible pattern.

Consider the following sequence:

- Doing what mom and dad tell you to do (i.e., childhood)
- Doing what you and your high school friends want to do (while
  often rebelling against mom and dad—i.e., adolescence)
- Doing what you think is right on your own terms, as a free and
  responsible adult (i.e., adulthood)

Or this one:

- Slavery
- Segregation
- Civil rights

Could we say there is a stage-sequence of emerging higher consciousness in these examples? Would we ever want to go *backward* in either of
these sequences?

Again, some people don't like talking about levels because they don't
want to put anyone down or create an excuse to treat people unfairly.
This is an entirely valid concern. But in some cases, we clearly *need* to
make judgments between greater and lesser levels of complexity and consciousness. Sometimes it's important to assert a higher stance. Is it higher
or lower consciousness to hate gay people? Higher or lower for a society
to grant equal rights to its citizens? Higher or lower to see the world in
either/or, polarizing terms (e.g., us versus them), as opposed to being
able to value relative shades of truth on all sides?

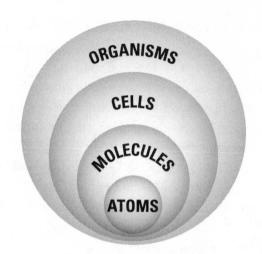

Figure 5.3

Simple levels of physical and biological evolution.

We can also look at biological evolution as an example of levels (see figure 5.3).

As the circles show, molecules are "higher" than atoms because they transcend atoms, yet also embrace them in their own makeup. Cells go beyond molecules in a similar manner, as do organisms with respect to cells, and so on. When a higher level transcends and includes a lower level, a qualitative emergence occurs, which means that something new comes into being that wasn't there previously. This "something new" signifies an evolutionary level.

When the Big Bang birthed the universe into existence billions of years ago, all the stars and planets and life forms didn't pop out fully formed, but had to *evolve into existence*. First, there were various forms of energy and subatomic particles; then atoms; then molecules; then single-celled organisms; then multi-cellular organisms; then various forms of plants and animals; then, early hominids; and then, poof, us amazing human beings! Reasonable men and women can disagree about the details of this miraculous process, but regardless of how exactly we got here, we can still reasonably say that a human organism is at a higher, more complex, and more conscious level of existence than, say, a carbon atom. (And the nice thing is, we don't have to worry about hurting a carbon atom's feelings, because it doesn't *have* any—or at least not the kind that could be offended by our arrogance.)

But notice: while we *transcend* carbon atoms by doing all sorts of things and possessing all kinds of qualities that they can't do and don't possess, we also *include* carbon atoms in our physical makeup. In fact, we *depend* on them. They're more *fundamental.* If carbon atoms were eliminated, there would be no human (or other living) beings. We include aspects of almost the entire evolutionary sequence, from atoms to molecules, to single cells, to neural cells, to limbic systems, up to our complex neocortex, which enables us to do things like use symbolic language and contemplate Kosmic evolution. This deepening from simpler to more complex, less conscious to more conscious, can be traced across the billions of years of Kosmic evolution. Each new level transcended and included all that went before, always growing into ever-greater degrees of creative novelty and awareness.

All 4 quadrants show evolutionary levels. The left-hand quadrants measure development in terms of *interior depth, or awareness.* The right-hand quadrants measure development in terms of *exterior complexity.* However, because all 4 quadrants "tetra-arise," an increase in interior consciousness corresponds, at least generally, with an increase in exterior complexity.

The emergence of the complex neocortex in the Upper-Right quadrant corresponded with the arising of higher intelligence in the Upper-Left quadrant. This, in turn, aligned with the flowering of human cultures in the Lower-Left quadrant and the development of civilizations in the Lower-Right quadrant. All four dimensions evolved simultaneously (and continue to do so!) into higher waves of consciousness and complexity.

What this means for our *personal evolution* is that we can intentionally focus on **harmonizing development across all 4 quadrants** in order to reach higher waves of consciousness and compassion. In fact, this is a primary function of Integral Life Practice. Because the 4 quadrants are profoundly intermeshed, overall development *must* occur in all 4 quadrants. If any one quadrant lags behind, it will tend to exert a *downward pull* on the other three. For example, if you are attempting to reach a state of clarity in your Upper-Left interior awareness, it will not help if your Lower-Right surroundings, such as your home or office, are a mess. That's why we tend to instinctively clean our (exterior) room when we're trying to focus our (interior) mind.

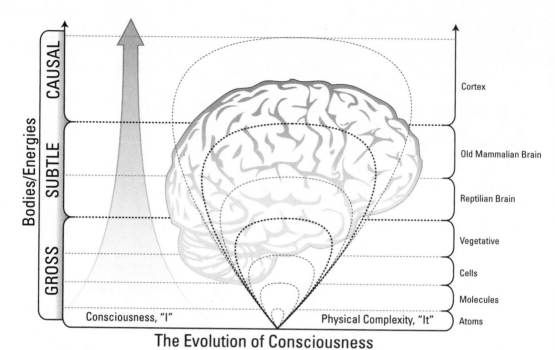

Bodies/Energies

CAUSAL · SUBTLE · GROSS

Cortex

Old Mammalian Brain

Reptilian Brain

Vegetative

Cells

Molecules

Atoms

Consciousness, "I"   Physical Complexity, "It"

The Evolution of Consciousness

Figure 5.4

Increasing consciousness = increasing complexity.

The same dynamic works in the opposite direction. If, for example, you are attempting to achieve a higher level of physical health and well-being (Upper-Right quadrant), you can be *pulled upward* by associating with people who value exercise, eating right, and healthy living (Lower-Left quadrant). And round and round the quadrants we go.

Growing into higher levels of consciousness and health involves transcending and including who you once were. The old you develops into a *new* you. The new you keeps some *enduring* characteristics from the old you, while shedding the *transitional* aspects of the old you. From each higher, deeper vantage point, what was once invisible becomes visible. You've experienced this, yes? You're not the same person today as you were ten years ago and you know it. You can look at the old you and describe the many ways you've grown beyond your previous self, as well as the many characteristics that have remained.

To further show what is involved, let's use a very simple model of moral development possessing only four levels or stages. An infant at birth has not yet been socialized into the culture's ethics and conven-

> Developmental researchers, such as Robert Kegan of Harvard University, describe the process of adult growth and development into more complex awareness as a matter of becoming aware of what previously shaped perception: the *subject* of one level becomes the *object of the subject* of the next higher level.

tions; this is called the **pre-conventional stage**. It is also called **egocentric**, in that the infant's awareness is largely self-absorbed. It cannot take the perspective of others and thus cannot regard them as similar beings deserving of moral regard. But as the young child begins to learn its culture's rules and norms, it grows into the **conventional stage** of morals. This stage is also called **ethnocentric**, in that it centers on the child's particular group, tribe, clan, or nation, and it therefore tends to exclude care for those not of one's group. But at the next major stage of moral development, the **post-conventional stage**, the individual's identity expands once again, this time to include a care and concern for all peoples, regardless of race, color, sex, or creed, which is why this stage is also called **worldcentric**. If the individual then keeps on growing (perhaps by taking up an ILP), they will progress to a **post-postconventional** or **kosmocentric** stage of moral development, thereby becoming capable of identifying with and caring for *all sentient beings*.

Thus, moral development tends to move from "me" (egocentric) to "us" (ethnocentric) to "all of us" (worldcentric) to "all sentient beings" (kosmocentric)—a good example of how the unfolding stages of consciousness surpass narcissism and grow into the capacity to take wider and deeper perspectives.*

---

*Keep in mind that a person is never simply at one level. Instead, people tend to fluctuate around **a particular level**, sometimes acting higher, sometimes lower, and hopefully edging our way upward over time. To say that someone is *at*, say, the worldcentric level in moral development means that *most often* they will take all people into account when confronting moral dilemmas—but *sometimes* they'll be "ethnocentric," and other times they'll be "egocentric." So when a person develops up to any given level, it means they have a *higher probability* of operating from that level on a good day. This is why sometimes we refer to levels as "waves," to emphasize their fluidity.

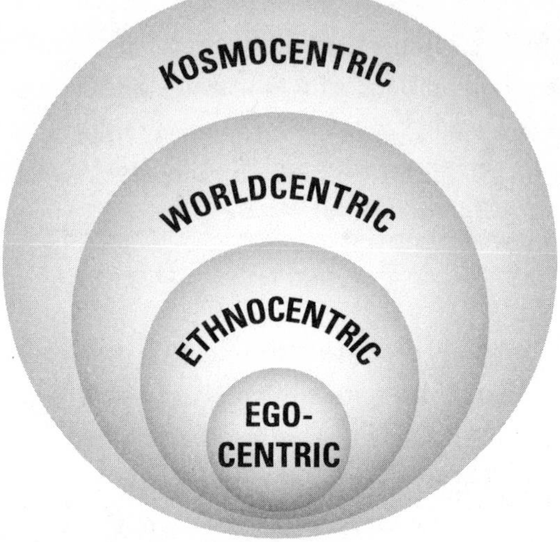

Figure 5.5
Stages of moral development.

- Egocentric = me
- Ethnocentric = us
- Worldcentric = all of us (all people and the planet we live on)
- Kosmocentric = the whole sentient, unfolding Kosmos

The *limited perspectives* of lower levels are happily left behind in the process of development. A lower-level aspect of consciousness can no longer pretend it's the center of the universe. With an understanding and acceptance of levels as *progressive* and *permanent* milestones along the evolutionary path of your own unfolding comes an implicit drive to grow into *higher levels and help others do the same*. Integral Life Practice provides a comprehensive, yet elegant method to live this inherent evolutionary urge.

That said, there is also (and very importantly) a sense in which we *are* wherever we are — and that's totally okay. Would you ever harshly judge a newborn baby for not knowing how to walk yet? Or a 5-year-old for not understanding calculus? No level of development is bad or wrong. Every single one is part of a natural sequence and has a right to exist. Each is *partially* true, but higher levels are (by definition) *truer*, because they transcend and include the lower levels.

There is no *absolutely highest* level, because there can always be *even higher* levels that have yet to emerge—and which certainly will, whether we like it or not! So we should be kind to ourselves—there's no need to be a developmental fanatic. Our job, as Integral practitioners, is to work with *all the levels we're aware of*—because all are real, all belong to this magnificent Kosmos, and the better we can understand them, the more effective and loving we can be in our lives—gently, naturally, and at our own pace.

Being aware of levels can influence our practice in many ways. For instance, we often have choices about the level at which we respond to experience. Choosing responses at our highest and truest levels will support our practice (as well as our ordinary life success). We are also constantly communicating and interacting with individuals and groups who are operating at a broad spectrum of levels. Practice often takes the form of meeting people where we find them and learning to speak in a language they will understand. See page 115 for more on Integral Communication.

Lines of Development

We've discussed levels of development in a few different ways—socially, biologically, morally—across the 4 quadrants. Does consciousness develop monolithically in all areas at the same time? According to AQAL, not at all. While there may be correlations among growth in different areas—and while growth in some areas may be necessary for growth in others—we can distinguish multiple **developmental lines** through which growth occurs in a relatively independent fashion. In fact, a level of development is always a level *in a specific line*. And just as levels are more like fluid *waves* than rigid ladder-like structures, lines are more like sinuous *streams* than straight and narrow tracks.

Over a dozen developmental lines have been found to exist, including the following:

- Cognition
- Needs
- Self-identity
- Values

- Emotions
- Aesthetics
- Morals
- Interpersonal relating
- Kinesthetic
- Spirituality

Each line is unique in that it can develop *relatively independently* of the others. In other words, you can be far along in one line, mediocre in another, and low in another. For instance, a person can have advanced interpersonal development but low moral development—like a smooth con man who uses his people skills to cheat others. Others may excel in emotional intelligence, but lack computer savvy. You can be extremely advanced in your cognitive line—you're an encyclopedic smarty-pants—but emotionally you're a wreck, or kinesthetically you can't even touch your toes.

Regardless of our particular highs and lows, developmental lines show us the many kinds of "smarts" available to us. Howard Gardner made a similar concept well-known through his research on **multiple intelligences** at Harvard University. The theory of multiple intelligences comprises a subset of all the developmental lines.

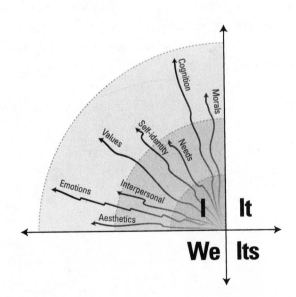

Figure 5.6

Some lines of development.

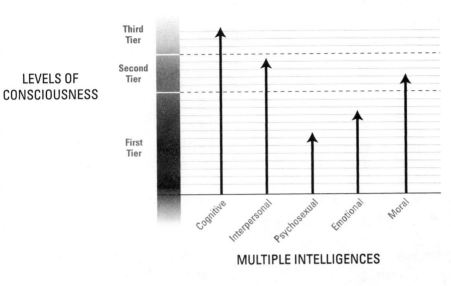

LEVELS OF
CONSCIOUSNESS

Third
Tier

Second
Tier

First
Tier

Cognitive Interpersonal Psychosexual Emotional Moral

MULTIPLE INTELLIGENCES

Figure 5.7
Integral psycho-
graph.

AQAL combines levels and lines (or waves and streams) to give us a more comprehensive, balanced, and precise view of overall development. A useful tool for seeing the relation of levels and lines in an individual is the **Integral Psychograph.**

The Integral Psychograph in figure 5.7 illustrates the relationship between levels and lines by depicting five important lines and their uneven development through three levels.

Figures 5.8–5.11 on page 84 represent some other sample psychographs. These are not meant to be seen in any kind of rigid way (remember: levels and lines are actually fluid like waves and streams!), but they give us a way of conceptualizing our overall development in a simple snapshot. Of course, it's always a lot more complicated than any graph can show, but having an orienting, big-picture view can help us immensely when it comes to working with the many tricky nuances of human development.

As you can see, every Integral Psychograph is a different zigzag of highs and lows, strengths and weaknesses, riches and (sometimes tragic) deficits. This helps us spot the ways that virtually all of us are unevenly developed, and thus prevents us from thinking that just because we're great in one area we must be great in all the others. Usually the opposite is closer to the truth. More than one business leader, spiritual teacher,

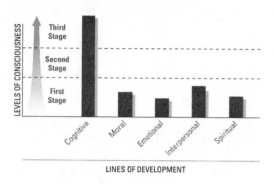

Psychograph:
Criminal Genius

LINES OF DEVELOPMENT

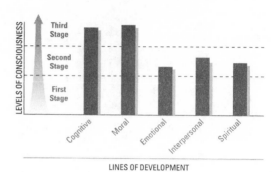

Psychograph:
Environmental Activist

LINES OF DEVELOPMENT

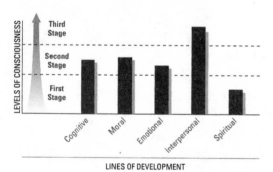

Psychograph:
Conservative Politician

LINES OF DEVELOPMENT

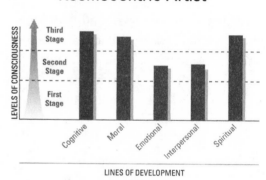

Psychograph:
Kosmocentric Artist

LINES OF DEVELOPMENT

Figures 5.8–5.11

and politician has spectacularly crashed because they failed to understand these basic realities.

Being aware of your own psychograph—cultivating a more Integrally informed self-image and self-understanding—gives you more freedom (and wisdom) to choose the best way to work with your own strengths and weaknesses, as well as those of others. In fact, *you can customize your Integral Life Practice on the basis of your Integral Psychograph.*

One simple strategy suggests that you focus on your highest lines (to leverage your strengths) and your lowest lines (to alleviate your most limiting weaknesses). By giving special attention to the one or two lines where you most excel and expanding your greatest potentials, you can

Types of Lines

- **Cognitive line** (necessary but not sufficient for other growth)
- **Self-related line**s (for example, ego, needs, morals, self-identity, values)
- **Talent lines** (such as, musical, visio-spatial, mathematical, kinesthetic)
- **Other important lines** (spiritual, aesthetic, emotional, psychosexual, interpersonal)

The many lines or streams identified by developmental researchers can be grouped together in these four major categories.

1. We put the **cognitive line** in its own category because research has shown that it provides the raw capacity to take perspectives that is "necessary but not sufficient" for growth in most of the other lines. This makes it (and hence the Mind module of ILP) extremely important. A major reason that the cognitive line is necessary but not sufficient for the other lines is that you have to be aware of something in order to act on it, feel it, identify with it, need it, or care for it.

2. The **self-related lines** or streams are especially associated with the self, its needs, its values, its identity, and its development through the major waves of consciousness. Although the many self-related lines differ from one another, they're also intimately related. A person's many self-related lines are typically close to the same level of consciousness.

3. Howard Gardner identified multiple **talent lines** or intelligences such as linguistic, spatial, mathematical, musical, and kinesthetic intelligence. Talent lines develop relatively independently of each other, meaning that some can be in full bloom while others are just sprouting, and still others remain dormant.

4. Certain **other important lines** are not listed among the self-related lines, but are more central to overall maturation than the talents. Among them are the spiritual, aesthetic, emotional, and interpersonal lines of development.

more fully offer the world your deepest gifts. Directing practice energy to your weakest lines may overcome potentially debilitating problems that would otherwise hold you back from fulfilling your highest intentions. Whatever lines you choose to focus on, the AQAL Framework makes sure you're at least *aware* of them all—both within yourself and everyone you encounter.

Integral Life Practice does not require (or even recommend) that you become hyper-developed in every single available line, like some kind of decathlete of consciousness, or developmental jack-of-all-trades. You can become a levels-and-lines decathlete if you want, but you probably don't have the time. It's certainly not required to have an Integral Life Practice. You don't need to master all the lines of development; just be aware of them. *This awareness itself will exert a balancing force on your life* because you'll naturally begin to adapt your behavior to leverage your strengths and compensate for your weaknesses. For example, you can add or subtract practices to remedy any imbalances. By understanding the AQAL Framework—a map whose territory is You—your self-awareness will naturally grow and deepen, so that you can make better decisions in your personal life, at work, and in your contributions to the world.

Answering Life's Questions

We can look at developmental lines as unique questions that life poses to us, again and again. Life asks us these questions, and we answer them.

- What am I aware of? (cognition)
- What do I need? (needs)
- Who am I? (self-identity)
- What is important to me? (values)
- How do I feel about this? (emotional intelligence)
- What is beautiful or attractive to me? (aesthetics)
- What is the right thing to do? (moral development)
- How should we interact? (interpersonal development)
- How should I physically do this? (kinesthetic ability)
- What is of ultimate concern? (spirituality)

Each of these questions has a long history. Some longer and more developed, others shorter and less developed. People have been chewing on them as we have evolved. And precisely because they are presented to us by life itself, our ways of answering them have developed. We develop *horizontally*—answers at each level can be healthier or less healthy—and *vertically*; the levels are hierarchies of how "intelligently" we can answer life's questions.

Look for a moment at your own history and notice how you've answered these questions differently throughout your life. Are you aware of more now than you were ten years ago? Do you have a broader self-identity now, than as an adolescent? Have your values shifted since you left college? Have your ultimate concerns deepened through the years? When we put it all on the table and take a good look at how we've answered these questions over time, it's easy to see the evolving nature of our developmental lines.

Keep in mind, we did not just make up these lines and the levels through which they unfold. AQAL incorporates the research done by hundreds of scholars from around the world.* Essentially, each researcher asked thousands of people—sometimes in one culture and sometimes across cultures—a set of questions, noticed the underlying pattern or structure behind the answers, and followed the responses over time. This is how we know that each developmental line has its own levels of accomplishment—from low to medium to high to very high (with no indication of an upper limit so far). An AQAL "all-levels/all-lines" approach puts all the different puzzle pieces together to give us a more comprehensive picture of human potential to date.

---

*Some important researchers in developmental psychology who have theorized and/or measured lines and levels include: cognitive—Jean Piaget, Robert Kegan, Michael Commons, and Francis Richards; needs—Abraham Maslow; emotional—Daniel Goleman; self-identity—Jane Loevinger and Susanne Cook-Greuter; values—Clare Graves, Don Beck, and Chris Cowan; moral—Lawrence Kohlberg and Carol Gilligan; spiritual—James Fowler. Cognitive psychologist Howard Gardner pioneered the concept of multiple intelligences and has posited eight: linguistic, logical-mathematical, spatial, bodily-kinesthetic, musical, interpersonal, intrapersonal, and naturalist.

Levels and Lines: Many Paths, One Mountain

Let's take a step back now and look at the big picture. Is there a common denominator between all these developmental lines and their levels? Is there a similarity between development in one line and development in others? According to AQAL, there is. The common denominator for all development in the interior of an individual is **consciousness itself**, and the rough equivalence that all levels share is their **altitude** of consciousness.

Picture a large mountain with, say, ten paths representing developmental lines. The mountain, of course, looks quite different depending on which path you're on—and these unique paths cannot be equated. Yet you can say that all the paths progress up the same altitude gradient— 3,000 feet, 5,000 feet, 7,000 feet, and so on. The altitude markers themselves (4,000 feet, 8,000 feet, etc.) are *without content*—they are "empty," just like consciousness per se—but each of the paths (developmental lines) can be measured in terms of its altitude on the mountain. The "feet" or "altitude" means degree of development, which is another way of saying the "amount" of depth and complexity that consciousness can inhabit.

Using altitude as a universal marker of development allows us to refer to general similarities across the various lines. But again, altitude, like "feet" or "inches," **itself has no content**; it is empty. No one says, "I had to stop building my house today because I ran out of inches." Or, "I better go out and buy some feet." These are just abstract units of measurement—but extremely useful. Likewise with "consciousness" when used in this fashion. It is not a thing or a phenomenon. It has no description. *Consciousness is not itself a line among other lines, but the space in which all lines unfold and all levels emerge.*

How do we represent this? We could do it in any number of ways. We've chosen a series of colors, arranged according to their order in the natural rainbow spectrum, as an easy-to-remember system of shorthand (see figure 5.12 following page 102).

Each color represents a general level or altitude of consciousness that applies to any of the lines we've discussed.* Each line still unfolds in a relatively independent fashion, and your Integral Psychograph will still be a mix of high, medium, and low altitudes—**Turquoise** cognition could conceivably appear in an individual with **Amber** values, **Green** needs, **Red** moral development, **Magenta** kinesthetic ability, **Teal** emotional intelligence, and **Orange** spirituality, (a brilliant, sociopathic, fundamentalist paraplegic, for example!)

The colors give us a simple and useful language to talk about levels of development in reference to any particular line. So from which altitude are you answering life's questions? Each time a situation presents itself in which you must implicitly answer one of life's questions, you are in effect speaking from your altitude of development in that line. Most people answer life's questions automatically: What is the *right* thing to do?—**Amber** answer; What do I *need?*—**Orange** answer; What do I *value?*—**Green** answer; How should we *interact?*—**Red** answer; and so forth.

An awareness of levels and lines opens a possibility for choice, however slight. Insight into where you stand on the psychographic map gives you a little more space to respond differently than your automatic reactions and answer from a little higher place. And the more you can do this, the easier it will become. Eventually it will become a permanent trait. The more you can answer from a higher place, the greater you'll grow and the deeper you'll flow through every wave and stream.

The first step is to become aware that the lines exist! The next step is to bring your highest intelligence into play in any low, lagging lines of development that may be holding you back. Maybe you are cognitively

---

*Those familiar with the Spiral Dynamics model will notice that some of the colors correspond (Red, Orange, Green, Turquoise) and others do not (Infared, Magenta, Amber, Teal). The Altitudes of Consciousness model introduced here includes the Spiral Dynamics values line in addition to all other lines of development. So every Spiral Dynamics level corresponds to a particular altitude of consciousness, whether the colors directly match or not: Purple-Magenta, Red-Red, Blue-Amber, Orange-Orange, Green-Green, Yellow-Teal, Turquoise-Turquoise.

AQAL Lines and ILP Modules

Practice in the **modules** of Integral Life Practice stimulates growth in many independent (and related) **lines of development**. Modules are not the same as lines, but they are related.

For example, the Body module involves more than just development of the kinesthetic line. Parenting involves numerous lines in all quadrants. Many practices in all modules support growth in the cognitive and self-related lines of development.

Practice in each module of Integral Life Practice naturally engages and stimulates growth in particular capacities and thus promotes growth in a cluster of developmental lines. Integral cross-training takes place when there is practice in all the core modules simultaneously. This is especially powerful because the whole is more than the sum of the parts. The synergy among them turbo-charges and reinforces growth in *many* of the key developmental lines. This is why ILP supports *integrated* maturation.

and spiritually brilliant but bound up emotionally and interpersonally. How do your emotions and interpersonal dynamics constrain your ability to participate in life's full complexity? Just seeing the pattern can focus your practice and growth for maximum results.

A Spectrum of Worldviews

The color spectrum — Magenta, Red, Amber, and so on — makes it easier to talk about the various altitudes of consciousness. In conversation, it's often much simpler to say a shorthand color code rather than a level's technical name. Keep in mind, however, that the colors designate altitudes and can refer to *any line of development*. So in many instances, it's essential to specify exactly which line you're talking about.

One line that's particularly useful is the **worldview line** because it gets at a person or culture's most fundamental assumptions about the

Worldview	Description
Teal/Turquoise	INTEGRAL–kosmocentric, can shift between all previous levels and see relative truths there
Green	PLURALISTIC–multi-worldcentric, the stage of divinity within all beings, all paths are equal
Orange	RATIONAL–worldcentric, the level of universal regard, reason, and tolerance
Amber	MYTHIC–ethnocentric, the stage of absolute traditional truths, tribal/ethnic beliefs; myths
Magenta/Red	MAGIC–egocentric, the world of magical powers, sacrifices, and miracles

Figure 5.13
Major worldviews.

world.* Since we do not live in a pre-given world that everyone experiences in the same way, different worldviews exist—different ways of categorizing, presenting, representing, and organizing our experiences. A person's worldview underlies the way he orients himself in his environment and gives meaning to his existence.

Each basic altitude of consciousness has its own unique worldview, its own way of interpreting and making sense of things. As they unfold, each successive worldview embraces a little more consciousness and complexity, wisdom and compassion. All the worldviews described below are true . . . but partial. And each step up to a higher altitude marks a *truer* and *less partial* view than the step before. These worldviews usually manifest as complex hybrids, since individuals and groups are always learning, evolving, and thus making transitions to new perspectives. We all have a "center-of-gravity" worldview from which we operate the majority of the time—while sometimes, we operate from above or below. Let's look at

---

*Although closely related, the worldviews line is not identical to the values line (as tracked by the work of Clare Graves and Spiral Dynamics). It focuses on the evolution of "meaning making" and how the world is comprehended, rather than on the evolution of values (what we hold as important), especially what is most highly valued.

the most essential and extreme expressions of some key colors in the spectrum of worldviews. These descriptions are, in a sense, just caricatures, and nobody really works exactly as described. They don't pretend to convey the full complexity of each structure. However, you'll probably recognize many of these characteristics in people you know or have learned about, and perhaps even in yourself.

In the individual dimension, everybody starts at square one. **Infrared** functions as the worldview of newborn babies across the globe until they grow up through **Magenta**, **Red**, **Amber**, and hopefully higher. Who do you know who might have a **Magenta** worldview (a young child?), or a **Green** worldview (a humanities professor?), or a **Turquoise** worldview (a Zen business consultant?)? As you read the following descriptions, try to recognize those levels in people you know, including yourself. Again, this is not to judge, but to understand diversity better and to communicate more effectively.

> "No problem can be solved from the same level of consciousness that created it."
> —Albert Einstein

INFRARED – Archaic Worldview

Survival is the unrelenting mission and purpose of the archaic worldview. Basic survival instincts dominate to obtain necessities such as food, water, safety, and warmth. The world appears as an undifferentiated mass of sensory activity. Newborn infants—like the first Homo sapiens—have an archaic worldview with no separation between themselves and the world.

MAGENTA – Magic Worldview

In a magic worldview, subject and object partially overlap so that "inanimate objects" like rocks and rivers are directly felt to be alive or even to possess souls. Sacred places, objects, rituals, events, and stories can influence the world and so must always be relied upon and protected. Tribal customs are passed down from an ancient lineage, including rites of passage and seasonal cycles.

Safety and security are sought by bonding together and identifying (fusing) with a tribe in order to persevere and protect against outsiders. Allegiance and admiration are given to the chief, parents, ancestors, customs, and clan. Mystical signs and the desires of powerful spirit beings must be followed for the continued safety and well-being of the tribe.

RED – Power Worldview

This worldview marks the emergence of a sense of self (ego) distinct from the tribe, although it often acts impulsively on behalf of its favored group. Seeing itself as the center of the world (egocentric), the Red individualized self seeks to express and fulfill its wants and desires immediately. "It's all about me." People with a Red worldview don't plan for the future, but rather act impulsively to get what they want now.

Red sees itself as the center of its own hero's quest that includes powerful gods, goddesses, people, and forces to be reckoned with. Life is a wild jungle with predators and prey. In order to avoid threats and survive, Red exerts its own power or seeks to align with a powerful leader. Red lives and dies by the "survival of the fittest" maxim of the jungle. Intimidating and dominating others is how Red gets things done. But if you're a weaker individual or group, it often serves you better to submit to the warlord or chief, accepting your place in the dominating power structure in exchange for protection and a share of the spoils.

AMBER – Mythic Worldview

The god or gods of the mythic worldview rule as deeply felt powers that have a direct hand in the earthly affairs of men and women. Instead of being united only by blood and kinship, Amber individuals of different clans and tribes can believe in the same god and, therefore, all be united as brothers and sisters under that one god.

They can live peacefully together under rules that maintain the established way of life and promote stability. Each individual must make sacrifices for God and country, which gives order and meaning to life. Our sacrifices and sufferings ennoble us. The violence and chaos of Red impulses threaten this orderly world. Order and goodness depend on strict laws, strong police, and soldiers. These people are heroes. All of us who work hard, obey the rules, and fulfill our social duties are honorable.

Rules give life a clear, absolute meaning, direction, and purpose. There are higher principles that must be followed. Everyone has their proper place in society, held together by laws and religious command-ments. Conservative and traditional, the Amber worldview emphasizes order, consistency, and convention.

Polarized, black/white, ethnocentric perspectives prevail. You're a be-liever or an infidel, a saint or a sinner, with us or against us. The author-ity shows the true path to righteous living. Guilt controls impulsivity through disciplined allegiance to traditional, well-established ways of living. Sacrifice and stability today guarantees rewards in the future. A glorious heaven awaits those who diligently follow the rules of the One True Way.

ORANGE – Rational Worldview

Orange, the rational worldview of modernity, cuts across group loyalties and applies universal systems and principles to all humans—the first truly worldcentric view. The ideals of equality, liberty, and justice for all come from Orange. As the history of modernity demonstrates, Orange strives for progress, success, independence, achievement, status, and affluence. The future is not predetermined or locked into place by tradi-tions. A new tomorrow can be created through goal-oriented actions taken today.

Orange plays to win in a competitive market place of ideas and oppor-tunities. Winning occurs through strategy, planning, and testing for the best solutions. The scientific method exemplifies Orange's belief that the subjective realm is fundamentally set apart from the objective realm. The phenomenal success of Orange science and technology continually enhances the standards of material living around the world.

GREEN – Pluralistic Worldview

The Green worldview can stand outside the monolithic systems of Orange and see multiple points of view. Since Green cannot yet make judgments of depth, pluralism and egalitarianism become the most appropriate responses. Everything is equally interconnected in the holis-tic web of life. Green moves to "demarginalize" alternative, minority, and underrepresented voices. The pluralistic worldview attempts to give equal recognition to a diversity of perspectives.

Green first made itself known on the world stage in the 1960s. Indeed,
all the major social revolutions of that time have Green footprints from
the environmental movement to the holistic health movement to the
human potential movement. Green's strong sense of pluralistic sensitivity drives it to scan the horizon to make sure that nobody's feelings get hurt and nobody gets left out. Political correctness, an emphasis on community, and consensus decision-making processes often result.

TEAL – Integral Systems Worldview

As awareness keeps growing into Teal, it notices something essential: every perspective captures some important aspects of reality extremely well, and yet each also de-emphasizes, or marginalizes, other aspects of things (that is, each is true, but partial). Teal also realizes that some views are *more* true, and less partial, than others. In other words, every view is not equal; depth exists.

Worldviews are now seen together as a nested hierarchy (or holarchy) of developmental depth and increasing complexity. Teal recognizes that worldcentric views have more depth than ethnocentric views, which have more depth than egocentric views. The Green worldview cannot make that judgment.

Teal also recognizes that none of the previous worldviews will ever disappear. Since all of them naturally unfold in an evolutionary dance, each of them (and all existence) merits care and respect. Teal comprehends both depth and breadth. The Teal worldview has a capacity and an interest in taking wider and more diverse perspectives that allow it to see and work more effectively with complex, interconnected systems (whether they be located in the domains of psychology, relationships, organizations, or global institutions). This produces "a momentous leap" in clarity, creativity, efficiency, and communicative skill for individuals operating at a Teal altitude.

At Teal, *deficiency* needs are replaced by *being* needs—needs that arise from fullness and not from a lack. At this stage people often view "problems" as creative challenges and optimistically seek to create "win-win" solutions. They outgrow victim psychology and can empathize with others' experiences without getting identified or emotionally hooked in.

They hold a big picture view, while living fully and responsibly as who they presently are and who they are learning to become. Awareness is freed up to enjoy the magnificence of existence itself. Individuals acquire both healthy self-interest and selfishness, being concerned with both personal development and the welfare of all people.

TURQUOISE – Integral Holistic Worldview

The Turquoise worldview recognizes more deeply how all ideas are constructs, even one's own sense of self. As this level of awareness dawns, people realize the automatic limits of all conceptual processes. And they begin to become naturally sympathetic not with any perspective, but with the *space in which all perspectives arise*. Turquoise is capable of using a variety of complementary tools to interpret the inherent mysteries of experience. Turquoise compassionately appreciates the virtues of every level of consciousness, without being blind to their limitations.

Turquoise brings not just increasing systemic awareness but also the tendency to identify with these systems rather than the individual self. This is the beginning of transpersonal modes of awareness. Turquoise individuals, in the waking state, might feel identified with or "one with" nature, or Spirit, and feel motivated by that abundance.

Turquoise individuals often find it difficult to locate peers who are able to understand and sympathize with their full dimensionality and depth of awareness. Even their mundane thought processes begin to account not just for our multidimensional complexity, but also for the essential unity of all people, creatures, and living systems. They become even more interested and committed to awakening and to rendering service to others and the world.

INDIGO and Beyond – Super-Integral Worldview

Indigo is the first truly transpersonal worldview, meaning a person's self-awareness extends beyond the personal. It goes beyond an exclusive identification with the personality, while including the personality in its signature uniqueness. By its very nature the Indigo worldview begins to transcend the separation of the subject from the object. Both are seen to arise in an interconnected unity. This level is also marked by a shift to a highly intuitive, flexible, and flowing relationship with experience and phenomena. In the Indigo worldview, existence is seen as a radically interconnected fabric, an ecology of flows of light, life, mind, matter, energy, time, and space.

Wholes are seen in intuitive flashes. Turquoise thinks through vision (vision-logic), whereas Indigo just sees wholes without having to string things together. Systemic and transpersonal wholes are simply apparent, including ecological, political, and cultural wholes that transcend the individual. The personal self-sense opens into these larger systems, identifies with them, and often feels a profound sense of oneness, particularly in the waking state and the gross realm.

The Indigo worldview not only sees through but also lets go of the gross related ego-self as the center and anchoring reference point from which the complex dance of relations, processes, and experience is always seen. This relaxes the tension or stress between individuality and interconnected unity. Life is viewed on a radically elastic time scale, ranging from minutes to years to lifetimes to millennia to deep time to radical timelessness or pure eternity. Indigo individuals feel rested in the Kosmos, in the natural flows of birth, growth, aging, death, joy, and suffering.

Far from an exhaustive list, the worldviews described above include the most obvious stages that researchers have located, plus the highest ones for which preliminary evidence is becoming available. We must not forget to recognize and even honor each worldview level for the essential role it has played and continues to play in the evolution of consciousness. Each worldview functioned and continues to function with beautiful efficiency given its time and place along the developmental spiral. Just think, every single one of the worldviews described above were—at some point in humanity's cultural past—revolutionary, the leading edge, a brilliantly creative leap forward.

How We Participate in Co-Creating Worldviews

Each worldview, operating for the most part collectively and unconsciously, presents the world as if it were the case. Integral Theory (by incorporating key insights from postmodernism) explodes this *myth of the given*—the myth that one purely objective, pre-given world exists for all to see.

Worldviews have never been fixed or predetermined in a metaphysical sense. Instead, they've been painstakingly carved out by generation after generation of human beings traversing the same structural paths, laying down new Kosmic habits for future travelers to follow. And because more people have walked the path of the earlier worldview structures, those early levels are more worn and have deeper grooves than the more recent ones. So if Magenta is the Grand Canyon, then Turquoise is a furrow, and Indigo a line in the sand. When fully digested, this incredible insight—that *the Kosmos is not already complete and fixed, but continually evolving through us*—becomes powerfully inspiring and liberating.

The Integral wave has evolved naturally. Teal Integral consciousness has already spontaneously arisen among millions of people all over the world, and many thousands are beginning to move into Turquoise and some even into Indigo. Integral theory did not *create* these possibilities; it simply *accounts for* them with new clarity and specificity. This empowers further evolution; it doesn't pretend to replace it. But it helps you glimpse the amazing reality of this life as it is—on every timescale simultaneously.

Creativity floods the outer reaches of evolution in a moment-by-moment unfolding of new possibilities. As more people reach the leading edge worldviews, they are actually *co-creating* the particular forms that those worldviews will take. Integral Life Practice exists in a *post-metaphysical* context, where the practitioners themselves—including you—venture into new Kosmic territory as conscious agents of evolution itself.

The 4 Quadrants Reloaded

Are there lines of development in all 4 quadrants? Absolutely! *Evolution occurs within each quadrant.* There are multiple developmental lines that have higher or lower levels in *all 4 quadrants.* The right-hand or exterior quadrants have levels of *material and energetic* complexity (in individuals and collectives). The left-hand or interior quadrants have levels of consciousness (again, in both individuals and collectives).

In figure 5.14, the diagonal arrows represent the many developmental lines in each quadrant and the concentric circles signify the levels or altitudes of consciousness and complexity through which each line evolves.

Notice that no one quadrant is primary. You won't ever find an exterior without an interior or an individual without a collective. So we can't say that activity in one quadrant always comes first and causes activity in another. But we can study how the quadrants mutually impact and influence one other. Think *correlation, not causation.*

Take mind and brain states as an example (see figure 5.15). According to AQAL, one doesn't *cause* the other, yet there is a very real correlation between the two, as you can see in the following example using states of consciousness (interior, subjective experience) and their corresponding brainwaves (exterior, objective).

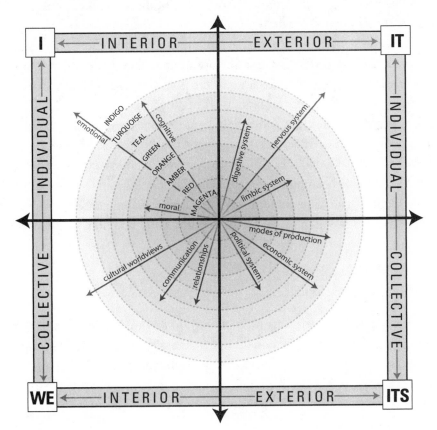

Figure 5.14
Lines of development in all 4 quadrants.

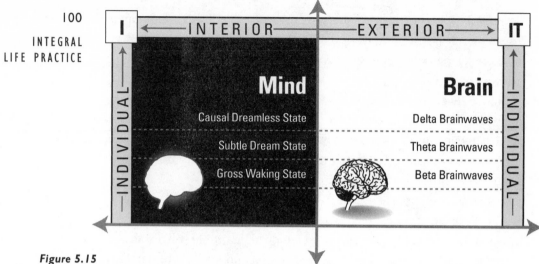

Figure 5.15

Correlation of mind
and brain states in
the 4 quadrants.

The mind/brain problem in philosophy is only a problem if we try to assert that only one quadrant is primary while denying the significance of the others. Once we accept that *both* the Upper-Left and Upper-Right quadrants (not to mention the Lower-Left and Lower-Right quadrants) are real and irreducible, we can quit the pointless argument as to which side—consciousness or the brain—is "really real," and instead focus on the fascinating questions surrounding exactly *how* these equally valid aspects of our being interrelate. Even more to the point is our own development in all 4 quadrants—ILP is not merely a philosophical exercise, but a means of becoming more integrated at our current level (horizontal health) *and* growing into higher levels of integration (vertical health). ILP includes practices that optimize the functions of the mind and the brain.

States of Consciousness

One of the most interesting areas of current research—and a ripe arena for practice—is **states of consciousness**. States come, stay for a while, and then pass. They are temporary and changing. We cycle through states every day—states of elation, boredom, fear, disappointment, irritation, arousal, curiosity . . . and these states go on and on.

Phenomena in all 4 quadrants pass through states—both the upper, individual quadrants and the lower, collective ones. When a company takes an economic nosedive and then recovers in a few months, it experienced a temporary state change in the Lower-Right quadrant. Or consider the Lower-Left quadrant and the shared hatred and fear that ripple through a culture after a terrorist attack. Transient state changes occur in each of the quadrants. Figure 5.16 gives a few more examples.

States can also function as personal windows into the extraordinary potentials of consciousness, brief glimpses into other worlds. Ecstatic or peak experiences are a powerful category of states. Have you ever made love so passionately that you felt completely merged with your partner? Have you ever played tennis in the zone and could hit the ball anywhere on the court you chose? While walking in the forest, perhaps you have experienced a radical oneness with the lush tapestry of radiant greenness

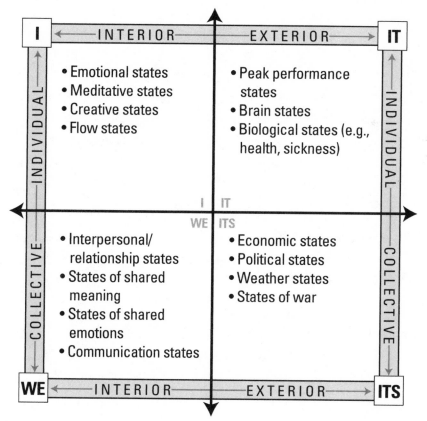

Figure 5.16

States in the 4 quadrants.

surrounding you. Have you ever listened to music so beautiful that it broke your heart wide open—vulnerable and exposed—allowing the raw ecstasy and pain of life to soak through? Think of the last time you had a peak experience that carried you beyond your normal perception of reality and gave you a snapshot of what's possible. These states are sometimes even intentionally cultivated by meditators and mystics, who learn to stabilize freer access to high states of consciousness.

The three most basic states—waking, dreaming, and deep sleep—are so common we experience them every day. Right now, you are in a waking state of consciousness and aware of physical reality. You can pinch

A Fourth State, and Beyond?

Some of the great meditative traditions describe two additional states that only very highly developed meditative practitioners are said to attain. Both of them go "beyond" the three primary states of waking, dreaming, and deep dreamless sleep.

In the *turiya* state (meaning literally "the fourth"), one's attention is neither fixated on gross, waking experience, *nor* on the subtler phenomena that occur in dream and visionary experience. In fact, attention is no longer fixated on *any* phenomena—not even the *very subtle* silence and stillness of deep, dreamless sleep. Things may or may not be arising—and yet, awareness remains steady. It is lucid and awake, resting purely as the subject or witness of all experience—through waking, dreaming, and deep dreamless sleep states. This witnessing awareness grows so strong that one's awareness remains stable 24/7! No matter what happens, and no matter what the body-mind is doing, awareness rests calmly in and as itself.

In the *turyatita* state (meaning "beyond the fourth"), stable witnessing strengthens and evolves until all separation between the witness and that which is witnessed dissolves. The sense of separateness between the "experiencer" and the "experienced" disappears. One experiences nonduality with all inner and outer phenomena, beyond any subject/object division!

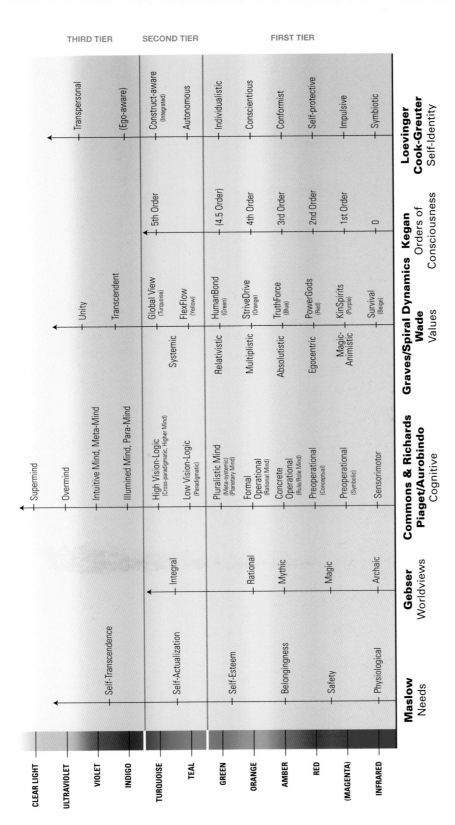

Figure 5.12

Altitudes of consciousness across some major developmental lines.

yourself to make sure. Tonight, when you go to sleep you'll enter a dream

state of luminosity where emotions and thoughts become vivid images. Then, after a while, you'll fall into a deep, dreamless sleep, devoid of any content.

Everybody is familiar with waking, dreaming, and deep sleep—the three major states of consciousness. But how *conscious* are you during each state? Being conscious while you're awake is the easy part. Awareness during the dream state is called lucid dreaming, and those who can remain fully conscious during deep dreamless sleep have realized formless emptiness. You can train yourself to maintain full awareness through waking, dreaming, and deep sleep states with practices such as meditation.

But you don't have to wait for bedtime to experience states of dream-like luminosity and emptiness. Because these states correspond to *energies* that are ever-present (though we typically don't fully engage them in our normal waking consciousness) they're open to everyone from babies to Buddhas. You can *feel into* these states right now because you have access to them anytime you want . . . if you know where to look.

State Training

Some states come and go spontaneously. A sudden, natural high. An unexpected drowsiness. A flight of fancy into a daydream state. However, you can also *train yourself* to enter higher states of consciousness and to make them a regular part of your life experience. In fact, this is what the masters of the great spiritual traditions have been doing for thousands of years, leaving a long record of experimental, cross-cultural validations.* Repeatedly entering into higher *states* for longer periods of time can

---

*Modern research seems to validate the ancient methods, showing that practitioners can stabilize access to certain higher states in a *stage-like fashion*—learning how to consciously and intentionally enter at will into dreaming, deep dreamless sleep and other states, including peak states of consciousness. We call these "state-stages" as distinct from "structure-stages," which mark the emergence of enduring capacities (e.g., a Teal worldview or a Turquoise emotional intelligence). State-stages are usually associated with contemplative training, where through practices such as meditation, one learns how to stabilize access to higher **mystical** states of consciousness. High state experi-

1-MINUTE MODULE
States of Consciousness (A Quick Tour)

Use your five senses to touch into the physical realm. Look around your environment. What do you see? What do you smell or taste? Listen to any noises that might be present such as the sound of your own breathing. Notice any sensations in your gross body. Is there heat . . . or pressure . . . or pain . . . or heaviness . . . or itchiness . . . or tension? Allow it all to be present as you witness the waking state of awareness.

Begin the transition to the more subtle states by turning your attention to the sensations associated with emotions. Is there sadness . . . or joy . . . or anxiety . . . or excitement . . . or irritation? How does the energy of your emotions feel? Do you feel a concentration of tingly sensations or vibrations or energy in any particular area . . . perhaps a few inches out from your skin? Can you feel the energy in the space around you?

Go subtler still. Turn your awareness to the mental plane. Are there memories . . . or ideas . . . or images . . . or impulses? Thoughts about the past . . . about the future? Now feel into your higher intuitive mind. Do you intuit even subtler energies swirling just above your head? Shift your perspective out further into the area around you . . . let you awareness expand even further.

Now notice how you can witness and feel physical sounds, sights, and sensations and subtle emotions, energies, thoughts, and intuitions, but you are not identical to any of them. Watch them closely and recognize that they're all impermanent, fleeting objects arising in the ever-present awareness that you truly are. Experience everything arising in the spacious awareness that is You. Feel how you are not in the universe; the universe is in You. Rest in stillness and be the empty space, the Suchness of the entire display. You are the one who has always been present: never changing,

> never moving, never wavering. Feel the still, silent causal state of formless awareness, unlimited and unbounded, radically free and full, complete, and perfect.
>
> Take a deep breath and enjoy it. . . . And now bring your attention back to the physical realm, but stay connected with the feeling of flow and openness associated with dreaming and deep sleep states as you go on about your day.

often (but not always) help to speed development into higher *stages*. One of the key benefits of Integral Life Practice is that it helps you develop your capacity for these *trained states of consciousness*.

Thus, Integral Life Practice draws strongly on the collective wisdom of humankind's spiritual traditions and schools. These traditions are the repository for our collective learning about every aspect of the universal paths into profundity and awakening. They have learned how to help people break out of the common tendency for attention to be caught exclusively in physical experience and a narrow range of thought and emotions. They understand how to cultivate a healthy, free, and conscious relationship to subtler experience. They understand how to cultivate and transcend the still, silent Witness of all arising experience. They even have a repository of deep understanding about the challenges and intricacies of the journeys and adventures through which different kinds of human beings traverse these depths—in relationship to self, God, others, and the world. And they have a rich vocabulary of tips and techniques for walking the path safely and effectively. ILP draws freely from this rich resource, such that advanced practice is steeped in the skillful means accumulated by our greatest spiritual traditions.

---

ences often tend to quicken growth into higher levels of awareness, but there's no absolute causal link. Meditative training does not necessarily alter the *level* of any other developmental lines. An excellent meditator might remain undeveloped interpersonally or mathematically, for example.

Red Pill or Blue Pill?

Some people use psychedelic plants or chemicals, sometimes referred to as entheogens, to experience powerful altered states of
consciousness. By modifying brain chemistry (in the Upper-Right
quadrant) we can induce an altered or peak state of awareness (in
the Upper-Left quadrant). Because of the problems and dangers of
drug use, including legal, cultural, and possible medical issues, we
don't recommend them. However, they are not invalid in principle,
and some practitioners use them as tools for state training.

Mind/brain machines—e.g., light and sound machines and audio
tone technology—can also induce higher states. However, it's important to complement any *exogenous* method of state-induction
(such as drugs and sound technology) with an *endogenous* method
such as meditation.

What's Your Type?

Not all differences are vertical or developmental. Two things can be radically dissimilar from each other without one being higher or lower than
the other. The AQAL Framework uses the word **types** to describe such
horizontal differences. Examples of types exist everywhere we look:

- Types of music: jazz, rock, classical, heavy metal
- Types of clouds: cumulus, stratus, cirrus, nimbus
- Types of languages: Indo-European, Sino-Tibetan, Austronesian
- Types of relationships: parent-child, sibling, friendship, profes-
  sional, romantic
- Types of hair color: blond, brown, white, red, black
- Types of geography: desert, forest, savanna, swamp, tundra, moun-
  tains

You may notice that you often prefer one type to another. For instance,
you might enjoy listening to jazz over heavy metal, prefer to live near the
ocean as opposed to the mountains, be attracted to blonds over brunettes,

or have a fetish for nimbus clouds. But again, we can't say that one type

is deeper, more evolved, or better than another. They're just different—
period. Each type has its own unique properties, its own strengths and
weaknesses, gifts and faults, yet none is more fundamental and none
should be ignored according to AQAL. Helium and carbon are two *types*
of atoms. In contrast, molecules exist at a higher *level* of complexity than
atoms because molecules *transcend* and *include* atoms in their own
makeup. Levels represent vertical differences; types represent horizontal
differences.

Take a look at this list of names: Napoleon Bonaparte, Helen Keller,
Henry Ford, Friedrich Nietzsche, Michelangelo, Pat Robertson, Marie
Curie, Jack the Ripper, Babe Ruth, Mark Twain, and Joan of Arc. Aside
from being famous, they make up a pretty diverse bunch, right? There's
no doubt that their answers to life questions such as "Who are you?" or
"What do you need?" or "What is of ultimate concern?" would be all over
the place. Yet even though their levels of consciousness differ, everybody
on the list shares a similar kinesthetic **type**: *left-handedness.* You can be a
left-handed savage, a left-handed scientist, or a left-handed saint. (Or perhaps, over the course of a lifetime, all three.) Your type remains essentially the same even as you evolve through higher and deeper levels in the
various lines of development.

Let's take a closer look at types by using the moral line of development, which, as you recall, unfolds from egocentric to ethnocentric to
worldcentric (and beyond). Researchers have discovered that both men
and women evolve through the identical moral sequence, but have also
found that they do so with a different emphasis, or a different voice.
Those with a more masculine orientation will grow through the *same vertical stages,* but with an emphasis on *rights and justice,* while those with
a more feminine orientation will put a greater emphasis on *responsibilities and care.**

Your type—whether it's masculine or feminine—describes the *texture,*
not the structure, of developmental growth. *Both men and women possess*

---

*Lawrence Kohlberg and Carol Gilligan are the best known researchers of masculine
and feminine moral development respectively.

Stages of Moral Development	Masculine Moral Development	Feminine Moral Development
Worldcentric	justice for all of us human rights	care for all of us responsible for global family
Ethnocentric	justice for us our rights	care for us responsible for group
Egocentric	justice for me my rights	care for me responsible for self

Figure 5.17

Masculine and feminine stages of moral development.

masculine and feminine sides (just like they both have a right and left hand). It's just that in men, the masculine pole tends to be more dominant, while in women the feminine orientation usually expresses itself more powerfully (just like one hand is usually more dominant than the other). Of course, some men could be more predominantly feminine, and some women more masculine. This indicates a horizontal difference in their energetic orientation.

As our Integral awareness grows, we are able to befriend all aspects of our being, including both masculine and feminine energies within ourselves and others. This does not mean that we must mute both sides so neither masculine nor feminine dominate. On the contrary! We can be *more masculine* or *more feminine*, depending on our sexual type and the needs of the moment. The difference is that if we're animating our masculine side, it's not at the expense of repressing the feminine—and vice versa. We could be more aggressive (or masculine) at work, for example, and yet come home and animate a softer, more nurturing, and more feminine mode. It just depends on how masculine and feminine tendencies are operating within us and how we choose to engage the world in any given situation.

Personality is another example of type. We each navigate life with our own personal style, our unique voice. Personality typologies make distinctions among the most common individual human patterns. They're just another tool to help us see the dynamics of the tendencies operating within us. In any personality typology, such as the Enneagram or Myers-Briggs, you'll most likely recognize aspects of each type within yourself. And indeed your personality contains countless facets and vast complexities—more than any single typology could possibly hold. However, one type usually stands out more than the others—and thus you could reasonably say, "This is my type."

The more nuanced and sophisticated the system of typology you are working with, the less it will feel like a static identity box—and the more insight you'll have into your dynamic and fluid individuality. Sometimes people even use two or more typological systems. The point of working with types (as with levels) is absolutely not to box anybody in, but rather to help us recognize the patterns operating within ourselves and others, so that we can facilitate greater communication and growth. Once you can *see* a pattern, then you are no longer completely bound by it—in fact, you are freer to change it (or at least work with it creatively), if you so desire.

Identifying Your Myers-Briggs Type

You can get a fuller sense of what we mean right now by briefly walking through the Myers-Briggs typology distinctions. This is a very quick summary, just to illustrate the "types" principle in AQAL

Myers-Briggs—one of the most widely used personality typologies in the world—has four pairs of type distinctions based on the work of psychologist Carl Jung. The first is introversion versus extroversion. If you get energized when dealing with other people, things, situations, and the exterior world in general, then you may lean more toward *extroversion*. Or, perhaps you give more attention to ideas, information, explanations, reflections, and your interior world, in which case you tend toward *introversion*. In short, do you like to "talk it out" (extrovert) or "think it through" (introvert)? In the Myers-Briggs typology, each type category is assigned a letter, which in this case would be: Extrovert (E) or Introvert (I).

The second distinction addresses how you process information. Do you attend to practical and factual details and like to follow step-by-step instructions? If so, you may be a *sensing* type and perceive the specifics first. Or, do you prefer to deal with ideas, generate new possibilities, find new patterns and meanings, and anticipate what isn't obvious? *Intuitive* types perceive the big picture first. These two types are known as Sensing (S) or Intuitive (N).

The next distinction addresses how you like to make decisions. If you make choices using a more analytic and detached approach based on objective logic, then you have a *thinking* orientation. Alternatively, if your decisions hinge more on personal values, sentiments, and relationships with others, then you're probably more *feeling* oriented. These types are referred to as Thinking (T) or Feeling (F).

Finally, consider how you organize your life. If you prefer a life that's planned, stable, and goal oriented, then your orientation is more *judging*. Those who enjoy a more spontaneous, unplanned, flexible life—adapting and responding to unexpected situations as they arise—are more *perceiving* types. Judging types want closure even if the information is incomplete. Perceiving types resist closure to obtain more data. These types are known as Judging (J) or Perceiving (P).

Your Myers-Briggs type is composed of your dominate preference in each category. Thus, your type can be expressed with four letters—for example, "ENFP" or "ISTJ."

How Personality Types Inform Your Practice

Understanding your personality type can be an extremely powerful facet of your Integral Life Practice. Resources abound that explain various personality types and how your personality preferences influence virtually every aspect of your life including your choices, your relationships, and your work in the world. Learning more about yourself in typological terms will help you design an ILP that works for your unique orientation to life.

Understanding the full range of personality types gives you insight into yourself, a greater appreciation for others who are different, and an enhanced ability to skillfully interact with diverse personalities. If you're aware of your type's strengths, then you can better apply them to your life goals and intentions.

Knowing where you go overboard is useful as well. For example, if you're hyper-masculine and your hero's journey for autonomy and independence has left you feeling disconnected and lonely, then relaxing your masculine orientation and cultivating feminine qualities such as receptivity, feeling, and communion could be a valuable practice. In contrast, you might feel fused with everyone you meet and have difficulty knowing yourself apart from other people or asserting your needs and desires. In this situation, you might want to practice getting in touch with your masculine side as part of your ILP. Whatever the case, neither masculine nor feminine is higher or better; they are simply two types at each level of consciousness.

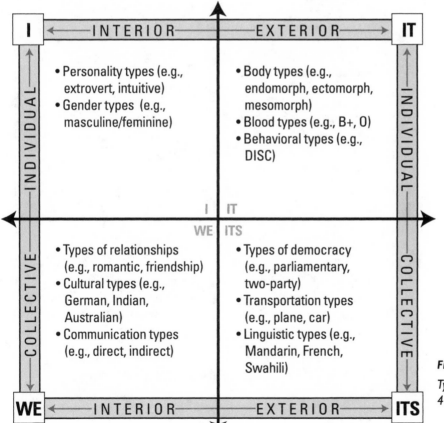

Figure 5.18

Types in all 4 quadrants.

Applications of the Integral Framework

Using AQAL to See a Bigger World

Like the tip of your nose, the AQAL elements are always intimately present, though you may not often be paying attention to them. But in addition to *dimensions* of your own being-in-the-world, AQAL also represents a set of *perspectives* you can take on yourself, on others, or on anything. AQAL's flexibility will surprise you as you discover and invent the many creative ways it can be applied to your life.

You can use AQAL to size up a situation as much or as little as you want. Running through the quadrants can be a quick and easy way to gain insight into any occasion—from a fight with your intimate partner

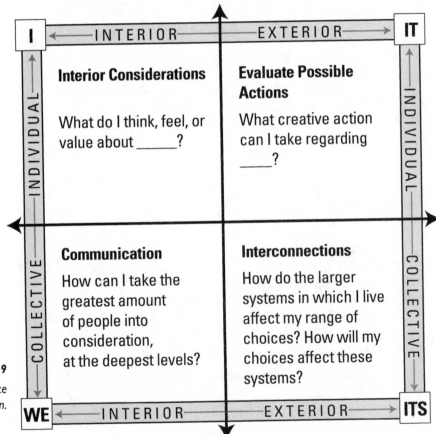

Figure 5.19

Use AQAL to size up any situation.

1-MINUTE MODULE
Quad Scan

A Quad Scan allows you to quickly get a sense of what you think/feel ("I"), the perspectives of others ("We"), interconnections with larger systems ("Its"), and possible actions you can take ("It") for any given issue. If you have a relatively minor decision to make, you can scan the quadrants in under a minute. Just touch on each quadrant for fifteen seconds—"I," "We," "It," and "Its"—and see what comes up. Practicing a Quad Scan will help you make *more* intelligent and informed decisions in *less* time.

to an international war—paying special attention to interior considerations, feedback from others, possible actions, and interconnections with other aspects of your life.

What Perspective Are You Coming From?

As a map of *unity-in-diversity*, AQAL helps us understand people and the seemingly crazy things we do to each other. With Integral vision, we can more clearly see the universal structures that we all share, in addition to the dynamics, textures, and developmental differences that make us all unique. Learning AQAL strengthens our ability to take multiple perspectives, to put ourselves in the shoes of another, and to answer the questions: *Where is this person coming from? Which quadrant-perspective are they focusing on? What altitude of consciousness are they operating with? Which lines of development stand out as strong or weak? What state are they in? What's their personality type?* The more we can understand where a person is coming from, the better we can relate to them, and the more harmony we can create.

In no way does this mean that we must agree with another's view. In this diverse, rainbow world, we're not always going to agree with each other or come to a nice consensus through dialogue. Although we can't always get to "yes," a more Integral understanding allows us to reach "no" with greater mutual understanding and openness to innovative resolutions. Sharpening our Integral understanding of where people are coming from won't necessarily make conflicts go away, but it can help us choose more intelligent and appropriate responses to the conflicts we do face.

Politics is a perfect example. In the American political system, Republicans tend to operate at an Amber-Orange altitude (more conservative, traditional, ethnocentric, and religious) and Democrats usually come from a more Orange-Green worldview (more progressive, worldcentric, and pluralistic).* Further, Republicans point to an *individual's* moral failings, poor decisions, and lack of motivation as the central reasons behind many social problems (Upper-Left quadrant) and Democrats often blame social ills on an unfair *system* (Lower-Right quadrant). A typical Republican/Conservative response to homelessness: cut free governmental handouts which will require homeless people to take responsibility for their own lives and get back to work. A typical Democratic/Liberal response: raise the budget for social welfare programs in order to create opportunities for those marginalized by an unjust economic system.

Even using just a couple of AQAL elements makes it immediately easier to see partisan politics as a dangerous duel of limited and partial truths. It also quickly becomes apparent why some policy recommendations diverge so much (Amber and Green party wings; different quadrant focus) and others appear quite similar (both parties share an Orange worldview). **Integral Politics** also highlights the glaring inadequacies of both parties, due largely to their lack of a view big enough to address the complex issues facing us today.

Whether it's your president or your next door neighbor, it's incredibly liberating to realize that if someone doesn't agree with you (e.g., in matters of politics, religion, art, economics, etc.), it might just be that they're at a different level of consciousness (higher or lower) in that particular line. This will help you to understand why you won't *get* them to agree with you, no matter how hard you try. Developmental disconnects occur

---

*Red, egocentric, strands of both parties complicate the picture.

when you communicate over the head of the other person, literally.* Try rationally discussing democracy with a tribal warlord or debating the finer points of quantum physics with a 5-year-old. Good luck convincing a fundamentalist that many different religions are paths up the same spiritual mountain. There are better ways to spend a Saturday night.

The more deeply you understand and practice the AQAL Framework, the more effectively you'll be able to communicate with others. When you truly recognize where another person is coming from, you can speak to that person's values and concerns in a language they can understand. **Integral Communication** involves adapting or *translating* the way you speak to the other's personality *type* (such as sensing language, intuitive language), *state* (ecstatic language, melancholy language), *quadrant* focus (We language, It language), *lines* (musical language, mathematical language), and *levels* (Amber language, Green language), while still being your authentic self—no easy task, we admit, but an extremely rewarding endeavor.†

Though skillful *translation* from one perspective-space to another is extremely important, there's also an innate impulse toward evolutionary growth or *transformation*, and that's where Integral Life Practice takes center stage. Trading one belief for another does not equal vertical growth. True development—from one stage to the next—ordinarily takes an average of about **five years** (and that's when people are actually growing—many are not). Just as an acorn doesn't become an oak tree in a day, human beings don't skip from egocentric to worldcentric morality overnight. Many debates cannot be decided with *objective* facts and evidence because the disagreements come from interpreting those facts from different *subjective* levels of consciousness. It might take an

---

*Of course, the opposite might also be the case; *you* might be the one at the lower level in a particular line. Given that possibility, it would be wise to hope that others will understand you at *your* level and act compassionately both to help you be healthier and happier where you are (since you're probably going to be there for a little while), and also to nudge you just a bit higher.

†For more information, access Adam Leonard's graduate thesis, "Integral Communication," at www.Integral-Life-Practice.com.

egocentric person ten or more years to develop to worldcentric and until then, he will never agree with worldcentric arguments, or even really understand them.

The real challenge, then, is to create room for everyone, including ourselves, to have safety—including safe passage from one life station to the next—from egocentric to ethnocentric to worldcentric to kosmocentric and beyond. Only from a post-conventional, worldcentric view or higher do individuals even recognize the global scope and implications of the environmental crisis, the AIDS epidemic, international poverty, or world hunger, and only if they have a healthy traditional foundation are they likely to have the moral fortitude to make a meaningful difference.

What Is Not Integral

Many people out there think that they've got *the answer*, that their approach is *the best*, that they have *the truth*. You've met some of them, yes? They can't all be 100 percent right, of course, because they'd contradict each other. Yet the opposite doesn't make sense either: *nobody's smart enough to be 100 percent wrong all the time!* Instead, everyone comes from a *perspective*, or point of *view*, which, by its very nature, is limited and partial. And the more perspectives you take into account, the better you can understand something, whether it be yourself, a relationship with another person, or a situation in the world. In contrast, the fewer perspectives you consider, the more susceptible you are to *fallacies* or misconceptions resulting from a limited view. A fallacy occurs when someone reduces what they understand to be "reality" by ignoring important perspectives, thereby arriving at misleading conclusions.

The AQAL Integral Framework attempts to incorporate as many perspectives as possible at this point in Kosmic history. AQAL uses quadrants, levels, lines, states, and types not only to identify, but also to fit together the innumerable partial truths available to us. In holding a place for everything, as much as possible, it becomes much easier to spot fallacies—partial truths that refuse to admit they're partial. In this section, we will briefly look at four such fallacies, how they attempt to reduce reality, and how AQAL can help bring about a more inclusive view.

The Absolutist Fallacy

This first and perhaps most pervasive fallacy occurs when a limited perspective bites off more than it can chew. A partial truth tries to play itself off as the whole truth, overstepping its realm of expertise and intruding into other areas. The absolutist fallacy can occur with any AQAL element, so let's take *quadrant absolutism* for starters. Extreme approaches take their favorite quadrant and triumphantly proclaim it to be all that exists! The graphics seen in figure 5.20 gives four extreme approaches that have reduced reality to their preferred quadrant.

An Integral approach, of course, recognizes and honors the important partial truths of all four perspectives—taming the extremes so they can work together. Such an approach honors and incorporates the valuable findings of all legitimate experts—even the absolutists. Every valid

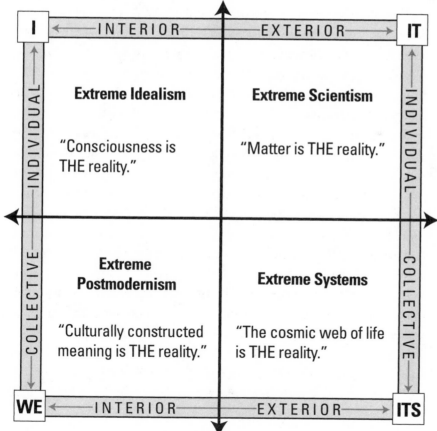

Figure 5.20
Quadrant absolutisms.

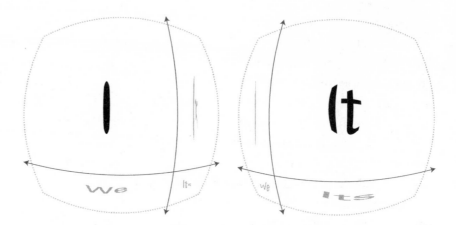

Figure 5.21. *Upper-Left quadrant absolutism.*   **Figure 5.22.** *Upper-Right quadrant absolutism*

methodology (or practice) reveals important truths. The Integral framework gives experts—from physicists to cultural anthropologists to systems theorists to mystics—a space to share the truth revealed by their methodologies and does so in a way that doesn't subtract from the truth revealed by other valid methods. In short, the quadrants *free* each approach by *delimiting* it to the specific area that it can most capably illuminate.

The same goes for all the AQAL elements. Early developmental researchers tended to assume that there was one thing called development, and they were studying it. So cognitive researchers believed that the cognitive line was the only fundamental line, and values researchers believed the same for the values line, to give two examples of *line absolutism*.

Level absolutism occurs when we fail to recognize the existence of levels of development, because we can't help but assume that our level (in any given developmental line) is the only valid one. Same with *type absolutism*: without acknowledging the diversity of personality types, it's easier to conclude that my style of approach to life is right or best. Finally, if you have a transpersonal state experience without understanding the nature of states and the full spectrum of state possibilities, you may falsely believe that your state answers all life's questions; this is *state absolutism*.

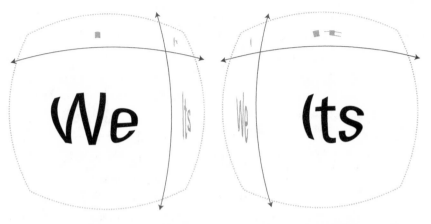

Figure 5.23. *Lower-Left quadrant absolutism.*   **Figure 5.24.** *Lower-Right quadrant absolutism.*

In all cases, committing the absolutist fallacy means inflating a partial perspective so it crowds out other important truths. AQAL puts a stop to it with a framework large enough for everything to have a place and for nothing to be left out.

The Pre/Trans Fallacy

Are babies enlightened? Are all college protesters motivated by "justice for all?" Answering yes to either question exemplifies the *pre/trans fallacy*, which occurs whenever a lower stage of development (pre-) is mistaken for a higher stage (post- or trans-), or a higher level is misidentified as a lower level. Let's take these examples one at a time.

Are babies enlightened? Romantic theories of human development claim that the infant at birth is fully in touch with Spirit—the divine ground of existence—and then, as the self begins to gain power, the growing baby somehow loses touch with this divine ground. Psychospiritual development, in this view, is the process of reclaiming what was lost in childhood: a return to egoless divinity. The Integral view, in contrast, sees human development as an evolutionary process, unfolding from pre-personal to personal to post-personal (or transpersonal) stages.

Pre-personal means prior to the development of the ego, or sense of "I"; personal means having developed a functional ego; and post-personal (or transpersonal) means having transcended and included identification with the ego, thus becoming transparent to greater degrees of ultimate reality. These levels are all touched by Spirit equally; the difference is the degree to which the self is *aware* of its ever-present union with the divine ground.

The Romantics mix up pre-personal (unconscious) with transpersonal (super-conscious). No baby ever enters the world at a transpersonal *level* of self. We all begin our lives at square one, with a pre-personal, unconscious, undifferentiated self, totally fused with the material world.* Self-development does not proceed from unconscious Heaven to conscious Hell to super-conscious Heaven, but rather from unconscious Hell to conscious Hell to super-conscious Heaven. In short, evolution moves forward toward sainthood, not backwards to babyhood.

Are all college protesters motivated by "justice for all"? In the past few decades, colleges and universities have been the site of student protests regarding issues such as international sweatshops, fair trade, ecology, women's rights, free speech, diversity, war, and so on. When looking at a group of protesters (Lower-Right quadrant) and the behaviors of individual protesters (Upper-Right quadrant), it usually appears that the activists are united in solidarity around a particular cause and engaged in similar actions such as waving picket signs, marching, and signing petitions.

Despite these similarities in outer behavior, the inner motivations of protesters tends to differ widely. Studies of moral development during the Vietnam War showed that only a minority of college protesters were motivated by post-conventional (worldcentric) reasons, such as care for the lives of Americans *and* Vietnamese or a desire to end an unjust war policy. Most protestors were at pre-conventional levels of moral development and were protesting in order to stick it to authority ("Don't tell me what to do!") or out of fear of being drafted themselves. The pre/trans fallacy can be difficult to spot because *pre*-conventional and *post*-conventional are both *non*-conventional, and so both push back against conventional ways of doing things.

---

*A baby can, however, access virtually any *state* of consciousness. See the "state/structure fallacy," page 121.

The State/Structure Fallacy

The *state/structure fallacy* makes the critical mistake of assuming that states of consciousness and structures (or stages) of consciousness are the same thing. States come and go as temporary flashes of fleeting experience. We can experience emotional, mental, or spiritual states at any given moment, and everyone cycles through waking, dreaming, and deep sleep states daily. Structures, on the other hand, are more long-term and stable, usually lasting for many years. You have to *build* structures over a series of stages, usually through committed practice, whereas you simply experience states. (The exception to this is meditative state/stages, such as from gross to subtle to casual to nondual, which also require practice to stabilize and tend to unfold sequentially in a stage-like fashion, although these are still more fluid than structures.)

So can a mystic and a fundamentalist experience a similar spiritual state? Yes—and no. *Yes*, because even the highest subtle and causal states are available to everyone at virtually any level of consciousness. Will a mystic and a fundamentalist each inhabit and interpret the experience in the same way? *No*, definitely not, because your structure-stage of consciousness (your Integral Psychograph) influences the meaning you give to your experiences. Meaning adds dimensionality to the intention with which you experience them. The lattice in figure 5.25 shows how *a state's meaning changes depending on one's structure-stage of development.* *

Every intersection represents an interpreted state experience (nine depicted in this lattice). A worldcentric, visionary artist and an egocentric 2-year-old both can have a subtle state experience, but they will give it completely different meanings. The 2-year-old may see "a golden angel" come down into mommy and through her shower him with light and energy. The visionary artist may experience his subtle body opening into profound communion with the exquisite light that he vividly perceives animating everything. And the interpretation is just as important as the experience, since how we interpret an experience determines to a great degree the long-term impact it will have on our lives. You can think of

---

*Both Ken Wilber and Allan Combs were instrumental in creating this diagram, which is also known as the "Wilber-Combs Lattice."

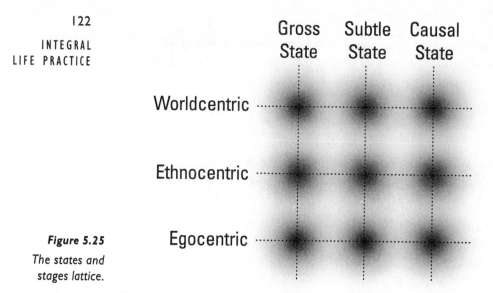

AQAL as an interpretive framework created from an Integral wave of consciousness for us to make sense of the many states (and structures, bodies, and shadows) that we can see precisely and exercise consciously through our Integral Life Practice.

The State/Structure Connection

The important distinction between states and structures (or stages) sometimes seems to blur. This is because spending time in high *states* of consciousness can turbocharge growth into higher *stages* of consciousness. Individuals at higher stages or levels of development are more likely to internalize the full implications of their high state experiences, and this reshapes their perspective-taking. In this way, practices like meditation that cultivate high trained states of consciousness become effective catalysts for *both* kinds of growth—into higher states of consciousness and higher structures.

The Level/Line Fallacy

Recall that the spiritual line of development asks the question, "What is of ultimate concern?" There's an entire spectrum of partial answers to this question—as there is with every developmental line—moving up the great evolutionary spiral towards greater awareness and compassion.

Each stage or wave of spiritual development has a different ultimate concern, from Amber to Orange to Turquoise and beyond. In the same way,
each spiritual stage has a different god as shown below.

A *level/line fallacy* occurs when a specific level (within a developmental line) is confused with the entire line itself. One of the most significant and dangerous level/line fallacies today concerns the spiritual
line. On the one hand, traditional religious believers (Amber) become
rigidly fixated at an Amber level of spiritual development—worshipping
a mythic, anthropomorphic god and ferociously defending it against all
potential detractors. Rational logic or mystical insights that don't align
with Amber sensibilities are rejected as offensive, heretical, and blasphe-
mous. In this way, religion is defined not as a personal spiritual quest of
continuous evolutionary unfolding, but as one particular level of development: Amber.

On the other hand, those who have reached a rational worldview (Orange) buy into this same level/line fallacy. Instead of defending the
Amber god, they reject it with the full force of logical and scientific rea-
soning. Yet Orange doesn't stop with trashing the mythic god. Because it

Figure 5.26

The spiritual line of development.

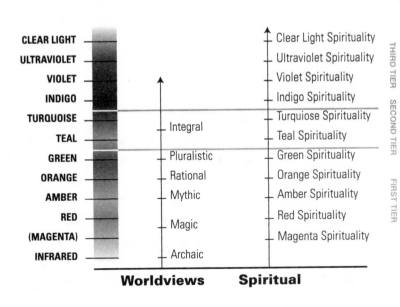

mistakenly views all religion as expressing an Amber perspective, Orange throws out and represses the entire line of unfolding spiritual intelligence—from Infrared to Indigo and beyond. So the level/line fallacy freezes Orange too because it mistakenly groups lower expressions of spirituality (Amber) with higher forms (Orange, Green, Teal, Turquoise) and rejects them all. This level/line fallacy fuels the classic battles between Orange science and Amber religion.

The way out: recognizing that religion and spirituality do not stop at Amber. Spiritual intelligence develops! The Orange deism of our founding fathers could be a profoundly spiritual way of life—and so could the Green existentialism of Heidegger—as well as Teal or Turquoise Integral awareness. Every level has its own version of spirituality with its own practices.

An Integral Operating System

We've talked a lot about AQAL throughout this chapter, but the question remains: what is it, really?

- A philosophy
- A framework
- A model
- A theory
- A map
- Dimensions
- Perspectives

The answer is all of the above. And why stop there? AQAL can also be thought of as an **Integral Operating System** or **IOS**. In an information network, an operating system is the infrastructure that allows various software programs to operate. The metaphor is simply that, if you are running any "software" in your life—such as your business, work, play, or relationships—you want the best operating system you can find, and IOS fits that bill. In touching all the bases, it allows you to run the most effective and cutting-edge "applications" available.

Once you've learned, or "downloaded," the Integral Operating System (as you have already begun to do by reading this chapter), it often begins to "upgrade" your mind by opening up new spaces and giving you a feel for more of the various perspectives we have available to comprehend our complex, hyperspeed world. The Mind module, however, cannot be reduced to mere intellectual study of AQAL. IOS functions as a **psychoactive** system that you can run through your entire body-mind to activate any potentials that you are not presently using or even aware of.

Once you download IOS, it automatically begins looking for areas that the Integral framework suggests you have, but that you might not have consciously realized—any quadrant, level, line, state, type, or body. IOS activates them, lights them up, and helps you realize that you have them all as possibilities of your own consciousness and being-in-the-world. By providing a wealth of crucial distinctions, all of which offer clear coordinates in our multidimensional Kosmic worldspace, it can infuse your mind and your important communications with precision, wide-angle stereo depth, and clarity. In some very substantial way, your world has changed—it's become bigger—and you'll never be the same again.

6

The Body Module

Redefining the Body Integrally

In this chapter we turn our attention to the Upper-Right quadrant—or individual-exterior—dimension of practice: the body. And what a complex, multi-functional, and miraculous thing this body of yours is! From birth to death, all your experiences, great and small, are made possible by your body—from eating to working to playing to making love, and so much more.

But of course, our bodies are also subject to illness, injury, pain, aging, and ultimately, death. In some traditions, the body has gotten a bad rap, for these very reasons. "Transcend the body," it is said. "The flesh is intrinsically evil." Yet an Integral view is eager to embrace our bodily existence. After all, it is the only earthly vehicle we have for living an enlightened life. And even though we can't eliminate pain or aging, nor make our bodies perfect, we can certainly make wise use of what we've got.

One of the most important values we hold, both culturally and as a species, is to be physically healthy, yet so often, we fail to cultivate our health. Being healthy in modern culture typically means only the absence of gross disease. And when disease (almost inevitably) occurs, we attempt to eliminate or control it with surgery or drugs. Sometimes, of course, *extrinsic* measures such as prescription drugs are necessary and are the only way to save a life or manage a chronic illness. True health, however, is balanced wellness, which results in large part from a healthy lifestyle—an *intrinsic* quality that requires practice.

An Integral approach to bodily practice aims both to establish a baseline of health and well-being and to open up potentials for *extraordinary* health—so we're not merely surviving, but *thriving* with intelligent vitality. An Integral body practice invites more of the conscious *juice* of life to flow through the body. In fact, it prepares the bodily vehicle to handle it.

How can you become an "ultimate driving machine" for life? *Integrally*, of course. It all begins with an extraordinary insight:

You actually have *three bodies*—not just one—and to be fully healthy, you must exercise all three.

It Takes Three to Tango

What are these three bodies? First, there is your physical or **gross** body— your body of flesh and bones, organs and cells, saliva and blood. Second, you have a **subtle** body of various kinds of energy, sometimes called chi or prana, and other subtle systems (such as the energy centers or chakras and acupuncture meridians) that are usually not recognized by Western physiology. Third, you have a **causal** body of infinite stillness, which is the body you get in touch with through meditative practice.

These *exterior* bodies and energies have an important connection with your interior reality. Recall the three major states of consciousness: waking, dreaming, and deep sleep. In fact, those three **states** and your

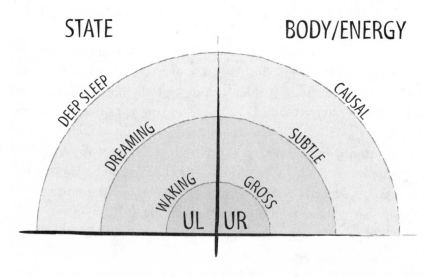

Figure 6.1
States of consciousness correlated with bodies and energies.

STATE   BODY/ENERGY

DEEP SLEEP   DREAMING   WAKING   GROSS   SUBTLE   CAUSAL

UL   UR

three **bodies** are interdependent and interconnected. Every major subjective *state* of consciousness has an objective energy or *body* associated
with it (see figure 6.1 on page 128).

Gross, subtle, and *causal* refer to the energies or bodies associated with
the three main states of consciousness (waking, dreaming, and deep
sleep). Correlated with the spectrum of states of consciousness in the
Upper-Left quadrant is a spectrum of bodies or energies in the Upper-
Right quadrant.

Waking consciousness corresponds to the gross (or physical) body.
Subtle or dream consciousness corresponds to a subtle body. And formless (or deep sleep) consciousness corresponds to a causal, or *very subtle*
body, as the Tibetans call it. Each one of your states of consciousness has
a bodily-energetic support.

Think about it for a moment. This is important information, isn't it? If
you actually have an *exterior* form for every *interior* state, the implications
are enormous. This means that by exercising or working out all three
bodies, you are simultaneously exercising your inner, conscious experience—you are *working in* or strengthening your natural states of awareness. Let's dive a little deeper into each of the three bodies and their
corresponding states.

Gross

The waking state is closely associated with the **gross physical body**. This
is the body that allows us to experience the natural world with our senses.
Empirical science studies the patterns or laws that this physical nature
obeys. When you're awake, you experience this gross sensory data: rocks,
trees, buildings, people, voices, sounds, smells, and so on. If someone
pinches your physical body, you feel it. When you kick a ball, you can
sense the equal and opposite reaction against your foot and leg. You can
see that ball obey the laws of physics and sail though the air before arcing
back to earth, pulled by gravity. Because the gross realm almost always
behaves according to the laws of science, it can seem like an incredibly
complex machine. This is the aspect of it that is predictable and orderly
(which not all of it is, for example the possibilities that exist in the quantum world). But this realm is also miraculous—*you* are an incredible, or-

ganic formation of countless parts and processes, all working together seamlessly to give rise to your physical reality.

Subtle

But when you fall asleep at night, it's an entirely different story: your gross body disappears from your awareness. No more physical rocks, trees, or buildings. Instead, you're aware of emotions, images, visions, ideas, dream worlds, and archetypes. You find yourself in realms where earthly physics goes out the window and down the rabbit hole.

In dream states, your energetic support vehicle is not a solid, gross body, but a spectrum of relatively fine or dense subtle energies of radiance, mind, sound, emotion, and life force. This is the **subtle body**. Bands of this spectrum have been traditionally associated with the *chakras*, and the subtle body is sometimes subdivided into different levels that are called by such names as *vital, etheric, sexual, emotional, astral, mental, and psychic*, referring to the Upper-Left states with which they are correlated.

Your dream body can change shape, walk through walls, and even fly. The subtle body flows freely through fluid domains, through ecstasies and nightmares, and through different times and places. It may be associated with gross sensory realities but it is not tied to them. It is closely aligned with intuitions, feelings, ideas, intentions, desires, and emotions. The subtle body is, in a sense, *more free*, because it's not bound by physical circumstances. And not only while you're sleeping. You can have a dream or idealistic vision that inspires you and others to action. Your subtle body charisma can lead the way for revolutionary changes—in your life, your creative expressions, and even in a whole society.

Your densest subtle energies are more closely associated with the gross physical body, and you encounter them in auras, acupuncture meridians, and bodily sensations of flowing life force. Subtler bands of energy are associated with sexuality and emotions; subtler still with the mind and insight; and the subtlest bands of energy are associated with supramental, blissful, intuitive intelligence—a kind of crowning glory to the radiance of your subtle being.

Causal

When the dream ends, you fall into formless deep sleep. In this and any *causal* state, both gross and subtle experiences subside. You are released into a still and silent realm. In this unbounded, vast, and spaceless space, nothing at all is happening.

Paradoxically, awareness is wide-open, present, and unobstructed. Consciousness simply *is*, without distraction by the moving objects of experience. Although there are no specific qualities or experiences arising, this nothingness is inherently characterized by utter well-being, the complete absence of suffering.

This almost infinite conscious expanse has an extremely subtle, almost indescribable body or energy—the **causal body**. Still and silent, infinite and infinitesimal, this body defies description and conceptual categories. It is the energetic embodiment of the ever-present Witness consciousness. It is the opening within which all experiences arise. The causal domain is the cause, space, and support from which your subtle and gross energies and bodies can arise. It's intimately present as the deepest source of *you*.

Your three bodies—gross, subtle, causal—exist simultaneously right now, in waking consciousness. Every time you enter subtle states through meditation, thoughts, visions, or emotions, you're animating your subtle body. Whenever you rest in the silence of pure awareness and release to infinity, you are attuning to your causal body.

Integral body practices help you pay attention to all three dimensions of bodily existence: gross, subtle, and causal. Through Integral body practices, you can consciously exercise all dimensions of your body-mind-spirit-shadow, including the highest aspects of your being.

As you take your Integral practice further, you can even *bring awareness into the dream and deep dreamless sleep states*. In other words, your physical body can be sleeping but *you* can remain "awake" while inhabiting your subtle and causal bodies. What might you learn from such an experience? How might your understanding of reality change? You'll find out if you pursue a 3-body practice far enough. But the benefits of an

Kung Fu or an MBA?

One friend of ours was on a serious business career track when he became devoted to studying a Chinese martial art. He came to the point in his career when he had thought he should take a sabbatical and get his Master's degree in Business Administration. But he realized that the time required for the MBA would force him to give up his martial arts practice. He decided his practice was too important at the time and didn't pursue his MBA.

Ironically, his career advanced even faster than he had hoped it would by getting the MBA. He just kept getting promoted. Looking back, he realized that even if his exclusive motivation had been to advance his career, his decision not to give up martial arts would still have been the right decision. "Kung Fu helped me advance in my career because it instilled qualities like agility, presence, adaptability, flexibility of mind and body, focus, discipline, and clarity. Bringing my practice to work is what got me promoted."

Integral body practice are also practical and immediate, so these are what we'll focus on first.

In the next section, we present the **3-Body Workout,** a Gold Star Practice that can help you jumpstart or deepen your Integral body practice. Then we will look at other forms of practice that you might want to include in your ILP, including traditional areas such as strength training, aerobics, sports, dance (and neuromuscular conditioning in general), and nutrition. Finally we'll explore some subtle body practices for increasing your *conductivity*, or the ability to conduct the energy of life. These include Integral sexual practice and conscious breath practice. We'll end with a brief discussion of causal body exercise and an invocation of your Witnessing awareness, which, in fact, you can maintain through *every* aspect of your Integral body practice (as you'll see).

One important point to keep in mind: Although we've divided the chapter along the lines of the three bodies, no practice involves *only* one body or another. You can lift weights, run, make love, or breathe while consciously engaging *all three of your bodies* simultaneously. However, the *emphasis* is usually on one body or another, and so we've placed each practice in its respective section according to its emphasis. See how much you can bring all three of your bodies into play, whatever practice you happen to be doing.

The 3-Body Workout

The 3-Body Workout enables you to engage all three of your bodies in one exercise program. How does it work? Just like Integral Life Practice itself—it's modular, scalable, flexible, and customizable to your needs. It's also a perfect morning routine, a way to wake up, focus, and energize before moving on to the day's activities. You can even do a 3-body 1-Minute Module as a quick way to connect up and exercise your body on all levels.

By approaching the 3-Body Workout as a **set of principles,** you can craft a routine that's right for you. These principles can be stated very simply: *Do **at least one exercise** that emphasizes each of your three bodies—causal, subtle, and gross—and maintain awareness and engagement of **all three bodies** while performing any exercise.* This may sound a little difficult at first (like juggling), but with some practice it can become second nature (like riding a bicycle).

You can do any exercises in any order at any time of day. Do whatever works best for you. There are gross, subtle, and causal aspects to *all* these practices (which is why you can do them all with 3-body awareness), but the *emphasis* is usually on one body or another.

Here are some examples of exercises you can do for each of your bodies:

Gross Body
   Weightlifting
   Running
   Aerobics
   Sports (skiing, basketball, tennis, volleyball,
      Frisbee, soccer, etc.)

Dance

Push-ups, squats, crunches (exercises using
    only your body weight)

Subtle Body
    Yoga
    T'ai chi
    Qigong
    Subtle Breath Practice (including micro-
        cosmic orbit and pranayama)
    Visualization
    Lucid dreaming

*Causal Body**
    Witnessing meditation
    I AM: Mantra Meditation
    Integral Inquiry
    Big Mind
    Centering Prayer
    The 3 Faces of Spirit

Some people prefer to spread their 3-Body Workout over the course
of the day and even do it in different places (for example, meditate at
home and weightlift at the gym). **However, it can be powerful to
combine your chosen exercises into one continuous exercise routine.** At Integral Life Practice seminars, and in the ILP Starter Kit†
3-Body Workout DVD, we teach a thirty-five- to forty-five-minute version of a full 3-Body Workout, which we also present in the following
pages. This routine unfolds in a specific order (beginning with causal,

---

*The causal body is explored at the end of this chapter, while the causal body exercises
are presented in chapter 7 since we contact the causal body through spiritual and meditative practice.

†The Integral Life Practice Starter Kit is a multi-media learning experience that includes five DVDs, two CDs, and three booklets with over 150 illustrated pages. You
can find out more about the starter kit and live ILP seminars by visiting *www.Integral
-Life-Practice.com.*

moving through subtle to gross, and then back to causal), which is meant to move you through a complete cycle of states (with causal witnessing as the foundation).

Here are the five basic steps:

1. Ground yourself in the **causal** body through your choice of an awareness/meditation practice.
2. Energize your **subtle** body through your choice of subtle energy practice(s). *Do this while remaining consciously grounded in your causal body.*
3. Strengthen your **gross** body through your choice of physical exercise(s). *Do this while remaining consciously grounded in your causal body and energized in your subtle body.*
4. Transition from **gross** body to **subtle** body awareness through some stretching and cooling down.
5. Rest in the **causal** body for a period of sitting meditation.

Go to www.Integral-Life-Practice.com to watch a video of this workout. This will help you learn it more quickly.

The Integral Difference

Most forms of exercise ignore the causal body. Many neglect the subtle body. It's extremely rare to find an exercise routine that trains *all three bodies at the same time.* This is the power of the 3-Body Workout. It's a condensed, efficient, and intelligent way of performing a truly *Integral* workout.

Moreover, it makes exercise more *interesting,* because you're no longer merely burning calories—you're bringing awareness and care to each movement and each moment. The more you practice, the stronger *all three of your bodies* will become. It's one thing to have big muscles or aerobic endurance; it's another to *also* have free-flowing energy and a conscious depth of presence.

Step 1: Grounding in the Causal Body

Begin by taking a few deep breaths and becoming aware of *you*. Use any form of meditation that evokes a state of pure witnessing or nondual awareness (see chapter 7 for several you can use). As an example, try quietly reading or reciting the following pointing-out instructions. They will help you access a state of *nondual ever-present Suchness*, which is open to the conscious reality of your deepest self and of all things. As you relax into this meditation, let the words gently guide you toward a disidentification with the immediate objects of your experience, such that you rest as the *Witness* of all objects. In this expansive state, feel your causal body.

Nondual Pointing-Out Instructions

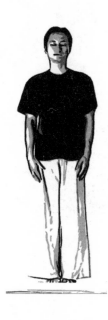

Notice the sounds around you and notice your bodily sensations.

Notice that you are not identical to these sounds and sensations.

All sounds and sensations are objects arising to the awareness that you truly are.

Notice your thoughts, feelings, memories, motivations, and impulses.

Notice that you are not identical to your thoughts, feelings, memories, motivations, or impulses.

All of them arise as objects to the awareness that is you.

You are the One who has always been present.

There was never a time when you were absent.

You have always been you.

So notice You.

Notice the Suchness that you are.

Do not pretend that you are seeking or finding or forgetting the One you truly are.

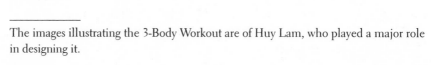

The images illustrating the 3-Body Workout are of Huy Lam, who played a major role in designing it.

Repeat this meditation as many times as you wish, or replace it with one of the Spirit module practices (chapter 7), for example, the I AM: Mantra Meditation (p. 242), Integral Inquiry (p. 243), or the 3 Faces of Spirit (p. 249).

Step 2: Energizing the Subtle Body

Now you can move into a routine based on any subtle body practice you enjoy, such as yoga, qigong, t'ai chi, or breath-work. Below is a suggested series of exercises, based on principles of yoga and qigong. For more ideas, please refer to the subtle body exercises later in this chapter (pp. 172–190).

First, a series of loosening movements to open up the body

- Roll your head, stretching your neck, and then turn it, looking left and right.
- Rotate your shoulders in circles forward and back.

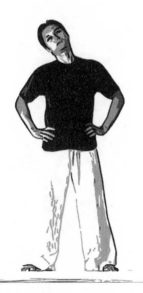 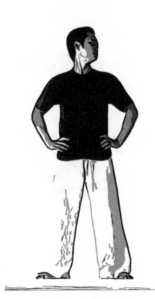 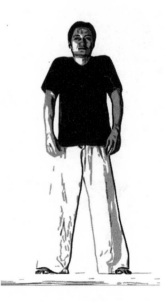

- Swing your arms up over your head and around in large circles, both forward and backward.
- Open your chest by bringing your arms out to the sides and swinging them forward and then back several times.
- Put your hands on your hips and circle them, clockwise and counter-clockwise.
- Do a forward bend with a straight back.
- Bend your knee and grasp your foot in your hand. Raise the foot upward toward your rear, stretching your quadriceps. Repeat with the other leg.

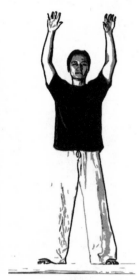
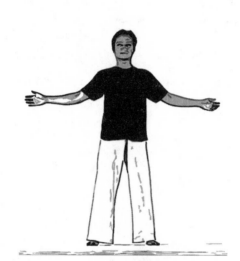
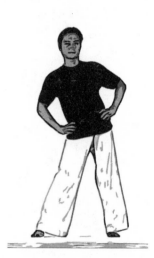

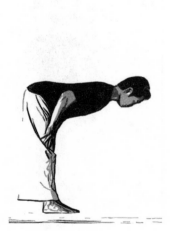
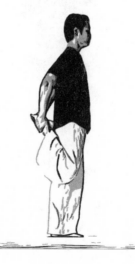
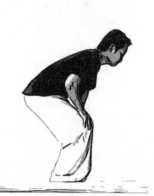

- Put your hands on your knees and bend your knees slightly up and down and then circle them gently.

Then, some enlivening exercises wake up the body's energy centers and channels.

Use your loosely closed fist or open hand to gently pat the entire surface of your body: arms, chest, abdominals, and legs. Be sure to include both the front and back of your arms and legs.

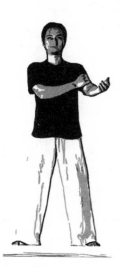 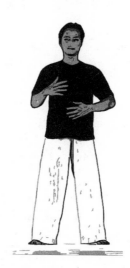

Finally, stand still for a couple minutes in a "chi-cultivating posture."

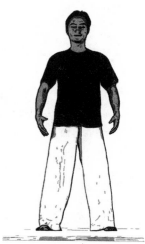

Stand with your eyes closed and with your feet in a shoulder-width stance, knees slightly bent, spine loose and long, and arms floating a few inches out from the sides of your body with your hands open. Gently touch your tongue to the roof of your mouth, right behind your upper front teeth. Breathe into the belly, expanding it on the inhale and then relaxing on the exhale, circulating and cultivating life energy throughout the body, while also resting in your causal body.

Step 3: Strengthening the Gross Body

Your 3-Body Workout can now move into a series of physical exercises. If you have a home gym, you can use it here as part of your 3-Body Workout (see pp. 150–160 for a discussion of strength training). If you don't have equipment, try doing a series of squats, push-ups, back arches, and crunches, as described below. The exercises are performed slowly and consciously, for just a few repetitions, holding the last two or three reps as long as possible. Be careful not to injure yourself; remember you are the only one who can be sensitive to your body's limits. Sometimes a period of cardiovascular exercise is included here (such as the 1-Minute Aerobic Module on p. 161).

Slow Squats

(Five slow reps; hold on last two)

- Place your feet roughly shoulder-width apart, or slightly wider.
- Loosely extend your arms straight in front of you.
- Slowly stick your butt out as you sit back into an imaginary chair. Keep your knees above your ankles, extending your rear and arching your back.
- Visualize and send energy from your vital core center down your legs.
- Hold the squat for a moment, and then as you exhale, push the ground away and return to a standing position, ready to begin the next repetition.
- As you do the squats, breathe slowly and evenly, inhaling on the way down, exhaling on the way up.
  - Hold the last two squats a bit longer, continuing to breathe evenly.
  - Stay in the sensations; become the sensations; let them arise and dissolve within your witnessing awareness.

Slow Push-Ups

(Five slow reps, hold on last two; either on feet or on knees)

- Begin in a "table" posture, on your hands and knees.
- Place your hands directly beneath your shoulders.
- Your torso should be kept straight, from knees to shoulders, or feet to shoulders.
- Inhale as you lower your body and exhale on the way up.
- Hold the last two push-ups at the bottom or midway long enough to safely exert your muscles (a little shaking is good!), while breathing evenly.
- Continue to bring energy and attention into the arms and chest.
- Stay in the sensations; become the sensations; let them arise and dissolve within your witnessing awareness.

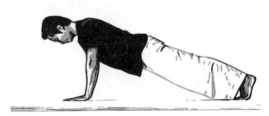

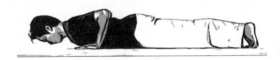

Back Arch

(Three reps, two holds)

- Begin by lying face down.
- Extend and lengthen the spine as you raise your shoulders and feet off the floor.
- Extend energy, drawing the crown of your head far away from your heels. Hold this position for a moment and then release it.
- Inhale on the way up and exhale on the way down.
- Try to keep your feet together through the whole movement.
- Keep breathing on holds.
- Stay in the sensations; become the sensations; let them arise and dissolve within your witnessing awareness.

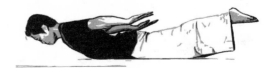

Slow Crunches/Sit-Ups

(Five slow reps, hold on last two)

- Begin lying on your back with your knees bent and your feet just below your buttocks.
- Put your hands on your abs to help you focus there.
- Flatten the small of your back against the floor.
- Inhale into your stomach and hold your breath.
- Exhale as you crunch up, trying to close the gap between your sternum and pubic bone.
- Empty the last air from your lungs, closing the gap further.
- Pause and notice the sensations in your abdominal muscles.
    - Lower flat to the floor on the in-breath. Repeat as soon as you have a full breath.
    - Stay in the sensations; become the sensations; let them arise and dissolve within your witnessing awareness.

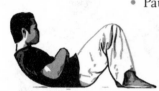

Step 4: Gross-to-Subtle Stretching and Cool-Down

When time permits, your 3-Body Workout can go on to a series of stretches (see examples below). They can range from very relaxed, pleasurable stretching to deeper, more intense stretching—anything from a few, light stretches to twenty hatha yoga sun salutations! Flow into your

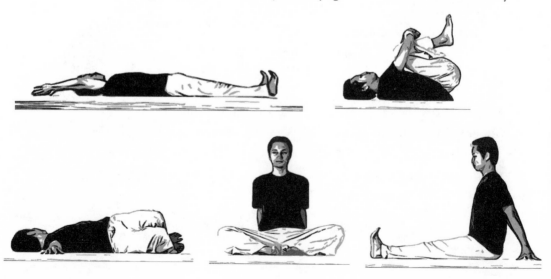

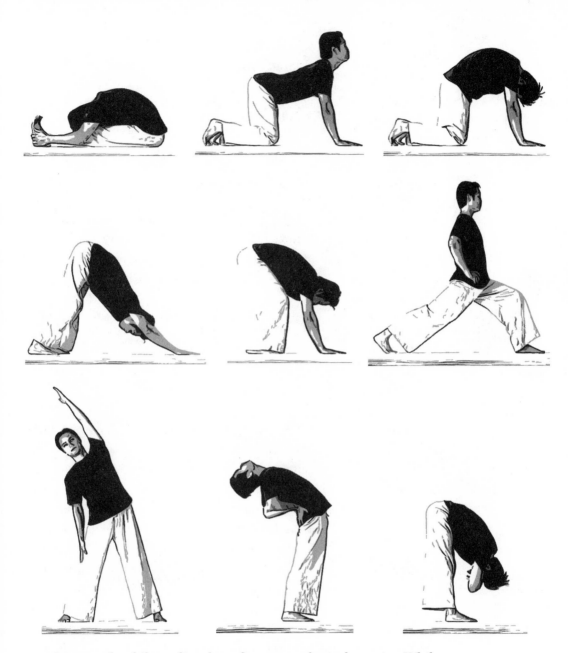

stretching gently while cooling down from gross physical exercise. While you do so, your attention will naturally move from an emphasis on the gross body back to the subtle body. An important key to this practice is to maintain feeling-awareness in and as all three bodies—gross, subtle, and causal.

Optional Step: Transitional Practices

This is sometimes the best time to engage in supplemental practices like affirmations (p. 310), subtle breath practice (p. 181), or reading a profound or sacred text.

Step 5: Resting in the Causal Body

The next to last step of the 3-Body Workout involves returning to its anchor in the ever-present Causal Body, through a period, however short or long, of formless sitting meditation. If you wish, this can segue into another kind of meditation, such as loving-kindness or Compassionate Exchange (see p. 252).

You can add the **Integral Dedication** here (as described on p. 148), before you close and go on with your day.

Summing Up: 3-Body Workout Principles

The 3-Body Workout can be done either free form or by following a routine such as the one above. The idea is very simple: exercise each of your three bodies—causal, subtle, and gross—and perform all exercises with full-spectrum 3-body awareness. The specific routine taught here is grounded, first, by noticing That which never changes, in which all things arise (the causal), and invoking the free relationship of consciousness to all things. It then proceeds to exercise all three of your bodies in an integrated way, using breath, feeling, and awareness. When time permits, it returns through the subtle and completes the circle with a causal body meditation. This prepares you to re-enter the world with presence, lightness, and clarity.

Here are some more 3-Body Workout tips:

- **Shorten or lengthen** the workout as appropriate for your schedule and needs.
- You can perform the **1-Minute Module** (p. 145) when you have very little time.

- You can perform a quick **10-minute workout** on a busy day.
- You can **extend the 3-Body Workout** to an hour, or even two or more hours, including whole exercise routines such as qigong, yoga, pilates, strength training, and/or a cardiovascular workout.
- **Adapt the level of difficulty** so your exercise program is both enjoyable and a bit of a stretch—thus increasing your fitness and vitality over time. Periodically refine your program to maintain your interest, challenge, and freshness.
- Use the **3-body principles** to craft a workout that you can perform at different times of the day, or in different places. Remember, all you need is one exercise for each of your three bodies—then perform each exercise with full 3-body awareness.
- You might want to follow a specific and complete **3-body routine** that cycles from causal to subtle to gross, and then circles back to the causal body. This can be an especially condensed and efficient way to get in great 3-body shape. Use the instructions above or visit www.Integral-Life-Practice.com for a video demonstration.

 1-MINUTE MODULE
3-Body Workout

The 1-minute, 3-Body Workout is a beautiful and powerful way to connect with and integrate your three bodies. It begins with noticing and anchoring the causal body, then activating the subtle body with breath and movement, and finally getting physically grounded in the gross body. A nice way to end is with the Integral Dedication.

Causal Body

1. Stand up straight and tall with your eyes closed. Breathe naturally. Place your palms flat together in front of your heart.

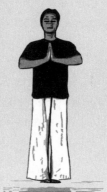

2. Speak these words in your mind: *Notice the Suchness, the is-ness of this and every moment.* (Pause, and do so.) *I am this Suchness. I am the openness in which all things arise.*

3. Inhale and exhale. As you inhale, slowly cross your open hands across your heart and upper chest.

4. As you exhale, uncross your hands, and raise your arms at your sides, with your open palms facing forward.

5. Speak these words in your mind:

I release to infinity.

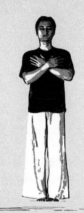 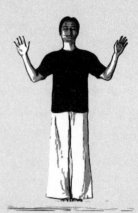

Subtle Body

6. Open your eyes. As you inhale, circle your hands outward and then down and finally, bring them together so that your fingers become loosely interlaced, facing upward just below your navel, and say: *I breathe into the fullness of life.*

7. Exhale as you bring your interlaced hands upward along the frontline of the body. As they pass your heart and shoulders, rotate your hands around so they face toward the sky, and then extend your arms fully over your head. As you do this, speak silently: *I breathe out and return to light.*

8. Breathe in as you circle your interlaced hands out and around and down until they return to their original loosely interlaced posi-

tion, face up just below the navel. As you make this movement, say silently in your mind: *Completing the circle, I am free and full.*

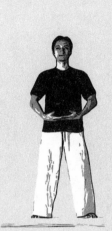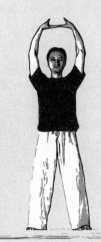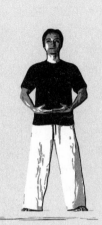

Gross or Physical Body

9. Touch your belly with both hands as you deeply inhale and exhale while speaking these words: *Infinite freedom and fullness appear as this precious human body.*

10. Gently squat and touch the ground with both hands as you say: *Touching the earth, I am connected to all beings.*

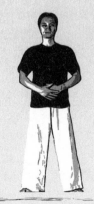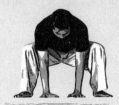

Integral Dedication

To finish up, you may dedicate the fruits of your practice to the benefit of all sentient beings. This dedication specifically invokes the intention of practice in all 4 quadrants of your existence, acknowledging all the dimensions of your being and embodying wholeness in a simple but profound way. Each quadrant will be evoked, for example, in the words of the dedication: *May my consciousness* (your individual interior, the Upper-Left quadrant) */ And my behavior* (your individual exterior, the Upper-Right quadrant) */ Be of service to all beings* (your collective interior, the Lower-Left quadrant) */ In all worlds* (your collective exterior, Lower-Right quadrant). The dedication concludes by invoking the liberation of all the quadrants of the conscious Kosmos into ever-present Suchness.

This same dedication can also be used to close a period of sitting meditation.

1. Stand with your feet together and your palms facing in front of your heart and bow, as you say, silently: *May my consciousness . . .*

2. Turn to your right and bow again as you say silently: *and my behavior . . .*

3. Turn to your right again and bow once more as you say silently: *be of service to all beings . . .*

4. Turn to your right again and bow. Say silently: *in all worlds . . .*

5. Turn again to your right (returning to the direction you originally faced) and open your arms and hands, face your palms forward, say silently: *liberating all . . .*

6. Bring your arms out and down to your sides with your palms still facing forward and say silently: *into the Suchness . . .*

7. Release and relax your arms and hands completely as you finish the phrase silently: *of this and every moment.*

8. With this, you have completed your dedication and are ready to step forward into the rest of your day.

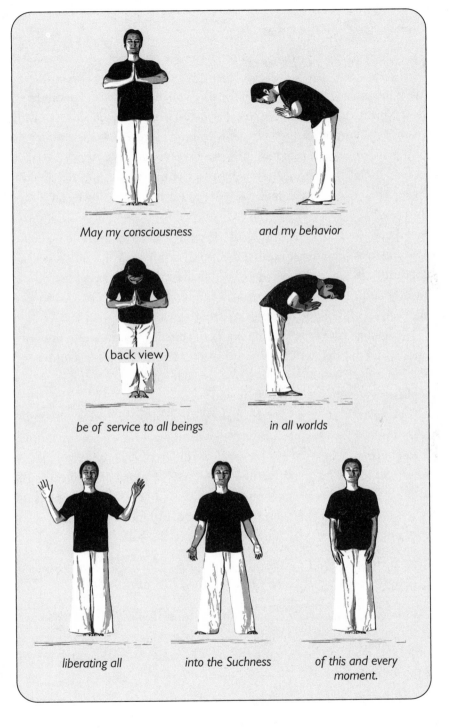

May my consciousness

and my behavior

(back view)

be of service to all beings

in all worlds

liberating all

into the Suchness

of this and every moment.

Gross Body Practices

Physical Exercise Is Essential!

We'll focus our attention now on the physical or gross level of bodily practice. New research continues to expand and underline the already firmly established importance of physical exercise. There is no question that physical exercise has profound positive effects on health, mood, cognitive clarity, longevity, and overall well-being. Human beings evolved while living an active lifestyle, and we seem to function best if we stay active and fit.

So good old-fashioned physical exercise—walking, running, strength training, aerobics, yoga, martial arts, sports, and so on—is still a central module of practice for optimizing physical health, with beneficial effects reverberating throughout every area of life. Therefore, your ILP should include regular physical exercise, perhaps even several kinds.

Customize your exercise program to fit you. You have unique strengths and vulnerabilities, so there's no substitute for exercising consciously and intelligently. Challenge yourself in order to be fit, but be careful to choose and engage exercises in ways that won't cause injuries.

Your exercise program can be as simple or complex as you want it to be. Simple can mean taking daily walks or lifting weights one to three times a week; complex can mean two or three different exercises every day or serious training for a competitive sport. We've provided a selection of Gold Star Practices and 1-Minute Modules as an excellent place to start when refreshing or upgrading your practice. But feel free to adopt whatever other activities you enjoy doing on a regular basis.

Strength Training: A Core Practice for Optimum Health

Building muscular strength is one of *the* most important results of physical exercise. A strength training practice that can be maintained with as little as one or two twenty-minute sessions a week can produce significant results.

Benefits of strength training include positive changes in:

- Lean muscle mass
- Muscular strength
- Strength of tendons and ligaments
- Hormone levels (improving levels of both "good" and "bad" hormones)
- Glucose tolerance
- Insulin sensitivity
- Body fat percentage
- Blood cholesterol and triglyceride levels and ratios
- Blood pressure
- And more

No other type of exercise has such impressive impacts on overall health as strength training. Metabolism changes as muscle mass increases, making it easier to lose weight and maintain health. Muscles can indeed be regarded as "the engine of youth." Strength training is the closest practice we have to time travel.

How it works: Whenever you work your muscles—whether the exercise is squats, push-ups, sit-ups, etc.—muscle tissue actually breaks down. Your muscle experiences a mini-death, and the more intense your workout, the more the muscle "dies." Soon after you stop the exercise, your body begins to rebuild the broken layers of muscle tissue, making that tissue stronger than before. Muscle growth results from overcompensating to protect the body from future stress. Through a regular practice of destroying and rebuilding, your muscles will strengthen and grow.

Your body already breaks down and rebuilds all of your muscles every fifteen to thirty days. Strength training speeds up the process with muscle regeneration peaking at twenty-four to thirty-six hours after training and continuing at increased rates for as much as seventy-two hours. When strength training, you actually burn fat and create muscle in your sleep!

Working one muscle group takes only a few minutes. If you work one major muscle group a day, you can create a strength training routine with a minimal time investment.

GOLD STAR PRACTICE
Focus Intensity Training (FIT)

Focus Intensity Training (FIT) is a state-of-the-art approach to strength training that makes conscious, coordinated use of the gross, subtle, and causal bodies.

When doing FIT we strengthen the gross, physical body by lifting weights or training against resistance; we strengthen the subtle body by focusing awareness and circulating energy throughout the body; and we strengthen the causal body by maintaining contact with the ever-present Witness that is aware of the sensations, sights, sounds, and feelings during each workout.

FIT works by flowing between focused intensity and deep relaxation.

Focus Intensity Training involves:

1. Pronounced periods of *tightly focused concentration* coupled with *high physical and emotional intensity* . . .
2 . . . alternating with deeply pronounced periods of *relaxation with low physical and emotional activation* and *broad, open, and receptive awareness.*

Health and fitness expert Shawn Phillips designed the Focus Intensity Training process to provide a more Integral approach to traditional weightlifting through a conscious engagement of the gross, subtle, and causal bodies. Resistance training is often considered a strictly physical practice (gross body), but the intentional generation of felt energies (subtle body), and resting in the Witness (causal body) can radically increase the effectiveness of something as apparently simple as lifting a weight and putting it down.

FIT Radically Expands Your Range of Functioning
Normally, people do not relax deeply, nor do they go all-out for intensity when they train. They stay within a narrow, habitual range

Pre-training Exercises	Core FIT Techniques	Post-training Exercises
Centering	Ground	Review/Record
Plan/Visualize	Elevate	Close/Dedication
Intention/ Dedication	Focus	Reflect/Integrate
Warm up	Recover	Journal (optional)

Phases of FIT.

of functioning. By radically expanding the zone in which you train, FIT enables you to amplify the results.

Compared to conventional strength training, FIT:

- Requires less time
- Creates better results for muscles and strength
- Offers multidimensional benefits (to all three bodies)
- Provides a more deeply enjoyable training experience

FIT gives us the precious opportunity to push past limits, connect with our deepest sense of human potential, and break through to the direct apprehension of something profoundly beyond the agitation and anxiety of daily life. As you practice, you'll inevitably run into many physical, emotional, and psychological barriers because you're on the edge of something that's pushing your growth boundaries. The Witness consciousness associated with the causal body doesn't fight or resist pain, but accepts and remains present with all sensations as dancing energy.

Resistance training can be a genuinely **transcendent experience**, because to truly transform the body, you have to endure a kind of mini-death in the muscle and the mind. In those moments of dying to one's idea of self and one's idea of what that self is capable of, one's Higher Self can stand forth. For an enormous number of people, strength training can be part of a truly Integral practice for touching their highest potentials in a deeply meaningful way. Sports fields and gyms function as churches for many men and women around the world.

FIT cultivates qualities such as focus, concentration, passion, commitment, receptivity, and presence. Like any practice, all the lessons and benefits of FIT carry over to other areas of life. Pushing through limits and barriers isn't just about lifting dumbbells, but about living life with dynamism and creativity, about taking risks to birth something new, about strengthening your awareness muscles, your heart muscles, your work muscles, and your service muscles. In the same way, practicing *being aware of what is* and *accepting what is* beautifully sums up the practice of mindful living. Focused Intensity Training brings meditation practice distilled from the wisdom traditions into 21st-century gyms.

In FIT, Each Training Session Is a Meditation

Before training, you set a conscious frame for your workout.

You can do this through *centering rituals* like mindfully driving and getting dressed while consciously breathing.

Through *planning and visualization,* you can specifically identify exactly what you are going to do during the training session and visualize yourself moving through your training session while embodying your highest consciousness.

You can set an *intention and dedication* by spending a few minutes in sitting meditation, connecting with your intention. You can even dedicate the practice session to someone or something beyond your separate self.

The core FIT execution cycle has four steps:

1. Ground: Take a couple of normal breaths in your belly and become fully present. Connect with your intention or dedication, with the energetic field of your subtle and causal bodies, as well as with the physical energy of the environment surrounding you. For instance, you can visualize energy circulating between your body and the earth below you, until you feel connected to a balanced and solid foundation.

2. Elevate: Rapidly take three to five short, explosive breaths into the upper chest to activate the sympathetic nervous system, increase oxygen, and intensify subtle energy currents. This is your chance, immediately before you begin your set, to charge the whole body, physically and emotionally, preparing for the exertion to come.

3. Focus: Begin your exercise set with single-pointed attention. Channel all 3 body-energies into a laser beam of focused concentration. Give special attention to the muscles being worked, subtle body currents, your breath, and the overall form of the exercise being performed. Keep your focus in the present moment and embrace all sensations that arise. If distracting thoughts come up, focus on the moment again through the breath or a repetition count (1, 2, 3 . . .).

CORE FIT CYCLE

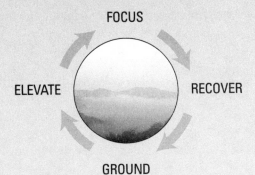

FOCUS

ELEVATE   RECOVER

GROUND

4. Recover: As soon as you finish your exercise set, relax. Breathe deeply from the diaphragm, open your awareness, and let go of everything. Notice the pleasurable release of subtle energy that naturally occurs and allow it to circulate. With each out-breath, visualize all tension in the body flowing out of the body, perhaps downward into the ground. Rest in the Witness, releasing to infinity. Feel deep relaxation as you immerse yourself in a spacious ocean of healing and recovery.

After training, bring this period of practice to conscious completion. You can do this by *reviewing and recording* your exercises, weights, rest times, and other variables you wish to track. You can also jot down a few words about your subjective feelings, sensations, and attention. It is important to do this *after* your training, because doing it during the core execution cycle diminishes your ability to recover and surrender deeply. Don't worry about not being able to track everything at first. As you become more familiar with your workout, you will be able to track everything easily.

Sit meditatively for a few moments and recall and *complete the intention and/or dedication* that you set before the workout. Notice what qualities this dedication brought to your training. Bring formal closure to your workout.

Finally, *reflect* on your experience of training. Notice anything that stands out: perhaps a period of distraction, a state of intensity, or a triggered memory or emotion. This integrates your training and clarifies its relationship to the rest of your life and practices. You may want to *journal* about your reflections. This helps solidify your learning

This same execution cycle can be used for any physical exercise, whether it is cardiovascular or muscle related, and whether the exercise lasts for one minute or two hours.

The extraordinary effectiveness of FIT derives from alternating between focus and release, concentration and expansiveness, full intensity and full disengagement, masculine and feminine. The higher and more intense the peak, the deeper and more expansive the valley. This undulating flow generates a 3-body synergy that allows your physical muscles to work harder, recover faster, and grow bigger. It is also a meditative practice, and one that helps integrate spirit, mind, and body.

1-MINUTE MODULE
Strength Training

In this 1-Minute Module, you strengthen your muscles by quickly but carefully challenging them to failure and then letting them recover. By taking this principle of challenge, failure, and recovery into account, workouts can be extremely short and effective.

Choose one muscle group to work on. You can use a barbell, dumbbells, a machine, or your own body weight (doing squats, push-ups, sit-ups).

Warm up. *Make sure to prevent injury.* This 1-Minute Module is very time efficient, but taking that principle to an extreme—like heavily loading a completely cold muscle—risks injury. So take care of yourself by warming up briefly but adequately! Also, it goes without saying, you should know something about proper technique when performing any exercise involving heavy weights. While we cannot provide detailed instructions here, resources abound, and you might also consider consulting a personal trainer.

Once you're warmed up adequately and making sure to use proper technique, perform the following steps:

1. Engage the FIT core execution cycle. Ground, Elevate, Focus and Execute, and then Recover.
2. While focusing and executing, repeat the exercise until you bring the muscle group to exhaustion.
3. Full exhaustion is reached when you can't do another repetition no matter how much you want to.

4. If you're using weights, this should take somewhere between eight to twelve repetitions.

That's it—you're done! One day, one set, one muscle group.

For your next strength training session, choose a different muscle group and repeat. Rotate through the major muscle groups over a seven-day period and then start over. To accomplish this, you can use exercises that train multiple muscles at the same time such as squats (gluteals, quadriceps, and hamstrings) or push-ups (chest and triceps).

Muscle Groups

When selecting exercises for your strength training practice, it's important to choose at least one exercise from each major muscle group for a balance. Below you'll find the major muscle groups and a few exercises that target them:

Abdominals – These muscles include the large flat muscle running the length of the abdomen and the muscles that run down the sides and front of the abdomen. Exercises may include standard crunches and curls, reverse curls and crunches (where the hips are lifted instead of the head and shoulders), and crunches involving a rotation or twist.

Biceps – The front of the upper arm. Biceps curls can be done with a barbell, dumbbells, or a machine. Other pulling movements like chin-ups and upright rows also involve the biceps.

Calves – The calf muscles are on the back of the lower leg. Exercises include standing or seated calf raises.

Deltoids – The cap of the shoulder. Exercises include push-ups, bench presses, front dumbbell raises, and rear dumbbell raises (done while seated and bent at the waist or lying face down on a flat bench).

Gluteals – This group of muscles (often referred to as "glutes") includes the gluteus maximus, which is the big muscle covering your butt.

Common exercises are the squat and the leg-press machine. The glutes also come into play during lunges and deep jumps.

Hamstrings – These muscles make up the back of the thigh. Exercises include squats, lunges, leg-press machine, and leg-curl machine.

Hip abductors and adductors – These are the muscles of the inner and outer thigh. The *ab*ductors are on the outside and move the leg away from the body. The *ad*ductors are on the inside and pull the legs toward one another and across the centerline of the body. These muscles can be worked with a variety of side-lying leg lifts, standing cable pulls, and multi-hip machines. Squats can be one of the most intense ways to work both, if they're done correctly.

Latissimus dorsi – Large muscles of the mid-back. Exercises include pull-ups, chin-ups, one-arm bent rows, dips on parallel bars, and the lat pull-down machine.

Lower back – Exercises include the back extension machine and prone back extension exercises. These muscles also come into play during the squat and dead lift.

Figure 6.2
Muscle groups.

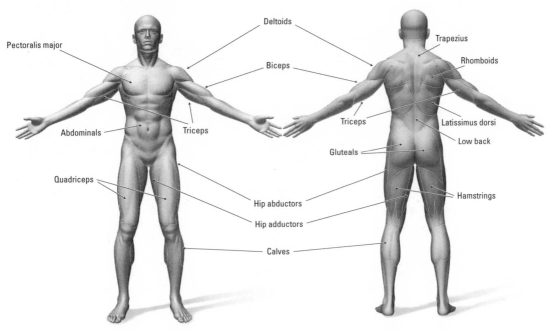

Pectoralis major – Large fan-shaped muscle that covers the front of the upper chest. Exercises include push-ups, pull-ups, regular and incline bench press, and the pec deck machine.

Quadriceps – This group of muscles makes up the front of the thigh. Exercises include squats, lunges, leg-extension machine, and leg-press machine.

Rhomboids – Muscles in the middle of the upper back between the shoulder blades. The rhomboids are worked during chin-ups, dumbbell bent rows, and other moves that bring the shoulder blades together.

Upper Trapezius – The muscle running from the back of the neck to the shoulder. Exercises include upright rows and shoulder shrugs with resistance.

Triceps – The back of the upper arm. Exercises include pushing movements like push-ups, dips, triceps extensions, triceps kick-backs, and overhead presses. The triceps also come into play during the bench press and military press.

Small Muscles – There are over 600 muscles in the human body, beyond the major muscle groups described here. Varying your form, many kinds of free-weight training, sports, and dance can help you strengthen these small muscles. Although it's fine to strengthen major muscles, don't neglect the others. They are important to balance, coordination, and whole-body health.

Flying High with Cardio

Cardiovascular or aerobic exercise can be a wonderful complement to strength training. "Cardio"—also known as "aerobics"—can take numerous forms:

Individual aerobic exercises: swimming, bicycling, running, jogging, jumping rope, step aerobics, cross-country skiing, elliptical training, power walking, and more.

Aerobic sports and activities: dancing, tennis, skiing, basketball, aerobics class, volleyball, rowing crew, racquetball, soccer, football, and many more. All of these are discussed in more depth in the next section.

Regular aerobic exercise can increase your lung capacity, so that it can process more oxygen with less effort. It can strengthen your heart so that it pumps more blood and carries more oxygen with fewer beats and less effort. It can increase the blood supply to your muscles and organs, lower your blood pressure, improve your cholesterol and triglyceride profiles, reduce body fat, and improve glucose tolerance and insulin resistance. It also helps your body release endorphins, producing the mood elevation often called "runner's high." All these benefits result in higher endurance and greater metabolic efficiency.

1-MINUTE MODULE
Aerobic Workout

The 1-Minute Aerobic Module is a *short* session of high-intensity interval training. It is particularly important to bring full consciousness and the principles of FIT if you are concentrating your exercise time in this way. The process is simple:

Choose any aerobic exercise that will raise your heart rate—it could be running, biking, or jumping rope.

- Warm up adequately.
- Ground.
- Elevate.
- Perform the activity at a high intensity with full focus. Exert yourself but don't overexert yourself. Keep it up for 1–3 minutes. If you're not sure how much is too much, then be conservative at first.
- Recover. Stop the activity and rest for a couple of minutes.
- If time permits, repeat this cycle two or three times or more.

High Intensity Interval Training is a particularly efficient approach to cardiovascular exercise that involves alternating short, high-intensity bursts of activity with brief periods of rest. Research shows that this approach to cardiovascular training is remarkably effective, significantly speeding up our metabolic rate, improving endurance, and increasing overall fitness with a relatively small investment of time. Why?

Intensity. *High-intensity* cardiovascular training produces more powerful physiological benefits than *medium-intensity* exercise. Since we can reach significantly higher levels of intensity if we only have to sustain them for short bursts, interval training makes high intensity possible.

Relaxation. Many of the key cardiovascular benefits derive from the process of *slowing down* our heart rate and breathing from a highly activated state. We get the benefits of this relaxation cycle again and again during interval training.

Efficiency. The key benefits of a cardiovascular workout can be achieved in much less time through high-intensity interval training. It's easier to stick with a program that requires only twenty minutes than one that requires an hour or more.

Also, this approach helps you sustain motivation. The high intensity bursts are intense (read interesting, challenging, and entertaining). They certainly spice up the workout, preventing boredom and keeping you coming back for more.

High-intensity interval training employs some of the key principles of FIT in an aerobic/cardiovascular context. By raising intensity and relaxing deeply, you expand your range of function.

In fact, the core FIT cycle—ground, elevate, focus, and recover—can be used with aerobic exercise, and it adapts particularly well if you're using high intensity interval training.

Sports, Dance, and Neuromuscular Coordination

We exercise another distinct dimension of the body when we engage in sports and other activities such as dancing that require split-second timing, balance, agility, and coordination. During these activities, we must continually make multiple rapid, unexpected adjustments in response to

Using 1-Minute Modules Creatively

As you custom-design a program to fit your needs and lifestyle, you may want to improvise on the basic 1-Minute Strength and 1-Minute Aerobic modules we have provided.

For example, you can take a middle path, concentrating the effectiveness of short workouts that use the principles of the 1-Minute Modules, but which take more time. You may choose to extend your 1-Minute exercises to twelve to fifteen minutes. This can give you powerfully effective workouts, while being enormously time efficient!

You can spread your strength training out into short workouts and still work more than one muscle group per day. You can also perform more than one set.

Generally, more frequent short strength training workouts work well when you have equipment at home, and less frequent, longer workouts are appropriate when you need to travel to a gym.

You can get an intense cardiovascular workout in just twenty or thirty minutes or so by repeating each interval as many as ten or twelve times. Or you can mix in different forms of cardiovascular practices: three sprinting intervals, three intervals of jumping rope, and three biking intervals, for example.

You can also extend the types and duration of aerobic exercises you do. For example, your aerobic practice might involve twelve minutes of high-intensity interval training every day plus a vigorous half-day hike once a week.

You can custom-design any kind of program. The possibilities are unlimited. The important point is to choose types of physical exercise that work for you; so design a program you enjoy—and really *do it*!

the movements of opponents and/or teammates, partners, the ball and/or the environment (including changes in the music, in dance).

When the brain confronts the unfamiliar, the nervous system receives and carries more messages than during a predictable workout. With consistent practice, the nervous system becomes more efficient, which is an essential dimension of total health.

The wide variety of postures and movements involved in sports activities allows us to exercise many of the body's more than six hundred muscles, not just the large ones that we target with strength training. This enhances the strength and responsiveness of our small, intrinsic muscles and connective tissues. Many of these same benefits can come from running, climbing, walking, dancing, hunting, fishing, fighting, gathering food, or farming—the ancient human activities that honed the structures of our bodies.

There is a dialogue between the nervous system and the musculo-skeletal system. The brain, spine, and nerves engage in coordinated learning together with a nearly infinite array of different muscle combinations. This sharpens neuromuscular coordination. Like other forms of exercise, this also tends to benefit the endocrine, respiratory, digestive, circulatory, and excretory systems, which all contribute to optimum fitness.

Sports injuries are common, so it's not wise to participate in sports indiscriminately. Check with a doctor if you're unsure of your ability to participate in a particular activity. A low-impact form of exercise might be better for you. Even ping-pong has wonderful benefits!

Whatever you choose, try to participate in the spirit of *play*. Be safe and enjoy yourself. Sports are not only healthy, they're also good fun. Often they're an opportunity to bond with others through the rituals of teamwork and healthy competition—or just going out for a beer after the game. Also, notice the *shadows* that come out of the woodwork when you enact the drama of winning and losing—tasting the ecstasy of victory and suffering the agony of defeat. Your on-the-field reactions and antics can make great material for a 3-2-1 Shadow-Process session. (A great time to do this is while you're having that beer.)

Sports or dancing can even be a spiritual experience. Your body's movement in sync with the other bodies and the rhythm of the performance suddenly feels like a spontaneous, divinely choreographed, flow of beauty and awe. This is when your gross, subtle, and even causal dimensions shine forth with unified glory—all in one magic moment of leaping, racing, throwing, scoring, sinking a putt, or swooshing down the mountain.

Stretching

Virtually all fitness experts—from professional football trainers to hatha yoga instructors—agree that stretching is the best way to prevent injury and increase your kinesthetic flexibility. It's something you can do anywhere—in your home, the office, or even while traveling—no gym required. Stretching comes quite naturally to all of us. Recall the last time you stretched automatically after sitting for a long time in the same position. It feels good!

In addition to feeling good, decreasing the chance of injury, and enhancing flexibility, stretching has a number of other benefits:

- Reduces muscle tension
- Improves circulation
- Reduces anxiety, stress, and fatigue
- Improves posture
- Enhances muscular coordination
- Increases range of movement in the joints
- Enhances kinesthetic intelligence
- Reduces muscular soreness

Fitness trainers usually recommend stretching before and after strength or cardio workouts. After a short warm-up, stretch each major muscle group. Relax into the stretch and breathe as freely and deeply as possible, opening into the stretch as you breathe, particularly during the exhalation. (Don't hold your breath!)

Integral Nutrition

Now that you've worked out your muscles hard, you'll need to feed them. One of the most important aspects of a body practice is nutrition. Food is a primal survival and psycho-emotional need, and our typical way of relating to it is rooted in our earliest, most primitive psyche. It is also a key social ritual, full of cultural meaning. But it is also a very important health practice with profound effects on our levels of fitness and energy.

Our ability to practice depends on eating a diet that supports that intention. Eating wisely is a practice that can have an especially dramatic positive impact on all other aspects of our life.

We live in a culture that makes it very easy to eat poorly and more difficult to eat well. This may be due to evolutionary factors. For most of humans' thousands of years of evolution we were hunter-gatherers. Living close to the edge of survival *helped* our overall health to crave concentrated calories, sugar, salt, and fat, and to be inclined to graze all day! But today, with tasty food conveniently available everywhere, advertised through media to which we're exposed many times a day, we suffer the degenerative "diseases of kings" that come from eating too much of what we crave.

It takes a very serious and continually renewed commitment to eat consciously and well. It's especially hard to develop a disciplined relationship to food without adopting rigid and/or extreme dietary prescriptions.

The ILP nutrition philosophy is therefore very simple: No one diet is right for everyone. Diet is individual and requires self-knowledge and self-responsibility. The calculation is very personal, which is why we're happy to give some broad recommendations and leave it to your own best wisdom to choose what's right for you.

The 4 Quadrants of Integral Nutrition

Factors in all 4 quadrants contribute to how we eat. We consume the foods we do for psychological, biological, cultural, and social reasons—the areas represented by the 4 quadrants. Eating habits, for the most part, have been conditioned and reinforced over a lifetime by all these factors, to the point that they've become automatic and unconscious. It's no wonder eating patterns are hard to change!

Taking an AQAL view of nutrition helps you step back and really look at your nutrition habits, so you can turn what's been automatic into a conscious practice. By adding perspective, each element of AQAL sheds additional light on the what, how, and why of nutrition. Taking a tour of the quadrants will give you a more comprehensive look at your nutritional life. It can also help you formulate an overall approach to your dietary practice that goes beyond merely avoiding certain foods or following the latest nutritional fad. Let's look at the 4 quadrants of breakfast, lunch, and dinner (see figure 6.3).

Upper-Left Quadrant (Intention): Eat Mindfully

This interior perspective focuses on the *why* behind eating. What motivates us to consume the way we do? Why do we have certain nutritional patterns?

The practice of **mindful eating** cultivates the ability to tune in to the present moment while choosing foods, preparing them, and eating and drinking. The act of eating involves a number of interior experiences— from deciding what to eat, to preparing or ordering it, to smelling the

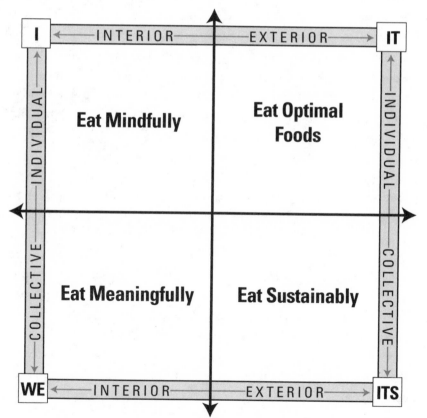

Figure 6.3

The 4 quadrants of nutrition.

food, to first tasting it, to savoring it as we chew it, to feeling it slide down the hatch and into our stomach. You will also notice food's impact on your subtle energetic states. This means being honest with our responses to various foods and acknowledging the felt-experience of how foods interact with our body (for example, indigestion, tiredness, enhanced vitality).

Strictly speaking, the subtle energies present in the foods you eat are an Upper-Right quadrant affair. However, it is in the process of cultivating a mindful relationship to eating that you will tend to pay attention to this very real dimension of your total nutrition. Fresh, living foods are full of life-energy. Processed and refined foods have less. As you continue to develop a more conscious relationship to food, you'll be able to make discriminating choices that take into account both the gross and subtle dimensions of what you eat.

A practitioner of mindful eating finds satisfaction in the *quality*, not the *quantity* of the eating experience. For example, an attuned awareness will notice the diminishing returns of taste states (technically called "taste specific satiety"). Our taste buds are like chemical sensors that get tired quite easily, so our experience of the first bite will generally be more flavorful and enjoyable than the last. (This is why free samples work so well!) At the end of a big meal, we may have very little taste experience left. Check it out for yourself. In a mindful eating practice, *less* food can equal *more* satisfaction.

Lower-Left Quadrant (Culture): Eat Meaningfully

The We of nutrition includes the shared meanings surrounding food. *Culture influences your food choices.* A culture's history and preferences favors certain kinds of foods over others, raises certain health concerns and ignores others, and attaches group identities to people based on their nutritional patterns (for example, "a traditional meat and potatoes kind of guy," "as American as apple pie," or "a granola hippie"). Practicing Integral nutrition includes being aware of how different cultures collectively interpret and relate to food.

Eating communities share particular meanings and worldviews that evolve—from traditional religious festivals to national identity foods to cosmopolitanism. Each cultural worldview has its own conversation about nutrition—its own food discourse. What do "we" agree is good to eat? When you eat meaningfully, you're consciously choosing foods in alignment with your community's worldview, value system, and ethics. Before purchasing or eating a particular food, check in to see if you feel a resonance with the company that produced the food, the store where you buy the food, or the person or restaurant preparing it. Pay attention also to who you're eating with! Sharing a meal with family, friends, co-workers, or a romantic partner is one of the most universal and pleasurable ways of creating a meaningful cultural "We" space. We break bread together. You can do so consciously and joyfully.

Upper-Right Quadrant (Behavior): Eat Optimal Foods

This quadrant asks the question, What do you *do?*—or, in a nutrition context—*What do you eat and drink?* Ultimately, your nutritional health depends on your behaviors—on *what* you actually allow into your physical body. This is often a highly personal matter, relying on your own research, food awareness, self-knowledge, trial and error, and listening to your body.

Nutrition science is an extremely complex, controversial, and often self-contradictory field. We can't possibly cover it all here, and a full Integral account of nutrition remains to be written. However, we can make some broad generalizations. An Integral nutrition practice points to the many scientifically validated approaches to diet that advocate paying attention to your proportions of protein, fat, and carbohydrates. It pays attention to *how much* you eat and when you eat it. It can even account for how you combine foods.

It also acknowledges other dietary criteria. Many people thrive, and swear by, eating fresh, whole foods rather than refined, processed, or synthetic foods. Some people thrive on vegan, vegetarian, or meat-rich "paleo" diets. There are numerous philosophic approaches to supplementation, most emphasizing some vitamins, herbs, antioxidants, enzymes, super-foods, or amino acids. No one diet fits everyone. Personal experimentation is often necessary because we must each account for our unique physiology and metabolism.

Some things are universally agreed upon:

- Minimize bad fat (particularly trans fats).
- Minimize simple carbohydrates.
- Minimize low-quality processed and fast foods.
- Control portion size.
- Minimize snacking (unless deliberately choosing frequent, small meals to regulate insulin).
- Drink enough water.

Nutritional practice involves eating consciously, learning from experience, and periodically experimenting. It also involves transforming our *relationship* to food, softening the neurosis surrounding food that we often feel in modern life. Sometimes, it's *okay* to eat that piece of chocolate cake, and we should allow ourselves to truly savor it. And sometimes, we need to be more disciplined. The key is balance—and not just for the sake of our physical health. Because food so powerfully affects emotions, diet is an opportunity for continual growth in emotional intelligence and self-awareness. Nutrition is a central area of life-long study and practice.

Tip: Keep a Nutrition Journal
It's difficult to change your eating habits before you know what they are. Keeping a daily *nutrition journal* serves as a useful practice for tracking your consumption behaviors. By objectively observing and recording all the foods, beverages, and supplements you consume throughout a day, you'll be able to see what's really happening.

By recording the foods you eat, you'll immediately be able to see your true eating habits. Knowing *what* you eat, *how much* you eat, and *when* you eat gives you a starting point for making more conscious behavioral choices about your diet.

Lower-Right Quadrant (Systems): Eat Sustainably
Food serves as a direct link between the human organism and its natural environment by providing the raw materials that construct our physical body. The Its perspective of nutrition looks at the natural and man-made systems supporting food's long journey from the earth to your plate. Every

But How Do I Integrally Lose Weight?

Weight loss is always a thorny issue due to the legions of "experts" offering (or usually selling) advice, the strong opinions of their followers, and the many body types and food preferences. Trying to find a diet that works can be so overwhelming that you lose your appetite. While that might ironically help, you may want to look at some of the most basic and widely agreed upon discoveries that nutrition researchers have found.

Perhaps the most foundational weight loss practice involves paying close attention to the *amount* of food you eat. For many foods, you can use your fist as an easy way to measure portion size: any serving bigger than your fist means too much. (As a matter of fact, reducing the total amount of calories you take in will probably increase your lifespan.)

A more technical (yet still basic) weight loss practice suggests restricting either fats or carbohydrates to less than 10 percent of your calorie intake.* In other words, reduce the amount of food you eat from the fats and the carbohydrates circles—from both or either, whatever works best for you—and continue to make healthy food choices. Research has shown that each approach (reducing fats or reducing carbs) works better for a certain proportion of the population. So before jumping off a cliff into the next crazy weight loss fad, experiment with these basic practices first. Then, when you reach a weight that's optimal for you, maintain it by sustainably balancing protein, carbohydrates, and fats.

---

*Be careful about *radical* reductions of fat or carbs. Most reputable experts who recommend restrictions still suggest small amounts of "good" carbs and fats.

food or beverage you consume has a hidden history, an unwritten account of the resources, materials, and impacts it took to bring them to you.

What's the hidden history of the foods and beverages you normally eat and drink? Where did they come from? How were they produced? How did they get to you? Factors to take into consideration include geography (grown locally or across the world), production methods (such as organic farming or using pesticides, natural or genetically modified), environmental costs, economic system (for example, fair or free trade), laws (such as packaging disclosure, inspection regulations), technology, company ownership structure, transportation networks, production facilities (such as free range or caged chickens), and so on.

Every time you purchase and consume a food product, or any product for that matter, you're implicitly supporting its hidden history. By becoming aware of the systems you're reinforcing with each swipe of your card, you can make more informed and conscious nutrition decisions, taking into account the interconnected ripples sent out with every food purchase.

In addition to the hidden history and systems of food, paying attention to the environment where you eat your meals can also be an important nutrition practice. Gulping down fast food in a traffic jam is a bit different from a quiet candlelight dinner with your intimate partner, don't you think? Compare eating in front of the television with eating across from a stimulating dinner guest or eating contemplatively at a silent meditation retreat. In each situation, a unique energetic exchange occurs among the environment, the food, and the person. The environmental context in which you eat significantly impacts your total eating experience.

It's not that one situation is more right than another, but each will influence you in a different way. Once you become aware of how different environmental contexts affect your enjoyment, digestion, mood, and so on, you can begin to choose more consciously when and where you'd like to eat. Now that we've exercised and nourished our gross physical body, let's consider our subtle body.

Subtle Body Practices

Subtle Body Exercise

It's common for practitioners to include *two major and distinct kinds* of exercises in their ILP Body module: exercises that emphasize the gross physical body, and exercises that emphasize subtle body and subtle energy.

What, Again, Is Subtle Energy?

Subtle energy generally refers to all energies beyond the gross phys-ical. Known in the traditions by such terms as prana and qi (ki or ch'i)—and, for example, said to be the mechanism through which acupuncture affects the body—these energies are often held to be the "missing link" between the intentional mind and the physi-cal body.

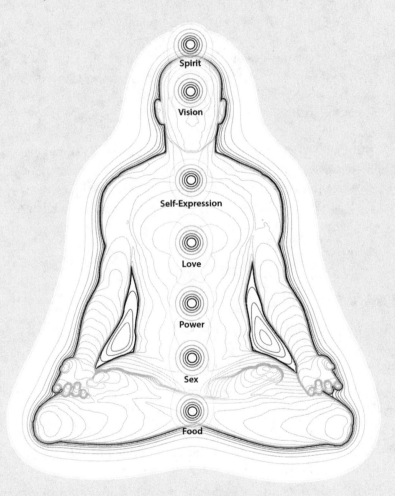

Chakras, sheaths, subtle energies.

The word *subtle* literally means "so slight as to be difficult to detect or describe," and compared to the physical, it is. Nevertheless, with practice and sensitivity, you can sense the spectrum of subtle energies that you are and that surround you all the time. So don't just believe in them—cultivate direct access to your own subtle energies and experience them for yourself.

Ancient traditions describe a whole *spectrum* of subtle energies. The grossest subtle energies (usually called *etheric*) are closely associated with the physical body. Subtler energies (*astral, mental, and psychic*) are associated with emotions, dreams, thought, and higher meditative experiences. These different degrees of subtlety are frequently discussed in terms of how they correspond to the seven *chakras*, which are an ascending series of energy centers in the body associated with food, sex, power, love, self-expression, insight, and spiritual realization.

Although these systems are both interesting and useful in certain circumstances, practitioners usually don't need to focus attention on the difference between the various levels of subtle energy. Generally, it is best to simply breathe and feel and consciously intend that subtle energy increase and flow as needed.

Yoga, Qigong, and the Martial Arts

Every type of exercise engages the whole being (so we're always using the gross, subtle, and causal bodies). Nevertheless, certain forms of exercise, like strength training and aerobics, emphasize the gross body. Others, including the ancient Chinese arts of qigong, t'ai chi, and other martial arts and the ancient Indian arts of yoga and pranayama emphasize the subtle body. The 3-Body Workout specifically exercises both the gross and subtle bodies and addresses the causal body through the inclusion of meditative practices.

Each subtle discipline is a unique tradition and corpus of expertise. They're definitely not all the same thing. Nevertheless, each of them involves specific practices of attention and discipline through which practitioners develop sensitivity to subtle energies. Through practice they learn how to breathe, feel, and move in ways that enhance strong and flowing subtle bodies (qi or prana), on many levels. Practitioners develop profound new abilities to manage their states of mind, emotion, and energy, often engendering new abilities and extending lifespan. Some highly refined subtle arts can even be cultivated as Integral practices, encompassing causal and gross body exercise.

Subtle energy practices increase equanimity, reduce stress, improve mental alertness, and have beneficial effects on physical functioning, too. They are also often practiced as subtle-body art forms and can exhibit a special grace and beauty in mature practitioners.

Human attention conventionally tends to become fixated in fairly narrow ranges of sense experience, thought, and emotion. Daily subtle energy practices can break these fixations of attention and transform the states and the range of function of the subtle body, helping us learn to ground, balance, and center.

Generally, practitioners find that the greatest benefits accrue after years of consistent practice in one of these subtle body disciplines. As a complement to gross physical exercise, such as FIT, subtle body practices help make ILP a seamless unity of body, mind, and spirit.

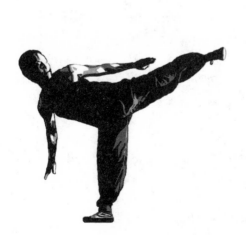
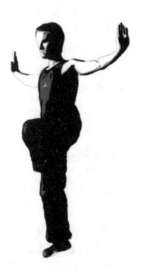

Figure 6.4
*Subtle body
practices.*

The Core of Energy Practice

Central to all subtle energy practices is learning to conduct more healthy life energy. Subtle energy pervades everything, so there's not a limited supply, but our capacity to open to it, circulate it, and release it can be extremely limited.

There are many traditional models of our subtle body and subtle anatomy, but they generally agree that the primary flow of life energy in the human system functions as a circuit of energy that goes down the front of the body, turns at the bodily base, and then ascends up the spine. It continually circulates in a natural circuit of descent and ascent.

The subtle life energy *descends* into the body where it is experienced more grossly as fullness of life, most associated with vitality and the *hara*, which is the Japanese word for the vital center in the body just below the level of the navel. We can emphasize this descent and fullness of life when we inhale and experience it moving down the front of the body.

Then the subtle life energy *turns* at the perineum (the bottom of the torso, the point midway between the genitals and the anus) and *ascends* up the spine and above the head, where it is experienced more subtly as freedom and light, most associated with brightness at the head center. We can experience this ascent into light and freedom as we exhale and experience it moving up the spine to the crown of the head and above.

This same fundamental structure is called the *sushumna* or central channel, with the *ida* (left channel) and *pingala* (right channel) in the Indian yogic traditions. The "microcosmic orbit" of Chinese Taoist traditions bears resemblances to this system as well. This same circuit was symbolized by way of the caduceus by the ancient Egyptians and Greeks.

Subtle Mastery

In highly developed yogis of any tradition the descending and ascending currents flow with enormous intensity. The head, heart, and hara all shine with life force. There is dazzling life-fullness, effulgent heart-feeling, and the radiant light of liberated intelligence. This only comes with mastery. Imbalanced or untrained human beings can tolerate only a comparative trickle of energy.

A great deal of the ancient wisdom traditions focus on strengthening the vehicle of the body-mind so that it can conduct more life force. This is what is meant by "opening the chakras." Learning to *conduct life energy* is a natural dimension of ILP.

One of the main ways we do that, in everyday terms, is to develop a capacity to tolerate sensations that ordinarily trigger us to throw off life force. For example, if we are feeling nervous or bored, we might find ourselves talking too much, fidgeting, or snacking mindlessly—all activities that tend to *discharge* the life-energy building up in us. Learning to tolerate subtle distress enables us to enjoy a fuller range of energy states, including different kinds of discomfort—physical, emotional, mental—by breathing and conducting all our daily experiences, especially of intensity and reactivity.

Integral practices enhance this conductivity by helping us develop a strong, energized, and unobstructed human system on all levels. Subtle energy practices involve freeing up feeling and awareness at the heart and engaging them through the breath. Part of this involves intensifying energy at the vital center below the navel, grounding the whole bodily system, and emphasizing presence and life-fullness. Another part of it involves conducting energy up the spine into and beyond the head, emphasizing contact with light and freedom.

The Microcosmic Orbit

The microcosmic orbit is a classic Taoist practice for conducting gross, subtle, and causal energies using the breath. This practice awakens, circulates, and directs energy through the orbit formed by breathing down the front line of your body from the top of your head to the perineum (the Functional Channel) and breathing up the back line from the perineum to the top of the head (the Governing Channel).

Basic Instructions for the Microcosmic Orbit

1. Focus on the sensations just above your head and inhale your breath energy down the entire front of your body.

2. Exhale and release your breath energy up the spine to the top of your head.

3. Repeat this orbit as many times as you choose.

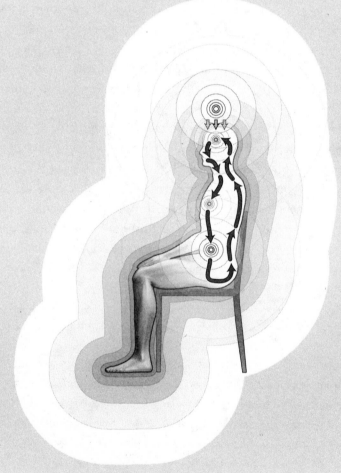

The microcosmic orbit.

Detailed Instructions

1. Sit in a comfortable position, relax your body, calm your mind, and regulate your breath. Notice your bodily sensations. Feel the weight of your body in your seat and the contact of your feet on ground. Bring your attention to the present moment.

2. Turn your attention inward and lower your gaze. As you breathe through the nose, feel, open to, and commune with the all-pervading energy within and surrounding you, especially above your head.

3. Visualize an especially intense concentration of energy above your head. Imagine that the top of your head is a blooming lotus flower, soaking up the light that's always falling upon you.

4. As you inhale, bring your energy and focus down to the area between (and behind) your eyebrows and draw energy forward toward this "third eye."

5. Press your tongue against the roof of your mouth behind your front teeth to enable more energy to circulate and let your energy sink down through the palate and tongue into your throat to the heart.

6. Move your breath down further and deeper within the body, about two finger widths below the navel until you feel a concentrated pocket of energy glowing there—a point of golden light—clear, bright, warm, and pure. Allow your breath to naturally become lighter and subtler.

7. When the feeling of energy in your navel is stable and full, use your mind to guide this energy down into the genitals, the perineum, and then back toward your tailbone. Steadily visualize this energy as a small snake gradually passing through the tailbone.

8. Now complete the second half of the orbit by exhaling and visualizing the energy moving up the back of your body to where the ribs meet the spine, then right on up the spine to the back of the head. Imagine energy traveling up your spine to the center and top of your head and even above the head.

9. Begin another cycle, breathing in as the energy moves down the front channel from the top of your head to your perineum and breathing out as the energy moves up the back channel from the perineum to the back of your head.

10. Repeat for as many repetitions as you feel comfortable.

The microcosmic orbit descends and ascends through the spectrum of body-energies, cycling the breath from causal to subtle to gross and from gross to subtle to causal—an orbit of energies. When practiced with intention, the microcosmic orbit seamlessly integrates movement through the three great energy realms.

Conducting Intensity

We experience increased levels of energy as intensity, and it often feels uncomfortable at first.

For example, if you hold your position and breathe when doing a squat or deep knee bend, you'll quickly feel intense almost painful energy in your leg muscles. (Pain in the joints is not good, but persisting through muscular pain can be a powerful practice.)

Can you practice conducting this intensity rather than reacting to it? Can you breathe into it, stay present with and as it, and allow it to change and move naturally? Such "conductivity" is a core subtle energy capacity.

At some point, you'll notice that it's just energy and intensity. And you notice what you're adding to it: emotions and thinking—your whole inner dialogue. Being completely present and open to what's arising in the moment requires only that you conduct additional intensity. How do you respond to discomfort? Do you see it for what it is, or do you resist it or react to it? Body practices give you a chance to practice free attention and flexibility even in the midst of intensity.

The ability to stay present with emotional intensity is very similar to staying present with bodily intensity. When your boss asks you to do the umpteenth thing beyond what you can realistically do, what happens? Your ability to conduct energy affects every area of your life.

Conducting Sexual Energy

The practice of conscious sexuality has many dimensions, most of them intimate and mutual, centering on the physical, mental, emotional, and spiritual relationship between partners. It also includes a dimension that is internal and individual—the development of the body's capacity to heighten, conduct, open, and deepen the natural flows of subtle energy. Yes, conscious lovemaking can help you get in touch with your body's subtle energy flows!

It is possible to conduct the highly impulsive energy of sexual arousal into a profound depth of open feeling and ecstasy. In doing so, you can learn to open and strengthen the body's subtle energy channels. Sexual practice can also help you learn what it's like to conduct a higher level of aliveness and charge through not just your genitals, but your whole body.

This process is often taught in highly technical terms, usually focusing (especially in men) on extending lovemaking by bypassing ejaculation and preventing degenerative orgasm and (in women and men) on re-laxing and opening to allow more powerful, conscious, and sustained regenerative orgasms. These can be valuable skills. However, all these techniques should be linked to a universal principle: in conscious loving, the whole body (gross, subtle, and causal) can come alive in the freest and fullest terms.

All techniques work best when they are rooted in the inherent happi-ness of an open heart. If you make love as a way of communing with Spirit in and as your partner, in a mood of loving service, intending to give rather than receive, you'll get the best results. Enjoy the natural pleasure of receiving life and surrendering yourself with each feeling breath—and delighting through all your senses. These are the core secrets of conscious sexuality.

Subtle Breath Practices

Both modern science and ancient traditions of self-cultivation point to the breath as one of the most powerful natural methods for balancing the body-mind and for shifting and deepening awareness. In yoga, the

3-Body Sex

In our schizophrenic sexual culture—whether sex is moralistically repressed as sin or hedonistically expressed as "fucking"—sex tends to be reduced to a mere physical act: Tab A in Slot B, or some variation thereof. This, of course, is only the **gross** dimension of sex. *But could you have sex—or really make love—consciously in all 3 bodies?*

At the gross, physical level, you and your partner's bodies could touch, rub, move, caress, kiss, and penetrate (or perform any other act) in accordance with your hormonal urges. Without you and your partner's conscious participation, this would lead fairly quickly to male orgasm and the end of the encounter. That would be easy enough. . . .

At the subtle level (which begins even *before* the gross and continues *beyond* it), you and your partner could share a deep emotional exchange. This could include a play of energies that you consciously conduct toward greater intensity—more brilliant subtle-body fireworks. By focusing your attention on the subtle dimension of sex, achieving orgasm might become less important, and the joyful play of energies up and down, in and out, and in every other direction, could become an amazing source of pleasure. Your heart centers could open and mutually resonate and perhaps even merge into a singular vortex of profound and passionate loving. You would still be free to have orgasms, if you wished, and those orgasms might even expand and intensify, but the play of energies and depth of emotion could themselves become free-flowing subtle orgasms.

At the causal level, you could rest in perfectly still, unobstructed awareness—the silent, conscious, spaceless space that's holding your gross and subtle bodies, and hearts and minds, throughout the sexual act.

And finally, **in the nondual union of all your bodies,** that

still and silent witness consciousness might reveal itself as inseparable from *boundless radiant love*. And that all-pervading love
might find itself *making art* out of the caress of two naked human
beings. In this art, you might gladly surrender to infinity, embracing
your lover with God's own arms, feeling right through your separate identities into the mystery of a Kosmos that allows such bliss.
Pure emptiness could hold the dance of undulating flesh and the
frolic of subtle electricity, and release them into an ecstatic lumi-
nescence that's utterly transcendent and yet tenderly intimate—
even in the sweetness of your lover's lips.

Could you let go into causal stillness, while allowing the subtle
bodies to swirl and play and the gross bodies to rub, lick, and penetrate, all in the spirit of radiant love?

Like every other aspect of ILP, it would take practice!

field of breath control, *pranayama,* was considered no less rich and important than the field of hatha yoga, or *asana,* the most familiar type of
yoga to most westerners.

As long as we are alive, we are breathing. The breath can always serve
as a natural reminder of the body and the mysterious spiritual source
of our breathing and heartbeat. Breath relates intimately with the state of
the subtle body.

The basic elements of many subtle breath practices are:

1. *Sitting* in a relaxed position with your spine as straight as possible,
   and, if you like, closing your eyes.
2. *Slowing the breath* as much as is comfortable, without straining.
3. *Tightening the throat and the muscles at the bodily base (around
   the anus, genitals, and perineum)* for a few seconds when the lungs
   are full, closing the body's subtle circuitry, and allowing energy to
   build up.
4. *Closing alternate nostrils* to balance the breath on the left and right
   sides of the body.

3-Part Breathing Practice

1. Stand, sit, or lie in a comfortable position. Take several deep breaths and relax.

2. Inhale through your nose and fill up your belly with breath. Fully sense what it is to breathe into your belly. Exhale and relax.

3. Inhale to your mid-chest region by allowing your rib cage to open outward to the sides. Fully sense what it is to breathe into your mid-chest. Exhale and relax.

4. Inhale into your upper chest, up to the collarbones causing the area around the heart to expand and rise. Relax and exhale.

5. Now combine them all:

   a. Inhale into your belly.

   b. Then expand breath into your mid-chest region allowing the ribcage to open outward to the sides.

   c. Then draw in just a little more air into your upper chest and let it fill all the way up to the collarbones.

   d. Now exhale your breath first from your upper chest, allowing the heart center to sink back down.

   e. Continue exhaling from the rib cage, letting the ribs slide closer together.

   f. Finally, exhale breath from your belly, drawing the navel back toward the spine.

   g. Repeat three or more breaths, following this 3-part practice.

Other keys to subtle breath practice are to bring attention to each breath, to relax and breathe naturally without straining, consciously allowing the body to fill completely on each inhalation, and to empty completely with each exhalation. The throat can be closed briefly between breaths, both with lungs full and empty. Do only what you can naturally do without forcing yourself or straining.

The Body Module's "Inner Game"

Body practices involve more than exercising and caring for the exterior organism as a 3rd-person "it"—one that will thrive with the right combination of nutrition, exercise, and rest. They also involve a deepening *integration* of 1st-person "I" awareness with and as the whole feeling body—gross, subtle, and causal.

Beyond exclusive focus on the body and exclusive focus on the mind is **Integral consciousness,** which unites them both in a body-mind synergy. Most practitioners, at some point in the journey, must work to consciously cross this key developmental threshold.

Integral consciousness is centered, balanced, and naturally aware *of and as* the whole conscious, feeling body. This stage allows us to see and take responsibility for the many ways we cut off the total body-mind from aspects and parts of itself, including patterns of emotional trauma, tension, armoring, numbing, and frozenness. This also includes the somatic dimensions of psychotherapeutic and shadow work. Through all these practices, the whole body-mind, layer by layer, is gradually re-integrated and restored to wholeness.

Head, Heart, and Hara

Integral consciousness notices and cares to heal the fragmentation of body, mind, soul, and spirit. Practices associated with this stage pay attention to all the key dimensions and centers of the total conscious body.

A simple and meaningful way to think of this is to use a 3-part model that includes the primary centers of the total body-mind: the *head*, the *heart*, and the *hara*.

The *hara* is the center of our native bodily intelligence, gut feeling, vital presence, and power. It is the source of our raw, primordial vital energy and our contact with our ground, legs, and center. In fact, in some systems this energy center is symbolized by the feet or legs. A healthy, open, conscious, and strong hara center enables us to hold our ground, to move with authority, to radiate vital intelligence and etheric energy, and to develop kinesthetic abilities and intelligence.

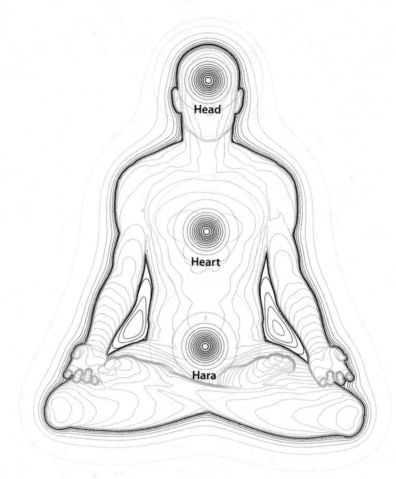

Figure 6.5
*Head, heart,
and hara.*

The *heart* is the center of our feeling intelligence, our intuition of Spirit, and our capacity to love and care for ourselves and others. A conscious, healthy, strong, and open heart enables us to breathe freely, feelingly, and fully—and to commune with our source and purpose and with others. It is the center of pleasure and appreciation, of care and service. Through the heart we radiate subtler energies to others and are inspired to service and self-transcendence.

The *head* is the center of our highest discerning intelligence and intuitions of the good, the true, and the beautiful. Through the head center, the light of consciousness shines out into space and down into the whole body, enabling us to penetrate illusions and free ourselves from limited or stuck perspectives. The head is the center of our highest mental and supramental energies and the source of the liberating power of conscious awareness.

Each of these centers is essential to health and wholeness. One of the key understandings that the human potential movement brought into popular awareness was the importance of cultivating a conscious and open head, heart, and hara. A common misunderstanding of this insight has been to emphasize the heart and hara and dismiss the head, which is no less essential to whole body health.

Various aspects of Integral Life Practice help to open and strengthen each of these centers of conscious bodily existence. When they're all lit up, integrated, and flexibly interconnected, we are whole, and we can function at our best.

Subtle Body Practice for Managing Your Inner States

Subtle body practices provide important tools for managing states of mind and emotions. They enable you to bypass your subjectivity and directly address the energetic signature of your states.

Subjective anxiety (Upper-Left quadrant) may interfere with your ability to function. However, if you can change the anxiety's energetic pattern to one of calm, then your state will also change, opening up different choices and making it more likely that you can act authentically and consciously.

For example, married people know that when they're at their worst they treat their spouse very differently from when they're at their best. Your husband can show up in exactly the same way on two days, and you'll behave totally differently.

Let's say he comes home full of complaints and anxiety, venting, and hardly asking about or noticing you. On a day when you've exercised and gotten enough sleep and had success at work, you'll more likely feel compassionate and affectionate. You'll help him calm down and get perspective.

On a day when you haven't gotten enough sleep or exercise, you've just been dumped on at work and gotten stuck in traffic, you'll be more likely to react or attack and far less skillful in offering support.

What if, on a nightmarish day, you could change your state so that it was more like your state on a good day? How would that affect your marriage? Your decisions? Your whole life?

Subtle body practices, if you persist in them to the point of mastery, teach exactly these skills.

No matter what *stage* you're at, you're always experiencing fluctuating *states* of emotion and mind. Your current state—both your subjective state and your bodily-energetic state—will help determine whether you function at your best or worst, your highest possible stage or a lower one. When life throws you challenges, your state can be as much of a determinant of how well you respond as your developmental stage.

Learning to manage your inner states through practices such as conscious breathing and conducting intensity will equip you to respond to those challenges from the most Integral consciousness available to you.

Breathe and Feel. Always.

Breathing is perhaps the most essential of all Integral Life Practices. Each breath is an opportunity to enjoy being alive. Breathing is a natural feeling link between awareness and the body. Through breath, we naturally enact the integration of body and mind, head and hara, via heart-feeling.

When we breathe, consciously or not, we open and *receive* sustenance, and also let go and *release* what's no longer needed. We are constantly re-enacting the foundational cycle of life—*reception and release*. We are always breathing, either consciously or unconsciously. We can participate in each cycle of reception and release—or not.

Holistic physicians often say that conscious breathing is the number one health practice. Spiritual teachers often call it the number one spiritual practice. No matter whether you focus on the exteriors or the interiors, you can't get away from it—the way you breathe has big effects upon your health, consciousness, and well-being.

Breath and feeling are inextricably linked. The heart center is nested right in the center of your lungs, and one of the most natural ways to activate the heart's feeling intelligence is by breathing consciously.

If you bring that heart-feeling through the breath into the whole body,

Stop and Take a Breath!

Consider:

- Anytime you want to bring more feeling or awareness into the present moment, the most effective thing you can do is to take a deep, feeling breath.
- Anytime you become frightened or angry, contracted, armored, or frozen, the first and most effective thing you can do is to take a deep, feeling breath.
- Anytime you become ungrounded or become dissociatively stuck in the head, the first and most effective thing you can do is to take a deep, feeling breath.

you energize every level of being, from toe to crown. This includes the full spectrum of subtle energies, from etheric to astral, to psychic and supramental.

Big Heart = Big Mind = Integral Feeling-Awareness

The breath is closely linked to both *feeling* and *awareness*, which are more closely related than you may realize. Zen students learn that a single Japanese word, *shin* (or *shen* in Chinese), is sometimes translated as "heart" and sometimes as "mind." Its real meaning is something like *heart-mind*.

This mirrors a profound truth. Free consciousness is not dissociated from heart or mind. It both thinks *and* feels. It is not lacking in feeling nor is it lacking in discriminative intellect. Feeling *is* awareness. Awareness *is* feeling.

Thus, the Buddhist practice of mindfulness might more accurately be called "feeling-awareness." Witness consciousness can perhaps more accurately be called "feeling witness consciousness." Unobstructed feeling (instead of being contrasted to thinking, as is common) is a natural dimension of discriminating intelligence. Clear thinking is a matter of profound feeling.

Feeling is inseparable from intelligence. The open, unobstructed mind is not separate from the open, unobstructed heart. It's neither useful nor intelligent to avoid or resist thinking. A more appropriate practice is to think intelligently, as the whole conscious body-mind, to liberate thought into its freest and fullest expressions.

What *is* useful and intelligent is to cultivate feeling intelligence, to practice it, and develop it. We do that through a whole life of ILP, and also in every moment.

And one of the best ways to initiate this central practice is—you guessed it—to take a full, feeling, intelligent breath, right now.

Resting in the Causal Body

As we become more at home in our gross and subtle bodies, and as we integrate the corresponding internal states, something special begins to happen—we begin to rest more deeply in the causal body, and we naturally become more grounded in ever-present awareness. This is a profound shift, but also an extremely subtle one (remember, another name for the "causal" is the "very subtle"). In fact, you may not even recognize it at first. While gross and subtle experiences can often be multifaceted and dynamic, a causal experience is not really an "experience" at all, but rather a state of *nothing happening*. This "no-thing-ness" is the nature of the causal body, and it's the stillness, silence, and emptiness of both meditative consciousness and deep, dreamless sleep.

We cover meditation practices in depth in the Spirit module (next chapter), so in this section we'd like to focus on the other way to exercise your causal body, namely, good old-fashioned sleep.

Sleeping to Awaken

Though perhaps not as obvious a practice as physical exercise or nutrition, sleep ranks among the most important practices to heighten the health and vitality of your three bodies.

Life's turbocharged intensity begs to be balanced with periods of rest and recovery. And if that balance isn't there, life will give you feedback.

An inadequate amount of sleep impairs your ability to think, to handle stress and anxiety, to meditate, to relate to others, to maintain a healthy immune system, to function kinesthetically, and to moderate your emotional states. There's more, of course, but we'll spare you the gory details because the point is pretty clear: not enough rest equals bad news.

The amount of sleep you need depends on many factors, from age to diet to meditation practice. Nevertheless, sleep experts generally recommend seven to nine hours per day for an average adult (although some people may require more or less). Some individuals are able to function at extremely high levels with just a few hours of sleep each night. Others need much more. You'll know if you're getting enough sleep by the obvious: Do you feel refreshed in the morning? Do you fall asleep when you're trying to meditate? Does drowsiness interfere with your mood or daily activities?

Despite the unambiguous findings of sleep researchers, regular, healthy, and restful sleep proves to be among the most difficult practices to achieve and maintain for many people. Approximately three-quarters of American adults experience a sleep problem a few nights a week or more, almost 40 percent get less than seven hours of sleep each weeknight, and more than *one in three* American adults are so sleepy during the day that it interferes with their lives and activities.

How can you improve your sleeping habits? Here are eight practices for better sleep:

1. Maintain a regular bedtime and wake-up time, including on weekends.
2. Establish a regular, relaxing bedtime routine.
3. Create a sleep-conducive environment that is dark, quiet, comfortable, and cool (that is, not overly warm).
4. Sleep using a comfortable and supportive mattress and pillow.
5. Use your bedroom only for sleep and lovemaking.
6. Finish eating at least two to three hours before your regular bedtime.
7. Exercise regularly, but complete your workout at least a few hours before bedtime.
8. Avoid consuming caffeine, nicotine, and alcohol close to bedtime.

But there's more to sleep than just getting enough of it. The passage through dream and deep sleep states is also a daily journey through the gross, subtle, and causal realms. It is an opportunity to bring feeling awareness to these transitions, not just for the sake of a healthy body, but also for the sake of a consciousness that fully inhabits all its worlds.

One of the experiences that some long-time (twenty-plus years) meditators report is an ability to *maintain witnessing awareness* through the dream and deep sleep states. To many people, this would seem impossible. But you may be familiar with the experience of lucid dreaming, where you are "awake" in a dream (or explicitly aware that you are dreaming) and even able to manipulate the dream. What if you could extend that same wakefulness beyond the dreaming state? What if you could cultivate wakeful consciousness even through deep dreamless sleep? How might reality be revealed to you then?

This is sometimes regarded as the quintessential definition of the highest spiritual state. Consciousness stabilizes; phasing ceases. Radical awareness persists through waking, dreaming, and deep sleep. The wakefulness of pure unchanging consciousness (embodied on the level of the causal body) becomes self-aware and stable. It persists through all three states and domains of experience—gross, subtle, and causal.

Ultimately, consciousness even finally notices its inseparability from everything that arises within it—it wakes up to the fact of its non-separation from the whole changing dance of experience. Ultimately there is nothing dividing consciousness from anything within or beyond the play of experience.

The highest stages of spiritual realization begin when the causal body ceases to be overshadowed by the gross and subtle bodies. It becomes self-aware. In the higher nondual realizations (sometimes called *turiya* and *turiyatita*) the causal body perspective grows so strong it cannot be shaken by experience and indeed comes to pervade all experience.

Thus, some of the highest stages on the spiritual path can be thought of as a third kind of bodily exercise. It is exercise of the causal body, the body of pure, unmoving consciousness—the Witness. This body is exercised by simply Being Itself—ultimately outshining anything and everything that arises.

Constant Consciousness

> That which is not present in deep dreamless sleep is not real.
>
> —*Ramana Maharshi*

The above quote is a shocking statement, because basically there is literally nothing in the deep dreamless state. That was Ramana's point. Ultimate reality or Spirit, Ramana said, cannot be something that pops into consciousness and then pops out. It must be something that is constant, permanent, or, more technically, something that, being timeless, is fully present at every point in time. Therefore, ultimate reality must also be fully present in deep dreamless sleep, and anything that is not present in deep dreamless sleep is not ultimate reality.

This radical statement has profoundly disturbing implications. Those of us who have had Zen satori-like experiences (powerful states in which we've felt our oneness with all existence) in the waking state appreciate how profound it would be for them to persist through dreams and deep, dreamless sleep. Most of what we care for exists in the waking state, which is impermanent. We pass in and out of the waking state every day. And yet, according to some great sages, there is something in us that is always conscious—that is, literally conscious or aware at all times and through all states, waking, dreaming, sleeping. And that ever-present awareness is Spirit in us. That underlying current of constant consciousness (or nondual awareness) is a direct and unbroken ray of pure Spirit itself. It is our connection with God and Goddess, our pipeline straight to Source.

Thus, the highest state of identity with Spirit involves surrender into this current of constant consciousness, following it through all state changes of waking, dreaming, sleeping. This will: (1) strip us of an exclusive identification with any of those states (such as the body, the mind, the ego, or the soul) and (2) allow us to recognize and identify with that which is constant—or timeless—through all of those states, namely, consciousness as such, by any other name, timeless Spirit.

Then, wakefulness persists in the midst of all experience, all day, and all night, even as the body and mind go through waking, dreaming, and sleeping. That wakefulness is unmoved in the midst of changes; there is no subject to be moved; there is only unwavering empty consciousness, the luminous mirror-mind, the Witness that is one with everything witnessed. Consciousness just reverts to the I AM of every moment and stays as that, more or less, stably. And Being itself, simple, conscious, is-ness, also intensifies. The silence becomes louder and louder until it is deafening. And when it crashes down so loudly that all existence is overwhelmed, it dissolves into the ordinary, rendering it with perfect clarity and unobstructed fidelity.

Causal body exercise builds causal muscles. The causal body becomes more and more robust, stable and intensely present. It is the intensity of conscious being.

When this constant nondual consciousness becomes obvious in your case, a new destiny will awaken in the midst of the manifest world. You will have discovered your own Buddha-mind, your own Godhead, your own formless, spaceless, timeless, infinite emptiness, your own Atman that is Brahman, your Keter, Christ consciousness, radiant shekinah— in so many words, One Taste, the single quality of all experiences, great and small, and also That which is beyond experience. It is unmistakably so. And just that is your true identity—pure emptiness or pure unqualifiable consciousness as such—and thus you are released from the terror and the torment that necessarily arise when you identify with a little subject in a world of little objects.

Once you find your formless identity as Buddha-mind, as Atman, as pure Spirit or Godhead, you will take that constant, nondual, ever present consciousness and re-enter the lesser states, subtle mind and gross body, and re-animate them with radiance. You will not remain merely formless and empty. You will empty yourself of emptiness: you will pour yourself out into the mind and world and create them in the process, and enter them all equally, but especially and particularly that specific mind and body that is called by your name. And then this lesser self will become the vehicle of the Spirit that you are.

And then all things, including your own little mind and body and feelings and thoughts, will arise in the vast emptiness that you are, and they will self-liberate into their own true nature just as they arise, precisely because you no longer identify with any of them, but rather let them play, let them all arise, in the emptiness and openness that you now are. You then will awaken as radical freedom, sing those songs of radiant release, beam an infinity too obvious to see, and drink an ocean of delight. You will look at the moon as part of your body and bow to the sun as part of your heart, and all of it is just so. For eternally and always, eternally and always, there is only this.

1

The Spirit Module

Spiritual Practice for an Integral Age

One of the main reasons many people engage an ILP is for *higher aware-ness*. While ILP encompasses numerous forms of practice and can serve a variety of goals and motivations, it is quintessentially about *waking up*. And for most of human history, waking up has been about realizing Spirit in the midst of ordinary life.

What do we mean by "Spirit"? What is "spirituality" and "spiritual practice"? These words all refer to "the matter of ultimate concern," the epitome of all that is meaningful, the essence of goodness, truth, and beauty. It is said that Spirit is love itself, without limitation. And it is said that Spirit is beyond description.

And yet, in our relationship with what is most essential, we find some of the most confusing and divisive issues. Certainly, if we look at the world's religions, we find a treasure of spiritual teachings and examples. However, we also find a history of cruelties, wars, and many other things that do not seem very spiritual at all. Further, some people do not iden-tify with the forms of practice, or worship, that the various traditions have handed down to us. For this reason, many people identify themselves as spiritual but not religious. They want to keep the baby of Spirit and toss out the bathwater of organized religion.

This still leaves open the question of what Integral spiritual practice looks like in the 21st century. Certainly, it is the heart of all religions, but it cannot be limited to the dogmas of any particular religion. It cannot leave out reason and science, but it cannot be reduced to them either. It cannot deny the body or cultural context, and yet it transcends (and includes) them. It cannot ignore the power of the unconscious and our shadow aspects, but it must place them in a much larger context.

But neither can spiritual practice jettison the profound contributions of our religious traditions. In fact, an authentic Integral spiritual practice is more than happily compatible with religious devotion. ILP can coexist with any spiritual tradition—Christianity, Judaism, Islam, Buddhism, the many strains of Hinduism, and Shamanism, or even any new religion. In fact, it illuminates the depth and richness of every path and practice—and can thus even revive and refresh our interest in our traditions—both for those who would consider themselves spiritual but not religious *and* for those who would consider themselves very religious.

The Spirit module of ILP focuses on what we might call "essential spirituality," which is to say, the core teachings, injunctions, and practices derived from the ancient wisdom traditions—*plus* the insights offered by modernity, post-modernity, and the AQAL framework.

This does not confine us to any one specific form of practice—it's not that we *must* meditate in a certain way, or pray, or even believe in a God. But the framework confronts us with the fact that we must practice or engage in certain activities to gain access to certain experiences, perceptions, and dimensions of awareness. It informs and empowers us to design our practice in a way that's personalized, relevant, and effective.

The Spirit module also allows us to discern important patterns of spirituality by using some key AQAL distinctions (introduced in chapter 5), such as:

- **States** of spiritual awareness, which come and go, versus **stages** of spiritual attainment, which we can experience in a more permanent fashion
- **Worldviews** and **developmental waves** and how they influence our understanding of the Ultimate
- The spiritual **line** of intelligence and the **levels** within it

- Our **1ˢᵗ-, 2ⁿᵈ-, and 3ʳᵈ-person perspectives** on, of, and as Spirit
- Spiritual practice in all **3 bodies**—gross, subtle, and causal

An Integral Spirit

For this new approach to spirit to be truly *Integral,* it cannot appear out of nowhere. Rather, it must draw upon the great spiritual traditions—from Christianity to Buddhism, Islam to Taoism, Judaism to Shamanism—*in their highest, most conscious, most ethical forms.* Consider them in detail and two things strike you: there are an enormous number of differences between them and a handful of striking *similarities.*

When you find a few essential items that virtually all of the world's religions agree on, you have probably found something incredibly important about the human condition, at least as important as, say, the few things that physicists can manage to agree on.

What are these spiritual similarities? Notice what it would mean if there were a handful of characteristics that regularly recur and connect humanity's attempts to know God (and presumably, God's correlative attempts to reach a slumbering humanity). These similarities would seem to suggest, among other things, that there are spiritual patterns at work in the universe, at least as far as we can tell, and that these spiritual patterns announce themselves with impressive regularity wherever human hearts and minds attempt to attune themselves to the Kosmos in all its radiant dimensions.

And that would *have* to mean that the standard-issue human being is hardwired for spiritual realities. That is, the human organism itself seems to be built for these deep spiritual patterns, although not necessarily for the specific ways that they show up in any particular religion, important as those are. The simple recognition of these deep spiritual patterns would be the glimmering of an Integral spirituality.

That recognition would also suggest that certain practices can help human beings attune themselves to these patterns of the universe. This attunement could occur through any of the great religions, but would be tied exclusively to none of them. A person could be attuned to an Integral spirituality while still being a practicing Christian, a Buddhist meditator, a New Age believer, or a Neopagan shaman. This would be something added to one's religion, not subtracted from it. The only thing it would subtract (and there's no way around this) is the belief that one's own path is the *only* true path to divinity.

Well, then, what are some of these spiritual currents or some of the similarities that recur in virtually all of the great religious traditions? Let's start with a short and simple list; not the last word on the topic, but an initial list of suggestions to get the conversation going. Most of the traditions agree that:

1. Spirit, by whatever name, exists, and it is good, true, beautiful, and loving.
2. Spirit, although existing "out there," is also found "in here," or revealed within to the open heart and mind.
3. Most of us don't realize this Spirit within because we are living in separation, sin, or duality—that is, we are living in an illusory, fallen, or fragmented state.
4. There is a way out of this separated state (of illusion, separation, sin, or disharmony); there is a path to our liberation.
5. If we follow this path to its conclusion, the result is an awakening, a rebirth, salvation, or enlightenment, a direct experience of union with Spirit both within and without (and neither), a supreme liberation.
6. This supreme liberation marks the dissolution or transcendence of illusion, sin, and/or suffering, and manifests in care and courage, service, social action, mercy, and compassion on behalf of the whole sentient Kosmos.

Does this list make sense to you? Because if there are these general spiritual patterns in the Kosmos, at least wherever human beings appear, then this changes everything; you can be a practicing Christian and still agree with this list; you can be a practicing Neopagan and still agree with this list. We can argue the theological details—but the simple existence of those broader currents profoundly changes the nature of the conversation.

"Spirituality"—What Are We Talking About?

If we accept that something like "Spirit" and "spirituality" are real, and can be found across traditions down to the present day, we still must clarify what we really mean when we use those words. Much of the confusion in conversations about spirituality is a result of not defining our terms adequately.

Like the word "love," the words "Spirit" and "spirituality" are used to mean so many things they often seem to mean nothing. But all of these words point directly at important realities. People along the diverse spectrum of perspectives regard spirituality as a central mental and emotional anchor, and it would be a shame to throw it away or dismiss it as cliché. So let's look more closely at some of the ways people commonly use the words "Spirit" and "spirituality."

1. Spirit is often used interchangeably with words like "God," "consciousness," "Suchness," "Is-ness," "the Self," or the "ever-present." Used in this way, Spirit refers to the ultimate identity of all things, the source or Ground of Being.

2. Sometimes it is used to mean **the conscious energy of life,** and in this sense it is interchangeable with words like "life-force," "prana," "qi," "Holy Spirit," "love-light," "God-light," and "divine energy." In this context, Spirit refers to the conscious current of being that moves and manifests all beings, phenomena, forces, and events.

3. Sometimes spirituality is used to refer to **an all-pervading caring presence,** the source of all care, love, and inspiration. More simply, it can be an **attitude** or **set of qualities,** including kindness, generosity, benevolence, equanimity, openness, compassion, and joyfulness.

4. Sometimes spirituality is used to mean a **line of development,** as in "spiritual development," "spiritual growth," or "spiritual maturity."

5. Sometimes spirituality is used to mean a **high state** of awareness that is usually extremely subtle, causal, or nondual.

6. Sometimes spirituality is used to mean **the highest levels of development in any line.** For example, when Michael Jordan played basketball at his most intense and brilliant, he manifested a fierce, masterful, and transcendent way of playing that seemed superhuman. Some people described it as *spiritual*. An artist who has reached the highest levels of aesthetic expression, a pianist who has cultivated extremely high musical intelligence, or a therapist who has developed the interpersonal mastery to say exactly the right thing at the right time, all might be described as spiritually gifted.

Which definitions of spirituality do you most tend to use? Which ones do you most resonate with? According to AQAL, as you might expect, every definition is true but partial, but it's enormously helpful to use all of these distinctions to clarify what we're actually talking about in any situation.

The Many Colors of Spirit

Here is another, particularly crucial, set of distinctions. Every altitude of consciousness will interpret Spirit differently. If we use the five major worldviews—Magic, Mythic, Rational, Pluralistic, and Integral—then we also have five very different "Gods," five levels of Spirit. Surveys consistently report that an overwhelming majority of people say they believe in God. But which color god? Believing in a magic Magenta god is light years away from a pluralistic Green god, which is radically distinct from an Integral Turquoise divinity. Many spiritual/religious conflicts spring from this exact issue. The debating (and sometimes warring) parties talk past each other because they're each referring to different altitudes of Spirit.

Worldview	Description
Teal/Turquoise	INTEGRAL–kosmocentric, can shift between all previous levels and see relative truths there
Green	PLURALISTIC–multi-worldcentric, the stage of divinity within all beings, all paths are equal
Orange	RATIONAL–worldcentric, the level of universal regard, reason, and tolerance
Amber	MYTHIC–ethnocentric, the stage of absolute traditional truths, tribal/ethnic beliefs; myths
Magenta/Red	MAGIC–egocentric, the world of magical powers, sacrifices, and miracles

Figure 7.1
Altitudes of spiritual awareness.

How does it show up in real life? Here is one example among many of how different levels, different interpretations of Spirit, can show up among Christians.

Magenta/Red Magic God: This level sees Jesus as a Magician, turning water in wine, multiplying loaves and fishes, walking on water, and so on. Jesus is experienced as a magical person who can miraculously alter the world. This stage is preconventional and egocentric. This Jesus is of interest because he can answer *my* prayers, meet *my* needs, and offer *me* blessings.

Amber Mythic God: This level sees Jesus as the Messiah, the Eternal Truth-bringer. This stage is *absolutistic* in its beliefs, so I must either believe and obey scripture as it is given or face damnation. This stage is also *ethnocentric*, so I am allied not just to God but also to my fellow religious believers. We are united against the heathens who resist and oppose our true faith. Only those who believe in Jesus Christ as their personal savior will be saved. This is, by far, the most prevalent level of spiritual consciousness, sometimes slightly altered as it begins to evolve toward Orange.

Orange Rational God: This level sees the Jesus of Nazareth, still fully divine but also fully human, in a more rationally believable way, as a teacher of the universal love of a deistic God. In relation to this God, I am free. I am able to exercise reason and personal responsibility. I care for myself and for my tribe and country but I also care for all people. I can find a good, true, and blessed life through Christ Jesus in my way with other Christians, but I allow that others might also find a valid spirituality through different forms of worship.

Green Pluralistic God: This level sees the Christ consciousness that exists within me and within all beings. I endeavor to discover and respect the divinity in myself and in all people. I deconstruct and reinterpret Biblical passages to speak to me in more universal terms and to champion issues such as ecological sustainability, social justice, fair distribution of wealth, nonviolence, and women's rights. I recognize the full validity of a wide diversity of spiritual paths. Christianity is merely one path among many—none better or worse than another.

Teal/Turquoise Integral God (toward Indigo Super-Integral): This level sees that the universal Christ consciousness can be found everywhere, in everyone, and in every perspective. Whereas the Green, Orange, and Amber-Red-Magenta Christians don't get along very well with each other, I find much in common with each and all of them, and I appreciate and resonate with the special strengths of each. For me, God is obvious and universal, present everywhere in every form, even though I see that some forms manifest more of God than others (cells manifest more of Being than molecules, which manifest more of Being than atoms—the greater the depth, the greater the divinity). I commune with God, as God, able to see God in every moment, alone or with others. I find fellowship with people of all faiths, while the special transmission of Jesus and my Christian tradition remain special, sacred, and an endless source of rich happiness. But I'm quite aware that I must do a lot of translating when I talk with Christians of lower altitudes, and because I'm able to do this, I'm usually generously willing.

The multidimensionality of Spirit tends to make conversation about Spirit difficult. After all, as we've just seen:

- There are different definitions of Spirit.
- There are also different interpretations of Spirit.
- These differences are rarely appreciated and even more rarely defined in spiritual debates.

One of the profound contributions of an Integral approach to spirituality is that it clarifies these confusions. Moreover—and most important—these clarifications can catalyze the experience of Spirit itself.

Can You Feel It?

Most of us have been touched by Spirit at some point in our lives. You may have had powerful experiences of . . .

Oneness
Love
Grace
Light and illumination
Ecstasy
Freedom, flow and Synchronicity ("the Zone")

. . . or a unique and individual intuition of something remarkable, and often indescribable. There are infinite varieties of spiritual experience.

From the first moment you recognized Spirit, things have been different. You've been touched by something wonderful. It may be vast, incredibly powerful, infinitely good, conscious, and/or loving. You may call it "God"—or you may not even think of it as "spiritual." It may have shown itself to you, embraced and infused you intimately, or even revealed itself *as* you—at least for a while.

You may or may not put it in these exact terms, but there is something basically spiritual about the very inspiration to practice. Most people have a subconscious or conscious sense of it, a vision of a happier, more loving, enlightened, and divinely human existence—an intuition of higher realities and possibilities fuels an interest in a deeper, richer way of life. And that intuition easily blossoms into an interest in spiritual practice.

There are countless spiritual practices: meditation, prayer, and gratitude; singing and dancing; breathing and worshipping and celebrating; building altars and places of worship; creating sacred art; and offering gifts. Traditionally, meditation or prayer has been *the* central dimension of practices that cultivate higher levels of awareness. It was called the "raja" or "royal" yoga. Even from modern perspectives, it's one of the best-researched and validated aspects of ILP.

It is also one of the ways that we can anchor and orient our whole practice. Having contact with Spirit involves cultivating experiences of Spirit. Most of these spiritual experiences are, in Integral terminology, *high* or *trained states* (or "peak experiences"). They don't last forever, but they bestow glimpses of transcendental perspectives, sometimes even the transcendence of perspective altogether. These glimpses change us. Over time, as we repeatedly enter high states, we become more fully and stably able to remain in higher states throughout the rest of our lives, whether we are waking, dreaming, or sleeping. Repeated "peeks" deepen

Visiting High States for Lasting Benefits

In Japanese Zen, powerful glimpses of freedom are called *kensho*. More lasting awakening is *satori*. In Sanskrit, practice is called *sadhana*.

It can be said that:

kensho begets *sadhana*,
and *sadhana* (over time) begets more *kenshos*,
and many *kenshos* beget *satori*—and freedom.

and stabilize these changes in us. They extend and deepen our aware-ness, enabling us to hold wider and deeper perspectives. Thus, they can accelerate our developmental growth into *higher stages*.

High states can be cultivated, but there's no one-to-one correlation between spiritual practice and spiritual awakenings. No set timetable dictates when high states will stabilize as permanent, higher *stages* of development.

To paraphrase Zen teacher Richard Baker Roshi, "Meditation won't bring about enlightenment. Enlightenment is a happy accident. A regu-lar sitting practice can't guarantee it. However, it will make you more *accident-prone . . .*"

That's why meditation, and other practices that cultivate high states, are a central dimension of the Spirit module of Integral Life Practice.

Practicing the Spirit Module

What practices should you do in the Spirit module? Most practitioners commit to a regular *meditation* practice. Others meditate only briefly and put more emphasize on other practices such as ritual worship, singing, or consenting to the presence of God. ILP makes room for all of this. You are free to select the practices that serve you best, or you can find a teacher or coach who can help you to make wise choices.

What is most important is regular (ideally, daily) practice—and en-gaging practices that are *authentic* and *appropriate*—well suited to you at this time. They do not have to be arduous or time-consuming. If you make regular, authentic contact with Spirit, your life and practice will be entirely different than if you do not.

Our religious and spiritual traditions offer a wealth of spiritual prac-tices, and in most cases, they are arranged progressively, with more ad-vanced practices coming only after a foundation has been built. So choose practices that are not too advanced but which engage you fully. They should be helping you deepen, open, and grow.

Your practices should *challenge* you and they should also *nurture* you. Challenges come from interrupting your habitual, unconscious patterns, and from requiring you to exercise and build various inner muscles of the heart and mind. Nurture comes from experiencing the attractive, healthy, essentially happy and life-giving qualities of Spirit, including receiving spiritual blessings, forgiveness, love, light, or bliss. In a balanced practice, both challenge and nurture are active and felt.

Spirit How?

As we've seen, there are many excellent forms of spiritual practice. However, we can distinguish **three general classes of practice:** *meditation*, *contemplation*, and *prayer* or *communion.* Let's begin with meditation. A recent survey of over two thousand scientific studies documents an enormous range of benefits from meditation.[†] These include physiological changes of state (such as in metabolism, respiration, and alleviation of pain); positive psychological and behavioral effects (including shifts in perception, concentration, brain physiology, and attention); and enhanced subjective experiences (including equanimity, extrasensory experiences, and illuminating dreams). Remarkably, meditators even have a significantly more youthful physiology than non-meditators, as measured by the classic biomarkers of aging. Most important, meditation is *the only factor* demonstrated to significantly accelerate growth through stages of development! The science is unambiguous: *meditation works.*

---

*There is an interesting history to these words and some important differences between them. For instance, in the medieval Christian tradition, what we now would call *meditation* (in the sense of a silent sitting practice of pure awareness) was referred to as *contemplatio*, while reflecting upon a specific theme in thought was referred to as *meditatio*. In our current usage, meditation involves silent sitting in pure 1st-person awareness; *contemplation* involves reflecting upon an object in the 3rd person; and *prayer* and *communion* refer to aspects of a 2nd-person *relationship* to the divine.

†Michael Murphy and Steven Donovan, *The Physical and Psychological Effects of Meditation: A Review of Contemporary Research with a Comprehensive Bibliography* (The Institute of Noetic Sciences, 2004), www.noetic.org/research/medbiblio/index.htm.

What Is Meditation?

Meditation usually involves returning attention, again and again to a primary object, whether it is your breath, a mantra, a deity, a loving feeling, or a mental image.

Meditation is a natural function of the human body-mind. When you meditate properly, this function kicks in and rapidly (within the first three minutes) produces a distinct psycho-physiological state, one that combines *low* levels of physical arousal with *high* levels of mental alertness.

It is usually practiced while sitting or kneeling on a cushion, chair, or bench in a relaxed posture with an erect spine. Meditation sessions can range from a few minutes to several hours (twenty minutes once or twice a day is common).

Meditative traditions often distinguish between *concentration* practice, (which builds the necessary "attention muscles" required to sustain focused attention) and *awareness* practice (which develops the inner spaciousness necessary to *release* attention into expanded subtle and/or formless causal states). Both of these practices free attention from its usual fixation on the discursive mind.

Integral Meditation is a general term for using the AQAL Framework as your launch pad for meditation. Although meditation ultimately goes beyond all mental forms, the traditions agree that "right view," or an adequate framework of understanding, is of crucial importance for interpreting and understanding meditation correctly. The more Integral your view, the more your experience of high states will speed your growth into high stages—and the more comprehensive and full will be your understanding.

Spirit Now

There is never anything between you and the boundlessness of Spirit, the ever-present Suchness of existence. In this very moment, Spirit is present and complete, no further away than your own awareness. You don't need to do anything for this to be real and true. You can just relax and rest in your own present awareness. *You can just wake up.* And if you do, you'll discover you were already resting in boundless awareness! This is what the "sudden school" of Zen Buddhism has recommended for centuries: "Just wake up, right now!"

Resting in the boundlessness of present awareness right now is the epitome of spiritual practice. You can do this spontaneously, right now, for however long it lasts—even though that's usually just for a brief moment. This is one of the highest and most noble spiritual practices known to humankind: notice and allow what already is. Let everything be as it is. Relax back into present awareness in which you were all along, in fact, already resting! Do this many times throughout the day, every day, until it begins to occur naturally and lasts longer and longer.

This simple instruction is true and complete. However, in practice, it is hard for most practitioners to progress with only the "perfect practices" of the sudden school. After sudden clarity, confusion returns. Awareness drifts. Clarity is now only an idea. Without the "gradual school" the sudden school can easily degenerate into the "talking school," in which awakening becomes something abstract and conceptual. Historically, it has usually been necessary for practitioners to have something more to do—to have a spiritual practice. And usually, the form it takes is influenced by this most direct method. It involves deliberately resting in present awareness *for particular periods of time during the day.* Another name for this is *meditation.*

The 3 Faces of Spirit

Integral Spirituality Engages All Three Faces of Spirit

- In 3rd person, Spirit is known as *It*. You *contemplate* and perhaps *serve* Spirit, the ultimate mystery of existence, and the total Kosmos, including the very Ground of Being, often through nature, mysticism, philosophy, and *action*.
- In 2nd person, Spirit is known as *You* or *Thou*. You open to and *commune* with Spirit or the ultimate mystery of existence, often through *prayer*.
- In 1st person, Spirit is known as *I*. You *awaken* consciously *as* inseparable from Spirit, the ultimate mystery of existence, often through *meditation*.

That which is Ultimate is ultimately beyond all perspectives. But it can only be pointed to *via* perspectives. Each of these perspectives offers something unique to our awareness and growth.

In 3rd-person contemplation, you see It. You open your eyes, mind, and senses to the ultimate mystery of existence, and thus notice details and distinctions (for example, the patterns, energies, colors, textures, and contours of natural places, creatures, and other living things, or even the perspectives pointed out in philosophy, including this discussion about the 3 Faces of Spirit). In contemplation you become aware of the fullness of Spirit and the Kosmos in more of its rich and miraculous multidimensionality—gross, subtle, and causal. Moved by this vision people often actively *serve* others and Spirit.

Familiar examples: art, nature mysticism, philosophical and mystical contemplation, service. The path of good works.

In 2nd-person prayer and communion, you open into intimate contact with the ultimate mystery of existence, letting *It* become *Thou*. You metaphorically face God, your ultimate Beloved, and become knowable to (not hiding from) that ultimate consciousness. In the process your

Yoga and Spiritual Life

As we deepen in contemplation, communion, and awakening, we co-incide more and more fully with Spirit. Our bodies and minds can only do this by offering less and less obstruction to the free flow of that infinite energy and consciousness. That's why mystical practice has always been associated with yoga.

Some of this yogic process was just described in chapter 6, as part of the Body module. But since all the modules interconnect, those 3-body yogas can't be totally separated from the Spirit module. In fact, meditation is the primary practice in some physically and ener-getically focused bodily yogas like kundalini, kriya, and shabd yoga. Keep in mind that all these interior states have exterior bodies. Natu-rally, then, there are practices that serve a unitive transformation by focusing on both inner *and* outer aspects of ourselves. Even those of us who focus on our interiors will progress best if we don't neglect the bodily transformation that makes interior transformation possible.

feeling heart and soul cannot remain untouched or immune. You allow yourself to receive grace, or the blessings of the mystery of existence. You open, deepen, and surrender.

Familiar examples: prayer, heartfelt consent to the presence of God, devotional singing, worship, ritual, and service. The path of bhakti yoga.

In 1st-person meditation, you come to know yourself to be the *I* of Spirit. You let go of all limited identifications with memories, thoughts, sensations, and desires, and awaken consciously *as* the I AMness of the here and now. You awaken into and as the total present moment, *as* the Self, the non-separate identity of the mystery of existence, and even beyond all conceptions, into what is sometimes called the Suchness or the emptiness that is not separable from anything or anyone.

Familiar examples: Big Mind, vipassana, shikantaza, dzogchen, nirvi-kalpa and sahaj samadhis; all approaches to formless meditation.

Many practices **combine** two or more of these perspectives.

Don't Throw Out the Baby . . .

These three faces or three ways of relating to Spirit are inherent to consciousness, even if they're not always recognized. It is possible for them to be expressed in relation to any and every level of divinity — Magical, Mythic, Rational, Pluralistic, and Integral. However, historically, certain faces of Spirit have tended to be emphasized and excluded at each stage of development:

Magic and Mythic Spirit tends to exclude relating to Spirit in the 1st person. (God is transcended, not imminent, and it's sinful to confuse fallen humanity with the divine.) Instead, it emphasizes a 2nd-person relationship (I pray to you, O Lord), but tends to relate to Spirit only as an objectified mythic deity.

Rational Spirit tends to move away from the 2nd-person relationship to the mythic deity. (I no longer believe in the old interventionist deity, so why pray or worry about my relationship to Spirit?) Instead, it emphasizes 3rd-person ways of relating to Spirit and Nature. (Spirit is a transcendental force or law of existence. I can contemplate the universe through science to know Spirit better.)

Pluralistic Spirit opens to discovering a 1st-person relationship to Spirit (I am waking up to see that I am not separate from Spirit!) However, it vigorously rejects rational and mythic versions of divinity. (Church religion is too dogmatic, and rational science is too reductionistic and limiting.) It is, alas, all too willing to accept exotic 2nd- and 3rd-person forms of spirituality without rigorous discernment.

Integral Spirit enters deeply into 1st-person awakening as Spirit (I am Spirit), deepens 3rd-person contemplation and service of Spirit (I see and serve Spirit as *It*), and resurrects 2nd-person communion with Spirit (I turn to face and love and be loved by *You*, Spirit of all).

A Crucial Insight:

Having left the mythic God behind, many Integral practitioners realize they had exclusively emphasized 1st-person awakening and had left behind their whole 2nd-person relationship to Spirit!

But Integral spirituality includes all three. A whole new dimension of fullness becomes possible when you restore the juicy, vital 2nd-person dimension of spiritual life.

Exploring the 3 Faces of Spirit:
The Essence of Contemplation, Communion, and Meditation

Let's dive into an actual experience of the three dimensions of the divine. The following exploration, covering Kosmic Contemplation, Integral Communion, and Awakening *as* Spirit, offers examples of the kinds of experiences that an Integral spiritual practitioner might have. Of course, every particular path will interpret Spirit in its own unique terms—and certainly your individual practice will yield its own distinct insights and understandings (for example, as a Christian, you may experience 2nd-person communion specifically in relation to Jesus, or as a Buddhist, you may interpret 1st-person awakening as a realization of Buddha-mind)—but an Integral practice will attempt to deepen one's relation to at least these three universal aspects of Spirit, by whatever names.

3rd-Person Contemplation of Spirit: Kosmic Contemplation

In Kosmic Contemplation, we notice and feel the entirety of this utterly vast and mysterious Kosmos: interior and exterior, gross, subtle, and causal. This includes the whole sweep of contemplative practices from nature mysticism to mystical philosophy (including much Integral philosophy). The paragraphs that follow embody this process of Kosmic Contemplation, describing in turn the gross, subtle, and causal bodies of Spirit.

Our whole existence—beautiful and terrible, full of logic and meaning, and utterly beyond knowing—is what human beings point to when they use words like divinity and God. Spirit, thus understood, is both transcendent and immanent—utterly beyond any experience, and simultaneously implicit and present in every shred of experience, in every particle of this amazing physical cosmos—gross, subtle, and causal.

Spirit can be found in the physical world—in the sky, the sun, the moon, the stars, the clouds. Spirit can be seen and felt in the grass, the trees, the earth, and the wind. Spirit is audible in bird and animal songs and is visible in the eyes and bodies of all our fellow creatures—as well as in all our fellow human beings and in all we do: our creativity and beautiful artistic expression, our science and industry, our stupidity and brutality, our trivial entertainment, and our most profound creations and utterances.

Contemplate the dance of this physical world across time. Across the vast epochs of evolutionary time, every living creature emerged naturally from and as the body of Spirit. The Big Bang flung forth our whole universe, spewing all space-time into being, including all the matter and energy of our cosmos, including what eventually became our sun and Earth and moon. Across billions of years of evolutionary time, our mother matter congealed as a planet with a hospitable atmosphere, a beautiful blue nest that gave birth, after a few billion years of unimaginable fire, remarkably, to liquid oceans and then to living cells. And across more billions of years of evolution, those cells evolved into more complex cells, and then tiny animals, and gradually, over hundreds of millions of years, into a vast, intricate, beautiful community of plants and animals, and then, over more millions of years into all the plants and animals we see today, including us, homo sapiens, all interacting in an immense, remarkable, unified community. This web of life reflects and displays the qualities of Spirit, the very qualities that gave birth to all of it. We can see Spirit all around us in the form of our whole natural world and everything we see.

The Subtle Energy Bodies of Spirit

Divinity is visible not just in the physicality of our world, but in the energy body of Spirit. Dynamic life-energy permeates all living things. You can see energy in every living being, rippling and flowing through their chakras and meridians and shining from their eyes. Seen in this way, even the most mundane moments of our daily life become a multidimensional dance of feeling-light. The animating energetics that bring nature to life are vast, intricate, and mysterious.

This divine light refracts itself into every form of subtle energy. This ranges across a great spectrum of subtlety. Perhaps the densest band is the etheric energy we can feel moving and buzzing in our bodies, flowing through our chakras and meridians, and radiating out into space from our skin, shining out in all directions like a great halo. Subtler than that is the realm of feelings, including all our range of good and bad feelings and emotions. Still subtler are the realms of mind, including every kind of ordinary thought and up into the sweetness of higher intuitive apprehensions. Subtlest of all are the finest transcendental intuitions of light, nectar, and bliss, more sublime even than the most elevated thoughts. And our subtle energies radiate up, out, and beyond the body, shining especially above the head, as pure radiance.

Divinity expresses itself as light. We can consciously participate in it. We can open ourselves and feel and breathe and conduct the force of life, also called the light, the subtle energy, or the Holy Spirit. We can breathe the Holy Spirit in, down the front of the body, and we can feel this divinity descending down as fullness of life, as vitality and presence. Then we can feel it turn at the base of the body and ascend up through the spine as we exhale, rising up to and into and even above the head where we can feel lit as radiant light and blissful freedom.

The Perfectly Still and Silent Causal Body of Spirit

But there is another vast dimension to Spirit's body, not the gross physical body and not even the subtle energy body of Spirit. The causal body of Spirit is that which is unmoving, unbroken, and eternal. All the conditions of our human lives come and go, just as we are born and die, but

Spirit survives, unimpaired, undiminished, unblinking, undistracted, undying, uncompromising, and absolute. Spirit is the One Who is unborn, undying, Who does not age or change. Spirit is the Ultimate Reality, the ultimate subject behind every conditional experience, the Self behind every conditional self, the I AM behind every I, the very Self of every being and all existence.

That One is beyond description—unmoving, silent, and perfectly present. This One is the very Space in which everything in the whole Kosmos arises and falls. Before the still and silent Heart gives birth to light and mind and feeling and embodiment, It simply *is*, perfect and sufficient. In that Presence, all that arises and falls is reflected for what it is, passing and secondary. This radical divinity is witnessing and, in essence, *living* you, all beings, and all events, alive in every desire and action, but especially and essentially as perfect Stillness. The empty spaciousness of Spirit is the clearing in which every perspective arises . . . and falls.

A 2ⁿᵈ-Person Encounter with Spirit: Integral Communion

It is a profound and paradoxical matter to turn and face the Unfathomable Mystery of Existence. How is it possible? How can you face the Ultimate, Unlimited, Almighty, and Omnipresent?

To practice Integral Communion is to open your whole body—gross, subtle, and causal—into communion with the Universal Mystery of Existence as one's most intimate Beloved. It involves unkinking the physical body, freeing the feeling breath, opening the emotions and turning them toward the Beloved.

Even if you've never considered it before, your relationship with Spirit must be one of love. After all, Spirit or God *is* love. What is it to open to a personal meeting with love itself, the very Heart that expresses itself in your heart and every heart?

In Integral Communion, we open and turn to face this Spirit who is love, the animating life of everything everywhere. We turn to face the being that has powered our every step, our every thought.

Spirit is incomprehensible—more uncompromising, more fierce, more enormous than mere words can say. Let yourself become humble and sober as you behold more weight, more power, more seriousness, more gravitas than any human mind and heart and body can open to meet.

Can you bring yourself to face and open yourself to intimacy with the most unimaginably huge, perfectly still presence? What would it require, what would it feel like to stop averting your gaze from that One?

In Integral Communion, you open your breath and feeling to commune with the very power that drives the universe. It's impossible; but the practice is to do your best, to open as fully as possible and to feel whatever limits you can't open beyond. The practice is to turn toward Spirit, to open emotionally to Spirit, to relax the automatic defenses of the mind and psyche.

Do your best to feel without limitations. Do your best to let feeling extend to Infinity. Do your best to inhale and exhale the holy breath. Do your best to face the boundless and universal presence of Spirit, to open to the perfectly still and silent absolute.

Such communion ennobles, enlivens, and empowers you even while it demands profound humility. It involves the senses, the emotions, the energy centers, the mind, and the higher mental functions. In such communion the energetic channels of the whole body open and flow with the Holy Spirit.

Let your emotions open intimately in communion with the same One who shines forth from the radiant eyes of every Beloved, whether your lover, your child, your parent, your pet, or yourself looking back at you in the mirror. That shining, Beloved God-Light—can you face Her, can you face Him, can you feel the One who has given birth to you? The One to whom you will return in your dying?

What does it take to open yourself to face your most Intimate Friend, Mother, Father, and dear Beloved, the only One who knows you by heart, the only One who has been there with you always? Here is the One with whom you have been in relationship every moment of your life, even when you have been oblivious. Every day of your life, you have only been swimming in the ocean of Spirit's Body, Love's Body, the Body of Light. So soften your heart, and open your breath and turn to face your wisest, most patient, most intimate, yet vastest, Friend. Before you is the

One who gave birth to you, the One who is living you, who has been Being you from the beginning.

Face the One Who is the Self of your very Self, the I behind your own "I." Face the eyes that gaze back at you from a place beyond the death of all your hopes, dreams, ideals, loved ones, and identities. Dare to gaze without blinking into eyes fooled by nothing, undistractable, unsentimental, gazing right at you, into you, and through you. Can you be present with the Presence who never flinches, Who has always been perfectly silent, still, conscious, and undeceived?

The overwhelming enormity and eternity of Spirit's perspective cannot be comprehended. The Perfect Infinite Beloved can only be glimpsed amidst your wholesale awe, humility, and surrender. Let yourself feel the weight, the potency, the purity, the consciousness of the divine. Let your heart be outshined, baked, transformed by a real encounter with the absolute.

Allow the grace.

Allow the humility.

Allow the awe.

Allow the surrender.

Let your defenses soften and your whole being open into sacred communion with the divine totality, with your deepest intimate, your Beloved, right here and right now.

1st-Person Awakening As Spirit

We can awaken directly as Spirit through various practices of formless meditation—or the experience of 2nd-person communion can deepen so much that all boundaries between you and God dissolve. You may even dissolve into oneness through ecstatic contemplation of the totality of being. In any case, you may begin to notice something mysterious: There is no separation, no difference, no radical distinction at the level of identity between you and that Heart and that Light Who dances into every kind of manifestation. The little "I" dissolves into the limitless I AM.

However you get there, the discovery is the same: You are all of it. This vast, incredibly complex, swirling and vast energetic dynamic, infinitely bigger than your body and mind, is nowhere more fully and actually itself than when it is showing up as you, as your very body-mind. This is first-person awakening *as* Spirit.

You Are the Light itself, alive, awake, and flowing. You are the life-force itself, alive everywhere, springing forth from the prior Ground of Being in every moment, dancing life into life in every moment, and surrendering itself back into the Unmanifest in every moment—but in all its dynamism, nowhere more at its center, nowhere more fully the Light, nowhere more fully released into synchronicity as Itself than Where you stand. You are the Light. The Light is being Light most quintessentially here and now—in the breathing of your body, the shining of your eyes, the radiance of your mind and feeling, the pulsing Life you Are.

Conscious in all her cells, Gaia is conscious nowhere more than here, as you. You are Nature. You are the web of life. In the rhythms and waves of your breaths the ancient pulse of the oceans can be heard and felt. You are not separate, not even separable.

Most deeply, let go into knowing yourself as you are, freshly being born and dying in every moment, birthed again and again as the body of Spirit. Birthed and dying like the grasses and the trees, the ants and the antelope. You are the body of the Mystery. This body in which you hear these words is the body of the Big Bang in one of its billions and billions and quadrillions of expressions. Not separate! The Big Bang is nowhere more itself than here, being you, enacting you, showing up as You.

You are all of it, yes. But, more fundamentally, the you behind the skin-encapsulated ego, the I behind the I, is the Awareness in which it all arises. You are the space in which the body-mind arises, the space in which the Big Bang arises.

Notice this page and the other objects around you. Notice your bodily sensations.

And notice: you are not these sights or sounds or sensations. They are all arising as objects of the Awareness you truly are.

Now notice your feelings . . . ideas . . . memories . . . desires . . . and sense of personal identity . . .

All of these are arising as objects of the awareness you truly are. You are not your feelings. You are not your ideas. You are not your memories. You are not your desires. You are not even your sense of personal identity. All of them are arising as objects in the awareness that is You.

You are the conscious Seer who is seeing all this. You are the conscious Feeler who is feeling all this. You are the conscious Hearer who is hearing all this. The Seer who you are is not separate or different from the One who is the Seer of all experience. Who you are is the Seer, the very Self behind the I in you and the I in me and the I in everyone. You are Empty and Free. And you always have been.

You have never moved. You have always been you. You have always been perfectly silent, utterly open, and infinitely deep. You are the ultimate depth that was before all birth and will be beyond all death.

Your mind and body and all the personality and locality of your individuality are reflected in the Consciousness, the Self Who you truly are. All of that is real and necessary and deserves to be honored. But do not forget that it is superficial to Who You Are most deeply; most profoundly you are not merely or even primarily that. You are the I AM whose center is everywhere and whose circumference is nowhere. Really.

So do not imagine that you are seeking or finding or forgetting the One you truly are, the One you've always been. . . .

Spirituality in Relationship

Spiritual Community

Although most of the practices described in the Spirit module are meditative practices that are performed alone, spiritual community has always been a central aspect of spiritual practice. A community of worship or practice can enrich the life of practice and one's commitment to it. Sustaining a practice, for example, becomes easier when your friends are doing it with you. Let's face it: practicing alone can be difficult. Participating within a spiritual community offers a caring network of accountability and support. The group can help you follow through on your commitments while you assist others to do the same.

Furthermore, by gaining additional perspectives from the group, you can make more intelligent discernments regarding your spiritual development. In many cases, a group can register changes in you more fully than you might notice yourself. Also, experiences that are shared with a group register more powerfully in your psyche than solo experiences, and they are confirmed by others as real. Feedback from a trusted friend often gives you the key insight necessary to recognize an area where you can grow. Sometimes when we do change, it is only when we experience ourselves in a new way *in our group setting* that the change becomes known to us as fully real and believable.

For all these reasons and more, spiritual communities often become powerful influences in the lives of participants. If they are healthy, this can be a natural expression of the great value they confer. But sometimes communities become unhealthy, and negatively influential. They can become cults in which either individual leaders or the group as a whole can abuse spiritual authority. Even under the best of circumstances, be aware that participation in a spiritual community has both costs and benefits. The dynamics of the community's life can both enrich and distract from practice and growth. Community is not inherently necessary to awakening, and yet for millennia many people have found it essential.

A healthy community enriches the life and practice of everyone involved. As much as they may benefit from the attention of a teacher, practitioners often can learn many things best from one another, informally, in the midst of sharing their lives. Some communities are extremely intense and even all-consuming. Others are less engaging, more relaxed and casual. Some are closed, others are open. Sometimes people convene as a community of practice through seminars, workshops, or ongoing groups lasting a weekend, a week, a month, or a year. Other communities last for decades.

Thus, your practice may be enriched and embodied through membership and participation in a congregation, sangha, or other community of practice—at least for periods of time. Participating in a community of practice itself can be a powerful spiritual practice. In groups we can hold and care for others and receive their holding and care. We can see them and be seen. We betray them and are betrayed, and we can repent and accept the repentance of others. We can forgive them and be forgiven.

And we can witness others and be witnessed in our practice, devotion, and awakening.

Community life is not a substitute for individual meditation and direct mystical awakening but rather a support, container, mirror, and training ground for individual spiritual practice. Understood and engaged rightly, spiritual community can be a rich field of practice in the Spirit module of ILP. To the degree that a community actively transcends what contemplative Christianity calls "the false self" (including the self-sense of the group) and to the degree that community members resonate together in ever higher, more inclusive harmonies, spiritual communities uplift their members' consciousness.

Integral Devotion

Integral Life Practice is naturally grounded in the experience of kindness, care, and compassion—and even love and ecstasy. Yogas of subtle body energies and feelings, along with worship and loving prayer, are part of almost every spiritual tradition—and they are a living dimension of a fully Integral spiritual life.

In fact, devotion naturally *integrates* practice by calling forth many of the defining characteristics of the awakened human body-mind such as:

- Feeling: Dissolving boundaries between the mind and the body, consciousness and sensation, via heartfelt feeling
- Breathing: Consciously breathing, as an integrated body-mind, with feeling reception on the in-breath and feeling surrender on the out-breath
- Head, heart, and hara: Continually conducting more and more life energy through head, heart, and hara, cultivating an open, strong, flexible, vital, and full body-mind

Each of these practices can produce results. But they need not be engaged methodically through effort. They are all natural and spontaneous by-products of a human body-mind that is consciously, feelingly living as love.

Opening to Devotion

One cannot just sit down and "do" devotion, mechanically, the way you can do push-ups. Devotion requires sincerity. A threshold must be crossed for devotion to be authentic. You must fall in love with existence itself (which can mean God, Spirit, Suchness, the Mystery of Being, or the Source of Grace). Until that threshold has been crossed, attempts at devotion tend to be slightly forced or self-indulgent.

Traditionally, crossing that threshold requires repentance—the universal precondition for receiving grace. "Repentance" is the English word used to translate the New Testament Greek *metanoia* (literally "a change of heart and mind"), the Hebrew Old Testament word *teshuvah* (literally "turning back," as in a U turn), and the Arabic Koran word *tawbah* (literally "turning toward the divine source"). Hindus too "hear" the word of God, and Buddhists recognize inherent suffering and "take refuge in the Buddha, Dharma, and Sangha." In every religion some kind of self-understanding and new, spiritually inspired commitment is necessary to take up the path.

In a trans-rational context, repentance can be understood as *insight* and *commitment*.

There are two simultaneous insights: (1) understanding selfishness to be a dead-end and (2) noticing and awakening to the transcendental, sacred, beneficent, and graceful nature of existence.

After these insights, the obvious stands forth: every moment of conscious life—especially this one—is a profound and wondrous gift. When that is feelingly understood, the heart opens naturally and authentically. Such gratitude is self-validating and obviously appropriate. It is self-evidently sane, while the *absence of gratitude* is not.

With this clarity comes a commitment to and responsibility for right action. Service occurs naturally with the feeling of spontaneous trans-rational devotion. Communion with the source of grace isn't an obligation, but a natural expression of one's feeling being. It is obviously good, true, and beautiful!

Integral Theism?

We are free to love and worship God in all stages of spiritual development. Our natural devotional impulse need not be suppressed, no matter
where we are in our spiritual growth. Our human neurology is wired to
enact relationship. Humans evolved while living together in hunter-gath-
erer clans and are neurologically structured to relate to others. We can engage our functions most fully when participating in relationships. Thus,
the authentic and powerful processes of theistic spiritual life—which enable us to enact the living drama of a personal relationship with Spirit—
are among the richest natural expressions of a truly Integral spirituality.

As spirituality evolves, it transcends "belief in" an objectified mythic
creator deity. Integral spirituality is sometimes identified as transcending
theism and arriving at panentheism, which is the view that divinity is
both immanent (in the world) and transcendent (beyond the world). Ultimately, Integral spirituality transcends and includes all categories. This
means that as it transcends old ways of relating to God, it re-includes
transformed versions of all ways of relating to God that are even fuller,
richer, more intimate and profound. Thus, among the free expressions of
Integral panentheism is a higher form of theistic mysticism.

Religion is considered theistic when it presumes a relationship with
God (or multiple gods). As we awaken beyond mythic conceptions of
God, "belief in" an objectified God falls away. Often at this point, people
lose touch with the feeling of devotion altogether.

But we don't have to lose a sense of devotion as we grow beyond magical and mythical thinking. A higher level devotional practice is still possible. We can always relate to God as our Ultimate Beloved—and even as
the nonobjectified Mystery beyond all perspectives. As we climb the ladder of development, this can naturally blossom.

Stages of Devotion

Theistic mysticism enacts a relationship with God. Like any relationship,
this ultimate intimacy unfolds through a drama. Mystics have found

countless ways to tell the story of this ultimate relationship, but all of them describe how the passion of the human heart is awakened and unleashed through a life-and-death struggle to unite with the ultimate Beloved.

Many of those stories go something like this:

1. **Ignorance.** The individual begins unconscious, unhappy, in crisis, or ignorant.

2. **Disquiet.** One becomes dissatisfied, aware of suffering, damnation, or alienation.

3. **Insight.** There is *metanoia*, repentance, recognition— awareness of suffering and contraction, and the willingness and will to transcend habits and engage in self-transcending practice. Sometimes insight is enacted as "conversion" to a religion and its founder(s).

4. **Surrender.** The heart opens, accepting a love relationship with Spirit and all things; here begins a life of devotion and service. Grace (the power of divine blessing) is discovered. Sometimes this is called *salvation*. Through surrender and humility it is possible to exercise will, tolerate discomfort, and practice discipleship in a way that transcends the commitment to the separate self.

5. **Transformation.** An ordeal ensues, which usually extends for years, even decades. Although it begins with purification of the ordinary gross life, it then encounters, illuminates, and purifies all the gradations of subtle experience, and even includes silent and empty "dark nights" of causal passage beyond any experience of light or bliss.

6. **Understanding.** There is a crucial transition in which there is awakening from the dream. This is spiritual realization, sometimes called "enlightenment."

7. **Unification.** At this point there begins the higher spiritual life, which includes worship of, embrace of, awakening as, service to, and celebration of and with the divine Beloved, seen in and as all people and things.

In the higher spiritual life, stage 7 can deepen by recapitulating stages 2–6, on larger and smaller scales.

There are many similar descriptions of this dramatic romance. One of the most authoritative is the mystical Christian, Universalist, or Theosophical passage described by Evelyn Underhill. Her model begins with *awakening* to Spirit (similar to stages 1–4 above). It then proceeds through an unpacking of stage 5 above into *purification*, especially of the body and passions and habits. This is followed by the *illumination* of various "stations" or "interior castles" of increasingly elevated subtle experience. Then it describes a causal "dark night" in which all subtle experiences of light or grace disappear. Only after all that does it culminate in nondual "unification" with God.

Another well-known structure for the story of spiritual growth is the "hero's journey," which proceeds through many dramas, including an underworld battle with a nemesis and a return into the light of knowing and claiming one's true inheritance.

These universal dramas all involve passion, longing, struggle, setbacks, and ecstatic union. The path is engaging, dramatic, passionate, personal. It inspires the heart and imagination thus mobilizing the most powerful human motivations. This is the path of the realizers and saints of all the great monotheistic religions. It possesses a special power, depth, and richness. It profoundly engages the nobility, tenderness, passion, and reflexes of our human nature. Even so, it also traverses the universal possibilities of gross, subtle, causal, and nondual states.

Integral spirituality transcends and includes all points of view. The paradoxical understanding at the heart of true nondualism makes room for the full range of all dualistic possibilities. It sees them (including the dramatic mystical romance with the divine Beloved) as radiant expressions of That which is beyond all dramas and changes.

Thus there can be insight, repentance, and practice. We can fall in love and commune, and deepen into mystical union. We can suffer a dark night of disconnection through which we are tested and deepened and prepared for a more profound realization.

We can live out our most moving archetypal stories *without* being bound by unconscious identification with them. The more Integral one's perspective the more access we have to the full richness of mystical life and awakening.

Trans-Rational Devotion

In traditional devotion, the heart opens to God, life is recognized as full of grace, and surrender and gratitude transform the inner life. It's a direct, juicy path, with profound synergies. But however effective and transformative, the ancient paths often tend to bind practitioners to fixed, literal or otherwise limiting beliefs and frames of mind. Is it possible to outgrow that without losing the spirit? Can we have both rigorous discernment and a heartfelt connection to divine grace?

The answer is a resounding *yes*! When devotion evolves beyond mythic belief, it gets *stronger* rather than weaker. Compared with pre-rational devotion, trans-rational devotion expresses a profoundly liberated consciousness—and thus it becomes more effectively *liberating*. There are trans-rational paths of devotion practiced by Christians, Jews, Hindus, Buddhists, Muslims, shamans, and many others. Trans-rational devotion (often in forms that embrace the traditions) is a natural expression of maturity in Integral practice, and it is fully compatible with ILP.

In the Tibetan Buddhist tradition, the most advanced practices (vajrayana) are grounded so firmly in nondual Suchness that they can serve high awakening by making skillful tantric use of all the relative aspects of life (samsara), including emotion, sexuality, imagination, art, and many subtle yogas. The highest expressions of Integral practice are similarly free to embrace all the juiciness of life. And love, or devotion, is the very heart of juiciness.

Devotional objects and rituals—statues, paintings, pictures, altars, incense, candles, bowing, singing, and praying—all can be used intelligently, mindfully, and tastefully, as opposed to being used inattentively, childishly, or fanatically, within an Integral Life Practice. They manifest differently than forms of devotion within a pre-modern metaphysics. Integral devotional practice can be a power tool for rich, communal participation in life.

A defining characteristic of trans-rational, post-metaphysical devotion is the simple relaxation of metaphysical beliefs as a necessary ground for devotion. We don't need to think about or believe in anyone's proclamations about the true nature or structure or name of God and the Kosmos.

The Integral practitioner pays attention to the only thing for which there is real evidence: practice. We pay direct attention to what happens when we fulfill the injunctions of devotional practice, when we respond to Spirit's deepest inner calling.

Over time, many of us observe that our body-minds function better and become illuminated when we live with an active, open, heartfelt awareness. Practice (entirely apart from whatever you "believe in") tends to support deepening, opening, growth, awakening, and love.

Integrating Life Practice through Devotion

This trans-rational devotional heart is not an *alternative* to intelligence in the mind, or vital presence in the hara. Devotion functions as a unifier and turbocharger of the open head, heart, and hara. It is one of the most efficient ways to be related to moment-to-moment experience. Devotional practitioners experience existence itself to be profoundly gracious and vast and lovable and awesome. And that very experience empowers intelligence, creativity, and openness.

Consider the experience of unlimited and omnidirectional love, not love only of specific beloved others or objects, but love itself, the very condition of love. In love, the heart opens and the body breathes, receiving and releasing and *naturally* communing with the universal subtle energy of life. All the body's contractions, gross and subtle, tend to relax and open. In this mood, it is natural and pleasurable to serve others. Awareness is magnified. A conscious practitioner who is serving and feeling and circulating the energy of life in love, and meditating sincerely and regularly, will also be well-situated to notice the still and silent heart-source of those energies. In the midst of profound communion, all boundaries can more easily dissolve.

The mood of devotion greases the way. The subtle body is harmonized in a way that frees up more energy and attention. It doesn't just support an open heart and a life of compassionate service. It also promotes unobstructed conductivity of the energy of awareness, and even supports the experience of high, formless causal and nondual states of consciousness.

Devotion is an extremely intelligent and pleasurable Integral practice that helps to integrate all body, mind, and spirit practices. All of Integral Life Practice can be engaged in the spirit of loving devotion.

Integral Meditation Practices

Meditation: Making Spirit Real

Fundamental to most forms of spiritual practice—whether they be contemplation, prayer/communion, or meditation—is a silent sitting practice. And among the universal elements of all such practices (which, although they certainly include prayer and contemplation, are often referred to collectively as "meditation"), four stand out:

1. A comfortable and healthy sitting **posture**
2. A basic ability to **concentrate** and maintain focused attention
3. A **healthy attitude** of openness, attentiveness, and curiosity
4. A **regular daily sitting practice**

Before learning specific meditation practices, let's take a look at all four of these universal principles that apply to meditation in general.

1. Meditation Posture

Sit comfortably in a chair or on the floor using a cushion. Any of the standard postures is fine—upright in a chair, in lotus, half-lotus, or easy posture, or with loosely crossed legs, or kneeling.

Two things are important: the hips should be higher than the knees, and the sitz bones and perineum should form a solid base under an erect spine.

The back should be upright, in its natural slight S-curve. Sit as if a string was running up your spine through your head and into the sky, but without straining or forcing. As you begin you can take a moment to stretch your back comfortably, opening your chest and shoulders, then relaxing. Allow your center of balance to be in your lower abdomen, with belly and shoulders relaxed and chest open. Be careful not to slouch. An upright and straight posture promotes alertness.

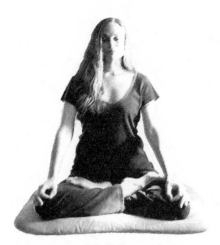

Figure 7.2
Full-lotus meditation posture.

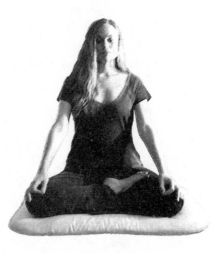

Figure 7.3
Half-lotus meditation posture.

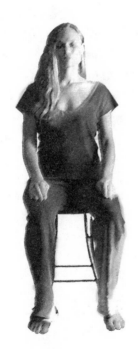

Figure 7.4
Seated meditation posture.

The palms of the hands can be placed on the thighs, palms open, facing up or down, or as in zazen meditation, you can bring the hands together, left palm face up underneath the back of the right hand, with the tips of the thumbs lightly touching, resting comfortably against your lower abdomen.

Breathing should be natural, unforced and through the nose. Breathe into your lower abdomen, feeling it expand and retract naturally.

Your tongue should be relaxed, lightly touching the palate or roof of your mouth just behind the teeth.

Your head should be tilted downward just a bit by pulling your chin in slightly while keeping the imaginary string running up your straight spine and through the top of your head to the sky. Your body should be completely relaxed. Pain is not a necessary part of the meditation experience. For many people, some pain is unavoidable, and it can be useful to learn to make peace with some discomfort.

Your eyes can be closed or you can meditate with slightly open "soft eyes" which makes it harder to drift into sleep. Each has different virtues, so you can experiment and choose what works best for you.

These tips can be helpful, but don't worry about them too much. The primary rule is: give posture just enough attention so that it doesn't distract your attention!

2. Concentration

Concentration involves training mental focus. A certain stability of attention opens many doors in meditation practice. It is often emphasized to beginners, but concentration practice is for everyone. Most experienced meditators find that their practice is enriched by regularly returning to the basics. It always helps to strengthen these all-important muscles.

These mental muscles can be strengthened by relatively difficult practices that involve one-pointed focus and which provide rapid feedback when attention wanders. Traditional meditators would cultivate the ability to maintain unwavering one-pointed attention for many hours or days on end. This is not necessary for ILP. But basic concentration is still valuable and can be learned in many ways, particularly through counting the breaths. We'll look at it in more detail in the coming pages (or you can skip directly to page 237).

3. A Healthy Attitude toward Your Chosen Practice
In spite of the wide diversity of meditative practices, a few principles apply almost universally.

Do it. All meditation involves the conscious use of your attention. Attend to the object of meditation—whether it's the breath or the mantra or the devotional feeling or the visualization. (When meditating without an object, release attention into formless contemplation—which is not the same as "spacing out" because you are still fully present.) Just bring your attention to the discipline as directly and authentically as you can.

Open to it. Meditation is all about the limitless potential of the present moment. Every time you bring your attention to your practice, you arrive here and now. Be open to the miracle of the present moment. Allow yourself to approach each moment with relaxed curiosity and a sense of possibility. Each new moment of meditation is at least potentially fresh and alive, not the same old, same old.

Don't judge it. Meditation is not a test or contest. Excess effort and struggle only get in the way. Berating yourself will only slow your progress. Meditation is a simple act of attention that, done properly, cuts through your neurotic self-preoccupation. To meditate is not to *oppose* the scattered tendencies of the mind, but to *do something else* with your attention. Just bring your attention to the practice.

Keep doing it. As a beginning meditator, you will notice your mind drifting away from the breath, through thinking or daydreaming. This is not a problem. It's part of the process. When you notice that you've drifted, just honor your intention to meditate. Return your attention to the breath (or whatever you've chosen as the object of meditation); actually continue to do the practice. Don't be concerned about the rate of your progress; just trust the process and apply yourself sincerely, continually releasing whatever expectations arise.

Wake up and enjoy. All valid meditative practices have one thing in common: Each presents a creative opportunity for awakening, strengthening, deepening, relaxing, or otherwise training awareness. Simplicity, or "beginner's mind," makes it possible to have an unobstructed encounter with each technique. This is enhanced by our vibrancy, radiance, curiosity, and enjoyment; we grow in *wakefulness* via our serene, essential, intelligent *playfulness*.

It's natural. Meditation is a natural functional capacity of the human body-mind. It is something that can be done by anyone who wants to. Most people can reach, within five minutes, a basic meditative state that is *physiologically distinct* from waking, dreaming, and deep sleep. In this alert, relaxed condition, people consume significantly less oxygen and their muscles relax more fully than when they sleep.

4. Establishing a Regular Sitting Practice

Many of the most important benefits of meditation only come over time, with regular practice. But many people find it difficult to establish a regular, sustained, daily meditation practice. How do you start meditating and stick with it?

It starts with a wholehearted decision to begin meditating. It's fine to try out meditation without making a commitment. But know that you probably won't stick with it and establish a regular sitting practice until you decide to make a real commitment. Once you're clear that you want to begin meditating, it is important to act on that commitment. One of the first things you can do is to create *time* and *space* conducive to your sitting practice.

It often helps tremendously to prepare a meditation space. You may want to do something, however simple (just straightening or cleaning the immediate area can be sufficient) to make sure you feel good about your meditation setting. This belongs to the Lower-Right quadrant of your meditation experience.

Then, set aside time for meditation. In the beginning, twenty minutes once or twice a day is often recommended. It's usually best to do it at the same time every day. Make sure you will not be interrupted during your meditation session. Note when you will be stopping with a watch or other timing device.

Many people find that they enjoy meditating more when they start with a personally meaningful ritual (such as a reading, prayer, lighting a candle or incense, and so on) that creates a good meditative atmosphere. For others, simplicity is empowering. Just sitting and meditating works fine!

Begin gently. Sit, adjust your posture, relax, and bring your attention into the present. Sincerely perform your practice throughout your meditation session. Then, at the end of the session, give yourself a minute to come out of it, move a bit, and gently transition before getting up and returning to your day.

Meditate every day if possible. If you miss a day or a week don't worry. Just begin again. If you don't have time for your full usual session, meditate anyway, for a shorter time. You'll find several **1-Minute Module** meditative practices in this book. Whatever intervenes, for however long, regard it like a distracting thought in the midst of a meditation session. Forgive yourself, honor your intention to meditate, and return to the practice.

As your practice develops momentum, you have the option to lengthen your meditation sessions. Serious meditators often sit for an hour or even several hours at a time, and many people meditate twice a day. Some people even go on meditation retreats in which they meditate all day for days or weeks at a time. Regard longer periods of meditation as an opportunity, though, and not as a burdensome obligation.

What is essential is not extended periods of sitting, but a living, growing, deepening, participatory relationship with Spirit. Engage it through contemplation, communion, and meditation. Refresh your practice regularly. Continually rediscover a living and dynamic relationship with Spirit during all your periods of meditation, short and long, and let this deepening engagement with Spirit inform your whole life.

Meditation Practices

There are many ways to meditate. In the West, some the of most widely practiced forms of meditation are Transcendental Meditation (TM), mindfulness meditation, zazen, and loving-kindness meditation. TM derives from ancient Hindu Vedic practices and uses a mantra (similar to the I AM: Mantra Meditation presented here). Mindfulness meditation cultivates open awareness and unobstructed, direct, and full contact with experience; it is the foundation of Theravadan and Tibetan Buddhist meditation practice. Zazen or shikan taza is the essence of Japanese Buddhist practice. These Buddhist traditions rest attention in the present moment, continually releasing thoughts into the essential formlessness of present awareness, most similar to the basic breath meditation practice and Integral Inquiry presented here. Loving-kindness meditation involves continually relaxing and opening the heart as we do in Integral devotional practices such as the 3 Faces of Spirit, which will be described below.

In the pages that follow, five meditation practices are presented:

1. **Basic breath meditation.** This is a way to build your concentration muscles while also enjoying the purity and clarity of a meditation practice.

2. **The I AM: Mantra Meditation.** This Gold Star Practice makes use of the ancient principles behind TM and other mantra meditation practices in a thoroughly Integral context, suitable for anyone, from beginners to advanced practitioners.

3. **Integral Inquiry (formless awareness).** This Gold Star Practice continually releases attention into formless awareness. Because it offers several stages of practice, it is appropriate for anyone. There is a 1-Minute Module as well.

4. **The 3 Faces of Spirit (meditation with form).** There are three Gold Star Practices based on the profound implication of Integral consciousness: We *contemplate* Spirit, *commune with* Spirit, and *awaken as* Spirit. The 3 Faces of Spirit can be enacted via a simple silent meditation, a several-part visualization, and a 1-Minute Module.

5. **Compassionate Exchange (meditation with form).** In this Gold

Star Practice, you visualize selfless sacrificial service to the whole world via every breath, ultimately dissolving even the distinction between self and other in non-separation. There is also a 1-Minute Module.

Basic Breath Meditation

Meditating with the breath is perhaps the most universal of all meditation practices.

We're always breathing, in every now. The whole body is always being breathed by an impulse into which we can utterly relax, with full awareness.

For beginners, it's a clear, direct, uncomplicated way to start a regular meditation practice. For more advanced meditators, it is still often appropriate—even advanced practitioners almost always benefit from revisiting, reinforcing, and deepening the foundations. Each time they return, they bring new depth to the process, transforming it into a higher and higher practice.

Breath meditation is one of the most elegant combinations of the two meditative capacities simultaneously: *mental focus* and *open awareness*. Concentration trains mental focus and stability, while open awareness relaxes, expands, and releases this mental focus into a free encounter with every present moment. Breath meditation thus stands at the border between formless and form-based types of meditation. It's a meditative *form* that readily releases into *formless* meditation. It helps to establish concentration while cultivating the ability to surrender into mind-expanding contact with the here and now.

Basic Breath Meditation Instructions

1. Sit quietly with an erect spine and breathe naturally.
2. Bring attention to the present moment and breathe, silently counting the breath. Begin counting your breath, counting the first inhalation as "one," the exhalation as "two," and so on.
   a. Breathe in while counting "one,"
   b. breathe out, "two,"
   c. breathe in "three," and so forth.

3. Start over after you reach "ten."

4. Between the in and out breaths, rest the mind. Pay special attention to the stillness between each breath.

5. Whenever your mind wanders, go back to "one" and continue to count the breaths. Set an engaging, gently challenging standard. It's your choice:

   a. You can go back to "one" only when you lose count.

   b. If you find you are adept at multitasking (that is, able to count while daydreaming), you may want to set a sterner standard, going back to "one" whenever thoughts take over the *foreground* of your attention and the breath, count, and present moment become *background*.

   c. You can return to "one" whenever *any* thought arises, even if it hasn't distracted you from the counting.

A Simple Summary

Follow the breath with the mind,
counting each breath,
resting the mind between the in and out breaths,
and return to "one" if your mind wanders.

Breath Meditation Is Always Right Now

Each breath and count returns attention to . . . what?

The present moment—*now*. This practice depends on cultivating your relationship to the present moment. What is it to be fully and consciously present? How do you "be here now"?

With every new breath, you have a fresh opportunity to open to the present moment. In every present moment you can consciously allow what is to be, and enjoy the expanding inner space and relaxation that may naturally occur.

As you count, each breath and each number is not data. It is just a reminder, a name for this living present moment. The numbers do not have to be dry, abstract, dead, and mechanical.

Regard each number as a name for this infinitely alive "now"—in which all enjoyment and depth—and Spirit and holiness—are found.

In that infinitely deep present moment, awareness can relax and open. In time it can learn to open profoundly. It can increasingly meet and be met intimately by the rich contours, textures, and infinite depth of constantly dancing, ever-changing present experience.

Enjoyment and feeling are the keys. As you practice, notice what you enjoy about meditating and counting your breaths, and what makes the practice become a lifeless obligation.

Your Mind *Will* Wander. Not a Problem!

When you notice that you have become lost in thought during meditation, return attention to the breath and count "one" as you inhale.

Wandering is inevitable, a natural part of the meditative process, not "wrong" or a problem. As you continue to practice, your ability to focus will improve. This is a good thing, and it makes deeper practice possible. But mental states are always changing. Everyone goes through phases in which their ability to focus waxes and wanes. Wandering attention is not a problem or an obstacle to meditation.

Don't forget: self-scolding and internal conflict interrupt the meditative process far more than wandering attention. When you discover yourself in the middle of internal criticism, the best way to minimize it is through gentle acceptance, and then simply returning to your practice.

When you realize your attention has wandered, honor your intention to meditate and return your attention to your practice. Yes, the wandering is perfectly okay. In fact, it all *is* meditation. Persistence is not just humble, but also noble and wise. Return to "one;" return to the breath; return to the infinite, mysterious, miraculous depth of the living present moment.

I AM: Guided Meditation

This guided meditation takes you to the heart of your witness consciousness, your native awareness, the simple feeling of being or "I AMness" itself.

Notice your present awareness. Notice the images and thoughts arising in your mind, the feelings and sensations arising in your body, the myriad objects arising around you in the room or environment. All of these are objects arising in your awareness.

Now think about what was in your awareness five minutes ago. Most of the thoughts have changed, most of the bodily sensations have changed, and most of the environment may have changed. But something has not changed. Something in you is the same now as it was five minutes ago. What is present now that was present five minutes ago?

The feeling-awareness of being itself, your most basic I AMness, is still present. You are that ever-present I AMness. That I AMness is present now, it was present a moment ago, it was present a minute ago, it was present five minutes ago.

What was present five hours ago?

I AMness. That sense of I AMness is an ongoing, self-knowing, self-recognizing, self-validating I AMness. It is present now, it was present five hours ago. All your thoughts have changed, all your bodily sensations have changed, your environment has also changed, at least slightly, but I AM is ever-present, radiant, open, empty, clear, spacious, transparent, free. Objects have changed, but not this formless I AMness. This obvious and present I AMness is present now as it was present five hours ago.

What was present five years ago?

I AMness. So many objects have come and gone, so many feelings have come and gone, so many thoughts have come and gone, so many dramas and terrors and loves and hates have come, and stayed a while, and gone. But one thing has not come, and one thing has not gone. What is that? What is the only thing present in your awareness right now that you can remember was present five years ago? This timeless, ever-present feeling of I AMness is present now as it was five years ago.

What was present five centuries ago?

All that is ever-present is I AMness. Every person feels this same I AMness—because it is not a body, it is not a thought, it is not an object, it is not the environment, it is not anything that can be seen, but rather is the ever-present Seer, the ongoing open and empty Witness of all that is arising, in any person, in any world, in any place, at any time, in all the worlds until the end of time, there is only and always this obvious and immediate I AMness. What else could you possibly know? What else does anybody ever know? There is only and always this radiant, self-knowing, self-feeling, self-transcending I AMness, whether present now, five minutes ago, five hours ago, five centuries ago.

Five millennia ago?

Before Abraham was, I AM. Before the universe was, I AM. This is your original face, the face you had before your parents were born, the face you had before the universe was born, the face you have had for all eternity until you decided to play this round of hide and seek, and get lost in the objects of your own creation.

There is no need to pretend that you do not know or feel your own I AMness.

And with that, the game is undone. A million thoughts have come and gone, a million feelings have come and gone, a million objects have come and gone. But one thing has not come, and one thing has not gone: the great Unborn and the great Undying, which never enters or leaves the stream of time, a pure Presence above time, floating in eternity. You are this great, obvious, self-knowing, self-validating, self-liberating I AMness.

Before Abraham was, I AM.

I AM is none other than **Spirit in 1st person**, the ultimate, the sublime, the radiant all-creating Self of the entire Kosmos, present in you and me and us and him and her and them and all—as the I AMness that each and every one of us feels.

Because in all the known universes, the overall number of I AMs is but one.

Rest as I AMness always, the exact I AMness you feel right now, just as it is, which is Unborn Spirit itself shining in and as you. Assume your personal identity as well—as this or that object, or this or that self, or this and that thing resting always in the Ground of it All, as this great and completely obvious I AMness, and get up and go on about your day, in the universe I AM created.

(*After this meditation practice, having grounded your understanding of the radical depth of your own I AMness, you might choose to engage a simple mantra meditation using those two simple words.*)

GOLD STAR PRACTICE
I AM: Mantra Meditation

(As a prelude to learning this meditation, consider the core of what I AM means through the I AM: Guided Meditation on page 239.)

Sit in a comfortable, upright posture, and let yourself settle. Then, use the word-sounds-meanings I AM or "Ayam." Recall it every few moments or whenever thought arises.* Let yourself be carried by it. There is nothing you need to accomplish. There is nothing you need to get rid of. Just recall this mantra, I AM. You can trust this process.

If you drift, just recall the mantra, I AM. You will naturally come back to the present moment. Recall this mantra or sound anchor whenever you want and always when you notice that you have been pulled away. If you notice that you are not involved in the meditation practice, remember I AM, returning attention to the present moment and returning to I AM every few moments.

If you begin to experience an expanded quality of consciousness, that is fine. If you don't, that is fine, too. Trust that it's all part of the process. Don't try to make anything happen, or wish anything to be different. You can be confident in the power of this extremely simple practice. Enjoy it, and let go into it. This meditation elegantly and effectively enables the body and mind to resonate very deeply, all the way to the subtlest levels of being.

If thoughts come, and if you get lost in them, don't worry. When you notice that attention has drifted, just honor your intention to meditate, and return to I AM.

---

*If your first language is not English, feel free to translate the meaning of this mantra. Or you can experiment with other phrases. For English speakers, I AM almost always works well.

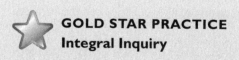 **GOLD STAR PRACTICE**
Integral Inquiry

What Is Integral Inquiry?

As we progress in meditation practice, new opportunities for self-realization and self-understanding open up. Integral Inquiry is an advanced 1st-person practice designed to penetrate to the core of your spiritual identity by inviting you to rest in *formless* or *pure awareness* and to notice the ways in which you habitually *contract* away from this primordial ground.

In its early stages, Integral Inquiry invites you to rest fully and deeply in this witnessing consciousness. As you continue the practice of Inquiry—both sitting on the cushion and in everyday life—the inquiry itself becomes more profound and radical. Eventually, as this absolute practice deepens and stabilizes, it becomes the context for relative practices.

Thus, within Integral Inquiry, you can bring all the tools of your ILP into play. These practices will help you further comprehend and ultimately transcend the patterns of contraction obscuring your essential nature, which is boundless, open, and free.

This meditation works on two sides: absolute and relative. On the *absolute* side, it invites you to relax your identification with passing thoughts and experiences and to rest in formless awareness, moment to moment. This is not a blank, mindless state, but your natural condition when you are free from self-contraction in relation to what is arising. Many approaches to meditation involve holding attention on an object—it could be the breath, body sensations, an image, or a mantra. Formless meditation involves *releasing attention from all objects* in order to rest effortlessly in pure awareness—a "non-practice" practice that is sometimes called "just sitting" or "pure presence."

On the *relative* side, Integral Inquiry invites you to dissolve the conditions that habitually distract you from pure presence, by facing and understanding them. Often these are personal shadow issues; thus Integral Inquiry incorporates the 3-2-1 Shadow Process. In addition, you can use other practices from your ILP toolkit (for example, the 3-Body Workout, the 3 Faces of Spirit, and the AQAL framework) in order to dissolve obstructions to your experience of the absolute.

How to Practice Integral Inquiry

Integral Inquiry helps us release attention into the present moment, neither identified with whatever arises, nor separate from it. This is effortless and free. When limiting mental activity arises, we ask a question, which helps us recognize and dissolve the extremely subtle and causal activity of self-contraction (often called "ego").

Over time, your Integral Inquiry practice may naturally progress through four stages. Stages 1, 2, and 3 are done while sitting in meditation and can be practiced for any amount of time, from just one minute (using the 1-Minute Module) to an hour or longer. Once you feel comfortable with one stage of practice, move on to the next one. Stage 4 invites you to take the Inquiry beyond the cushion, into your everyday life, and includes the full, flexible, and appropriate use of any aspect of Integral Life Practice.

Stage 1: Prepare by Becoming Grounded in Pure Presence

Stage 1 is about building your concentration. Using breath meditation (described above) cultivate concentration until you can maintain a stable focus for five minutes. Once you're able to do this, you should continue to strengthen these key contemplative muscles either periodically or as an ongoing practice. You may even want to practice five minutes of breath meditation at the beginning of each session of Integral Inquiry.

After you've reached the point at which you can sustain several minutes of stability during meditation (and this can take six months of practice!), you can drop the counting after a few minutes and begin to follow the breath with your attention. Just pay attention to the present moment of the breath cycle, without counting. Use the breath as an anchor for present moment attention. Use it to help you release or go beyond the thinking mind and rest in pure presence. Keep opening into your most natural condition of formless awareness.

Relax and release your attention into the amazing, always new, already free wonder of the present moment. Sit and breathe and be present in and as this always fresh, trustable, yet unknowable mystery.

Stage 2: Inquire

As you become comfortable with stage 1 of the practice, you might notice that when you sit in formless awareness, the mind often *contracts* from this blissful spaciousness, becoming distracted and absorbed by thoughts, emotions, or sensations.

The mind tends to contract chronically, in many different ways, again and again. When you meditate, this often takes the forms of thoughts, images, feelings, sleepiness—and every other form of distraction you experience while sitting. When you notice any of this happening, inquire, and relax. Choose a short question to help you notice this compulsive activity that takes place at the subtlest levels of attention. Useful questions include "Who am I?" "What am I doing?" or, more humorously, "Who am I kidding?" You can go deeper, addressing the subtlest activity of awareness, and ask "Avoiding?" or "Contracting?"

The inquiry is not meant to stimulate analysis of why your mind wandered—"What was I avoiding? Why?"—but to bring awareness to what is actually taking place through the mind's wandering, to actually *see* this activity as it occurs, and then let it go—while simultaneously and naturally returning attention to the breath.*

To put it another way, in inquiry one is asking, "What am I doing instead of being present as free attention? What is there to notice?" One answer given by sages is, "vast emptiness, and automatic contracting of the mind."

In practice, inquiry is quite quick. There's just an open invitation to awareness, while attention returns to the formless present moment and the breath. But the deeper you go into inquiry, the more you'll be able to see your activity of contraction and to understand and become responsible for the subtle dynamics through which the separate self arises.

As this process deepens, let the whole exercise arise in emptiness, in Big Mind. Then, allow thoughts to self-liberate spontaneously.

Stage 3: Freely Use Integral Life Practice Tools as Inquiry

After you have become proficient in the second stage of Integral Inquiry, so that the process of Inquiry is natural and real, you can move on to stage 3, bringing Integral Life Practice to bear more explicitly on your meditation.

What typically distracts you from pure presence? Sometimes it will be a shadow issue. So, for example, if a particular person or situation with an emotional charge keeps arising in meditation, you can Face it, Talk to it, and Be it, using the 1-Minute version of the 3-2-1 Shadow Process.

Shadow work is often most needed. However, you can use any Integral practice to release your attention.

---

*It's important to note, this is not the same practice as "labeling" (another popular form of meditation, which involves identifying different kinds of experiential phenomena as they arise: thought, memory, daydream, pain, tingling, etc. You actually ask a question and then simply notice what is the case while resting in present awareness.

- You might do a 3-2-1 Shadow Process on a situation that is bothering you.
- You might refresh yourself with Body practices, like breathing from the heart and conducting the circle of life force, and filling the body with energy, radiating from the hara, heart, and head.
- You might ask the questions "Avoiding?" or "Contracting?" or "Who am I?"
- You might remember Spirit in the 2nd-person perspective by internally speaking the word "Beloved."
- You might even inquire directly in a way that takes *no outward form at all,* just the restoration of free awareness.
- And finally, you might use any element of the AQAL map to identify and locate your attention—Are you having a particular state-experience? What is the context in which it is arising? And so on. . . .

Whatever form of Inquiry you use, it is the way you use it that makes it Integral Inquiry. Choose a question or practice you can use to release the compulsive contraction of energy and attention that tends to occur. Use it to relax the cramp within consciousness that divides the subject from all objects. Inquire and be free of the habitual fear that is superficial to the vast Suchness you really are. Inquire, and return to sitting in pure presence.

Stage 4: Practicing Integral Inquiry in Your Everyday Life

When Integral Inquiry is well established, you can begin to use it not just when you are sitting in formal meditation, but *in any moment of life.*

This brings meditation into the rest of your waking life, breaking down the artificial division between meditation and life activity. As consciousness more and more freely and fully encounters and pervades your waking experience, it can naturally begin to appear in your dream and deep sleep states also.

This is a fully flexible, fully Integral discipline. It is also a very advanced practice. It begins when you can release attention from its compulsive patterns into formless synchronicity with and as the present moment's spontaneous arising. As soon as you fall into objectification or opposition or otherness or thought, you can inquire, using whatever Integral practice seems best fitted to free your attention and energy. Whatever you choose to do, the point is to do it fully until you are freed of limiting contractions and restored to formless awareness of and as the present moment. Then, in that freedom, go about your day.

 1-MINUTE MODULE
Integral Inquiry

1. Sit quietly with an upright spine and breathe naturally.
2. Rest in the present moment, releasing attention into the Suchness or openness in which everything is arising. Relax into what Is.
3. If thoughts arise or your attention wanders, ask a question that helps you notice what has distracted you from unconditional awareness. You can ask, "Who am I?" "What am I doing?" "Avoiding?" or "Contracting?"
4. Let the question open you to a deeper understanding rather than getting involved in trying to answer it. Don't engage a mental story about your avoidance or contraction. Just touch the moment with open awareness and be present to the obvious.
5. When you inquire, you'll notice you relax and release your conventional mind. Relax into the present moment exactly as it is, and let the inquiry continue to arise randomly or spontaneously.
6. When your available time is over, complete and dedicate your session.

GOLD STAR PRACTICE
The 3 Faces of Spirit

Putting It All Together

Since 3rd-person *contemplation,* 2nd-person *communion* (or prayer), and 1st-person *meditation* are all inherent dimensions of an Integral spiritual life, something important is missing if any of them are not included. We can do specific 1st-, 2nd-, and 3rd-person practices, or we can exercise them all together in a single Integral meditation practice such as the 3 Faces of Spirit.

We are related to everything—including Spirit, the great Mystery, Suchness, and the ever-present—through perspectives. And, as described above, the perspectives through which we can relate to Spirit are very similar to the perspectives through which we relate to one another.

- We can contemplate, serve, think, know, and talk *about* Spirit (knowing It) as nature and through study and philosophy in the 3rd person.
- We can relate *with* Spirit (being with Thou) and *listen to, pray to, receive, or commune with* Spirit in a 2nd-person relationship.
- And we can meditate and awaken and feel and know ourselves and speak as Spirit (awakening as the I of all) in a 1st-person apprehension of our source and substance.

Meditating with the 3 Faces of Spirit

You can engage the 3 Faces of Spirit for just a few minutes or as long as an hour or more. You can also enter into deep engagement with the contemplations and meditations on pages 211–212 under 3rd-Person Contemplation, 2nd-Person Prayer or Communion, and 1st-Person Meditation.

All three perspectives can be brought to mind using short and simple words or phrases. Whenever attention drifts and it is time to return to the practice, a word or phrase can be used (1st person, 2nd person, or 3rd person) to help the whole body-mind reconnect with the Ultimate and thus return to meditation.

For 1st-person, a useful short phrase is I AM. We might also use "Myself," "Just This!," "Awareness," "Presence," or "Mirror Mind."

For 2nd-person, we can use the names of God when approached face to face: Thou, Beloved, My Love, Jesus, Allah, Amitabha, Mary, and so on.

Possible 3rd-person names or phrases are: Spirit, Kosmos, Reality, Is-ness, Perfection, Gaia, Evolution, and so on.

In this meditation practice, do the following:

1. Attend to the breath.
2. Anchor your 3rd-, 2nd-, and 1st-person relationship with the Ultimate using a word or short phrase for each.
3. Spontaneously, whenever you notice the opportunity and with full feeling-awareness of the Ultimate, recall any one of those words or phrases.

Begin by anchoring a relationship to the 3rd-person Ultimate in your body, mind, and feeling. Experience "It" while associating it with a word or phrase you have chosen to invoke and express this 3rd-person relationship. For example, Kosmos.

Then turn with full feeling to face the Ultimate, presuming your full 2nd-person intimacy, and letting that register in breath, body, mind, and feeling, while associating it with a word or phrase you have chosen to invoke and express this 2nd-person relationship. For example, Beloved.

Then deepen in that intimacy until you open into recognition of no separation at all—your 1st-person identification with and as the Ultimate, letting your breath, body, mind, and feeling register your Ultimate identity, and associating it with a word or phrase you have chosen to invoke and express this 1st-person apprehension. For example, I AM.

Then, just sit, noticing the breath. At random, and anytime your mind wanders, utter, with full feeling, one of three words or short phrases that express your 1st-, 2nd-, and 3rd-person relationships with Ultimate Reality.

The key is to choose words that resonate for you. Feel free to choose others besides those suggested here. The important thing is that you use phrases that are evocative for you.

Feel free to repeat a single phrase for several minutes if you like, or even a whole session of meditation. It is okay to continue until another word or phrase spontaneously comes forward.

When meditating this way, we resonate in relationship to the Ultimate, from one perspective or another, again and again. We sit in the silence, listening, opening ourselves up into the Ultimate through all perspectives.

 1-MINUTE MODULE
The 3 Faces of Spirit

At any moment, you can experience Spirit as a 3rd-person It, a 2nd-person Thou, or a 1st-person I. Repeat the following sentences quietly to yourself, letting each perspective arise gently and naturally.

- *I contemplate Spirit as all that is arising—the Great Perfection of this and every moment.*
- *I behold and commune with Spirit as the beloved infinite Thou, who bestows all blessings and complete forgiveness on me, and before whom I gladly offer utter gratitude and devotion.*
- *I rest in Spirit as my own Witness and primordial Self, the Big Mind that is one with all.*
- *In this ever-present, easy, and natural contemplation, communion, and meditation, I go on about my day.*

If you wish, you can replace the word "Spirit" with any word of your choice that evokes an Ultimate Being. It could be God, Jehovah, Allah, Christ, the Lord, or the One.

GOLD STAR PRACTICE
Compassionate Exchange

Touching Everything and Letting It All Fall Away

Compassionate Exchange is a way to use self-transcending and self-sacrificial care and compassion to move freely through all perspectives instead of staying chronically identified with only one. In this meditative practice, we consciously and deliberately exchange self for other. That is, we practice taking on the "other's" perspective and regarding the self as if it were the "other," benefiting other *at the expense* of the self, reversing the usual orientation of the ego.

Most creatures tend to move toward pleasure and away from pain. We move instinctually to defend the self from discomfort and harm, and to meet the needs and fulfill the wants of the self. In Compassionate Exchange, we dissolve the armor that builds up around this limited, survival-based orientation.

In fact, we reverse the self's usual orientation and *breathe in* suffering, and then *breathe out* the pleasurable release of suffering. We reclaim the tremendous energy and freedom that result from reversing the automatic tendency of seeking pleasure and avoiding pain.

To state it most simply, in Compassionate Exchange, the "I" moves into awareness and care for "you," and "us," and "them," and back to "me"—the self. Then the "I" rests in the Self of the self—the Witness in which all perspectives arise.

Meditating with Compassionate Exchange

Compassionate Exchange can be practiced for any length of time, from just two or three minutes (a 1-Minute Module) to an hour or more. Here are the essential elements and steps of Compassionate Exchange:

1. Bring attention and feeling to the heart via the breath, while recalling a memory that evokes the experience of care and compassion.

2. Picture someone dear to you and breathe this person's distress and suffering into your heart. Exhale the essence of freedom from suffering and direct it toward this person.

3. As you breathe in, take in the suffering and distress of more and more people. Each time you breathe out, breathe out the essence of release and freedom from suffering and direct it toward this growing group of people.

4. Over the next series of breaths, expand your care to include all beings. Take in their suffering and distress. Breathe out the essence of release and freedom from suffering and direct it out toward all beings. This complete reversal, even violation of the self's impulses to seek pleasure and avoid pain can be quite difficult. It can stimulate all sorts of resistance and negativity. A key to Compassionate Exchange is to keep accepting and releasing these reactions and to keep returning to the practice.

5. Then focus on one being among all sentient beings: yourself. Take in your own suffering and distress and breathe out the essence of freedom of suffering, directing it toward yourself. From this free perspective, breathe, feel, and naturally embrace and affirm your vitality and humanity.

6. As the final step in the practice of Compassionate Exchange, notice that you and all the people you have pictured and all the suffering and freedom from suffering are arising in the awareness that is witnessing all of this, and this is who you truly are. As you continue to breathe, notice that this Witness is present not just in you but also in all others. Their Witness is exactly the same as the Witness you are. There is only one Witness. Rest in that natural, open, effortless expanse of Awareness.

The Perfect Practice

Some spiritual traditions that have a tremendous range of meditative practices describe the very simplest and most radical of all spiritual practices as "perfect." Sometimes such practices have been reserved for initiates who have done spiritual work for decades. At their essence they all describe the same practice, the one with which this discussion of meditation began.

And it goes something like this:

No practice is necessary. You are already resting in the boundless ever present Suchness of your own awareness. So just rest. Abandon effort. Just notice the boundless and eternal space of awareness in which everything is arising. Rest there. Rest again. Don't worry if it only lasts for a short moment. Just rest again in spacious, empty, present awareness. And again. Brief moments are just fine. Effort is unnecessary. Keep resting in awareness (or notice that you are already resting in awareness) until it becomes permanent and obvious at all times.

What becomes permanent and obvious?

Nothing and everything.

Just this.

That about which nothing can be spoken.

Is-ness itself.

Spirit.

You.

This.

Always.

Already.

Now.

Yes.

8

Integral Ethics

The Need for Integral Ethics

Integral Ethics, like any decent ethics, is the art of *being a good person*. It's the practice of **goodness** in our everyday lives and includes all the ways of being truthful, authentic, caring, and courageous that constitute our basic integrity. Integral Ethics also refers to the dimension of our lives where we must make difficult and complicated choices and nuanced judgments about what is right and wrong, acceptable and unacceptable, and quite often, unavoidably ambiguous. It's where we must grapple with **moral dilemmas**, in politics, sexuality, health, relationships, work, money, and sometimes life and death situations.

Integral Ethics does not purport to tell us how to live or to give specific answers to our moral questions. Rather, it provides a *framework* for thinking about how we live and for making the best moral decisions we can. It also *makes sense* of people's different ethical structures by using the familiar AQAL distinctions—quadrants, levels, lines, states, and types.

Most of all, Integral Ethics is a *practice*—an evolutionary, open-ended, moment-to-moment endeavor to embody sincere care and actualize our deepest intuitions of "the good" in our lives and in the world at large.

But Isn't Ethics Boring, Stifling, Oppressive . . . ?

At one level, yes, "moral values" and "ethics" are not much fun. After all, they're buzzwords for enforced conformity to traditional "thou shalt" and "thou shalt not" injunctions. Do this, don't do that—and most of all, follow the rules. Ethics seems to ask for childish conformity. But this is merely a *conventional* level of ethics. As we develop, ethics soon becomes not so much about following preconceived rules, but about something higher, more intelligent, and more enlivening.

At Integral levels of awareness, ethics is no longer the fear-based, unintelligent selfishness of being a "good" or "bad" boy or girl. Morality ceases to feel like childish conformity to parental injunctions and instead becomes a creative manifestation of conscious freedom, a natural expression of enlightened self-interest (which yet sees beyond the self).

Of course, conventional morality can be a good thing and is especially important in the transition from *egocentric* to *ethnocentric* awareness—from a regard only for *me, me, me* to a care and concern for the larger group, like my family, tribe, or nation. But beyond hedonistic and traditional ethics, there are *post-conventional* forms of ethics, including *worldcentric, multi-worldcentric,* and *kosmocentric* stages.

Like life itself, ethics becomes more liberated—and more enjoyable—when we include more comprehensive perspectives. As we evolve ethically, we are able to embrace perspectives of increasing magnitude—from 1st-person "I" (it's all about *me*), to 2nd-person "us" (our family, our group), to wider and fuller perspectives including 3rd-person "all of us" (all human beings, the planet itself), and even "all sentient beings" (which accounts for multiple worldspaces, and ultimately, all beings in all space and time).

Integral Ethics includes all these levels. It aims to increase the health of any particular level wherever it is found, while also gently encouraging growth to higher, more encompassing levels.

In modern and postmodern society, we're most familiar with ethnocentric, worldcentric, and multi-worldcentric morality—in other words, Amber, Orange, and Green. We're witness, in fact, to the military and culture wars that result from the clash of these different perspectives—from "my country (or tribe or religion), right or wrong" (Amber) to "freedom and justice for all" (Orange) to "we must care for the entire web of life" (Green). Of course, each of these levels contains a slice of the truth, but since each thinks it has *the whole* truth and can't see *the other's* truth, they are perpetually in conflict. Only at Integral levels and beyond do we begin to see and appreciate how these multiple levels are all part of a

Level	Complexity of Perspective	Focus	Altitude
Kosmocentric	5th Person (up to nth person)	All sentient beings in all worlds	Teal to Turquoise, Indigo and beyond
Multi-worldcentric	4th Person	All human and other beings, pluralistically	Green
Worldcentric	3rd Person	All human beings, universally	Orange
Ethnocentric	2nd Person	Us, family, tribe, nation	Amber
Egocentric	1st Person	Me	Magenta to Red

Figure 8.1

Levels of ethics.

larger evolutionary unfolding. Those who practice an Integral Ethics naturally care for the health of the entire evolutionary process itself. They will attempt to *transcend and include* the important truths of egocentric, ethnocentric, worldcentric, and multi-worldcentric, while pushing the edge of their own growth ever further.

The Assault on Ethics

Sadly, our ability to engage an ethical practice has been under assault on three major fronts.

First, in the academic world, postmodern thinkers focus on the cultural construction of morality, without emphasizing its developmental history from pre-conventional to conventional to post-conventional and beyond. This pluralistic relativism flattens ethics into a false equality by giving every moral stance the same value. In an attempt to eradicate arrogant judgments, extreme postmodernism has assaulted our moral compass itself. This is commonly decried as "moral relativism."

Second, postmodern psychologists have raised concerns over the damage created by harsh and disempowering judgments. Yet they've failed to give equal emphasis to the importance of conscience and self-critical discernment.

Third, popular spiritual misconceptions of emptiness emphasize the "choicelessness" of formless awareness, without validating the other side of the highest realizations—the capacity to function (and make necessary and appropriate judgments) in our social and cultural reality—even while remaining grounded in the realization of emptiness.

Further, if you attend a course today in professional ethics (in virtually any given field) you're likely to be introduced to a rather technical and legalistic series of disclosures, non-disclosures, and other procedures. At their best these do help you provide your clients and colleagues with some important protections. But instead of being a means for expressing your conscious care, ethics in such contexts tends to become mostly about covering your backside in order to avoid lawsuits, formal complaints, or other allegations of impropriety. Such approaches engender so-called "ethical" behavior that is motivated not by authentic care but by fear of consequences. In fact, they tend to hold back ethical growth by reinforcing *pre-conventional* motives.

These inadequate perspectives on "ethics" are dominant. So the ethical choices we face are usually discussed in oversimplified terms, as if our only options are conformity to social conventions, amoral pragmatism, or "whatever's right for you" moral relativism.

We Must Discover a Higher Ethical Sensibility

Authentic, sincere, caring ethics has gotten lost in the shuffle. This is a serious problem, because ethics is one of the most essential virtues, one that has in no way become obsolete. On the contrary, without the authentic intention to behave ethically, Integral Life Practice cannot really begin. It's true, we don't list it among our 4 Core Modules. That's only because it would be redundant—the intention to relate to others with consciousness and care is implicit in the desire to engage Integral Life Practice in the first place. We can't schedule our ethical exercises for a certain time each day. They come upon us as life presents them. So ethical practice naturally shows up in every moment of life. And the way it expresses itself keeps changing and unfolding, because practitioners keep growing in their ethical awareness. While your Integral ethical practice may include specific guidelines or commitments, which you might take very seriously, it also becomes a way of being, an *attunement* to the demands and the energy of the moment. You can think of this as an **ethical sensibility**. Just as a talented jazz musician can *feel* in what direction the music wants to go, an advanced ethical practitioner develops a *sense* for what's the right action (or non-action) at any given time. Of course, this takes a lot of practice! An integrated, conscious practice of body, mind, spirit, and shadow is the basis for an Integral Ethics.

The Framework of Integral Ethics

Growing Ethically

Can you feel the **Eros** of the Kosmos—the natural evolutionary attraction toward greater depth, complexity, and consciousness? It draws us to higher and higher stages of development. Integral Ethics postulates Eros as a developmental gradient or force—the very same impulse that led

The Platinum Rule

The ability to take wider and deeper perspectives may lead you to higher expressions of traditional ethical dictums. For instance, the Golden Rule, recognized by most religious traditions, essentially says "treat others as you would like to be treated." Yet when you take another's perspective you may discover that the way you would like to be treated differs from the way the other would like to be treated. Hence the Platinum Rule: "Treat others as *they* would like to be treated." The Platinum Rule honors the rich diversity of human sensibilities and structures of awareness by asking advanced ethical practitioners to take the perspective of another and act from that awareness. The philosopher Karl Popper articulated the Platinum Rule when he said, "The Golden Rule is a good standard which is further improved by doing unto others, wherever possible, as *they* want to be done."

from the Big Bang to atoms to cells to human beings—but you need not see Eros in metaphysical terms. It is simply a way of interpreting one of the most essential, profound, and mysterious tendencies of the Kosmos. There could be other ways of describing this force, but clearly *something* is at work.

The important point is that as we tune into Eros, by whatever name, our circle of care and compassion opens and widens to include more and more perspectives. We grow from caring about self (*egocentric*), to family, friends, tribe, and nation (*ethnocentric*), to all people (*worldcentric*) and the planet (*multi-worldcentric*), to including all sentient beings and processes (*kosmocentric*). In the highest vertical stages of development, we recognize our interconnectedness with and inseparability from everyone and everything, and experience a powerfully felt sense of responsibility for the Kosmos itself.

Vertical ethical practice calls us to align with the evolutionary grain of the Kosmos, the inherent Eros that draws us to wider circles of compassion and care. You can encourage your own vertical ethical growth in many ways. One practice involves sharpening your moral discernment, your ability to balance competing values and make wise ethical choices. Another practice is to become more aware of different levels of ethical functioning and to take responsibility for functioning at your highest possible level. We will discuss both of these vertical ethical practices later in the chapter.

Horizontal ethical practice calls us to express our care and ethical concern more fully and consistently, by extending it into more areas of our life. The focus here is less on cognitive or spiritual advancement (although these remain important), and more on *applying* an ethical framework to your relationships, your job, your everyday activities, and so on. Wherever you are on the evolutionary spiral, you can always apply your ethical understanding more fully to your life, and walk your talk with a greater degree of integrity. Since you can always express your care more fully and effectively, there's always room for horizontal ethical practice. One primary horizontal ethical practice involves taking responsibility for all 4 quadrants of your being. Since the quadrants exist at every altitude, then no matter where you may tend to show up vertically (Green? Turquoise?), you can always be Integrally ethical in a horizontal sense (I, We, It, and Its). We will explore horizontal ethics more deeply also.

In practice, of course, we want to simultaneously behave ethically both vertically (attempting to include higher and more integrated perspectives) and horizontally (including as much of reality as possible at our current level of development).

The Basic Moral Intuition

A useful principle for practicing Integral Ethics is the Basic Moral Intuition. The Basic Moral Intuition is "to protect and promote the greatest depth for the greatest span." Depth refers to level of development—a baboon is deeper than a ladybug, which is in turn deeper than an amoeba. Span refers to the number of beings affected, regardless of level of development—as in the utilitarian principle of "the greatest good for the greatest number." The important value of this utilitarian formulation (which stems from an Orange altitude of consciousness) is its inherent egalitarianism; the problem is that it completely leaves out the crucial depth dimension.

Integral Ethics combines egalitarianism with a due regard for development. It's a vertically inclusive egalitarianism. Thus: *protect and promote the greatest depth for the greatest span.* Every being is precious. So is every species. But developmental depth is precious in a particular way. The extinction of dodo birds impoverishes the earth. But the extinction of Homo sapiens (along with music, arts, spirituality, and all human culture) would impoverish the earth more profoundly.

Protect and promote the greatest depth for the greatest span. Exactly *how* to do that is the great province of moral intuition and practical wisdom because there is no one single, best, instrumental answer. This is not calculus; it is the messy world of human flesh and its interaction.

Who Do You Throw to the Sharks?

One interesting ethical practice sharpens moral sensibilities and discrimination by asking difficult questions. Consider deeply how you would implement the *basic moral intuition* in the trickiest of circumstances. Life has a way of continually presenting unexpected situations to challenge your ethical assumptions.

A classic ethical conundrum is the lifeboat dilemma. Imagine that your mother ship has floundered, and you, as captain of a lifeboat in shark-infested waters, face a terrible choice. The boat now holds ten people but can only safely hold seven. To jeopardize everyone in order to avoid making a difficult choice would be morally indefensible. So you have to act—and fast.

But whom do you throw overboard? Obviously you must consider various factors. Einstein clearly stays on board over Hitler. So does Gandhi, or an innocent child. But other choices can be quite difficult. If only one can fit, do you save Mother Teresa, a young mother of five, or a brilliant, dedicated young trauma surgeon? Who do you value more highly—a swimming dog that has already saved three lives, or a cowardly criminal that stepped over others to save himself?

These are deep, paradoxical, and difficult questions to answer. Although there is no *one* right solution, some solutions are *more right* than others. Even if there are no absolute rules, it is easy to make mistakes, and our ability to make these choices wisely grows along a developmental trajectory. So there is most certainly a practice of vertical ethical discrimination.

Ground, Intrinsic, and Relative Value

Integral Ethics recognizes three distinct kinds of value that beings possess:

Ground value refers to the fact that every entity—from a quark to a blade of grass to a human being—is *equally* an expression of absolute Spirit, emptiness, Suchness, or God. In this ground sense, every being and natural system—and especially every *person*—is infinitely precious and equally deserving of ethical regard. In all of our talk of depth and span, we must keep this ground value in mind.

Intrinsic value refers to development depth. The more depth, the more intrinsic value. Remember, depth is not a simplistic ladder, for we must take into account all aspects of development when referring to depth.

Relative value points to usefulness in a specific context. For instance, in the lifeboat scenario above, the trauma surgeon may not have as much intrinsic value as Mother Teresa, but he is able to save more lives in a desperate situation. (You can see how tricky the balancing act between depth and span can be!)

Meeting Ethical Dilemmas

In living practice, we must frequently balance the competing ethical demands of a situation. We must sometimes choose among important, yet competing, personal, cultural, social, and natural values. And we are also sometimes confronted in 1st, 2nd, and 3rd person. Sometimes we must ask, "What should *I* do?"; sometimes we wonder, "What should *we* do?"; and sometimes we need to determine, "What should be done about *it?*"

Integral Ethics points us in the general direction of the evolutionary, upward-trending developmental grain of the universe (or Eros), but it grounds us in care for the entire spectrum, from top to bottom, with an *intention* to preserve the health and well-being of the whole (or Agape).

This practice of making normative judgments of relative goodness is a muscle often banished from polite, politically correct, postmodern society, but in many life situations it remains crucial. Thus, moral discernment is a capacity that needs to be exercised and developed, which takes courage, clarity, and practice!

Morality and Ethics

So far we've been using "ethics" to signify the whole realm of ethics, morals, laws, and behaviors. As you may have noticed, we've been using the words "ethics" and "morals" interchangeably. However, Integral theory does make a technical distinction between the two. In addition to sometimes describing the whole ethical-moral realm, ethics can also refer particularly to the common values and expectations of a specific group (for example, a professional group, such as doctors or lawyers), while morality refers to the judgments made by an individual. We can use the 4 quadrants to distinguish the two, as well as see their relationship to **behavior**, which is what an individual *actually does*, and **laws**, which are the systems of rules and constraints that govern collective behavior.

As individuals we make moral choices ("What should I do?") that result in our behaviors ("What I actually do"). As a culture, we debate the ethics of both individual and collective choices ("What should we do?"), and create enforceable rules or laws ("What we must do"), and consequences for violating them.

There is another, more general sense in which we use the word "ethics"—as an umbrella term for the *practice of basic goodness* itself. In this sense, there is an "ethics" to being an ILP practitioner, just as there

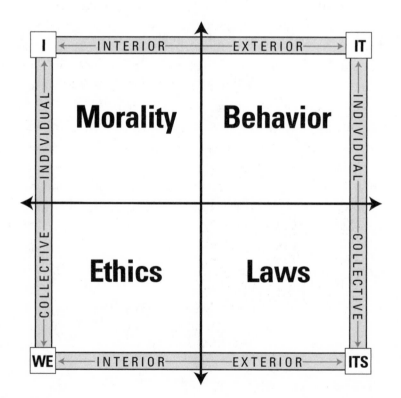

Figure 8.2
The 4 quadrants of ethics.

is one to being a doctor or lawyer or public servant. However, ILP culti-

vates a post- (and even post-post) conventional form of ethics, which implies a highly individual—and yet still universal—form of judgment.

What makes Integral Ethics universal is not that any particular rules
are applied in a totalistic manner, but that it acknowledges a universal,
evolutionary impulse (or "Eros") toward **greater depth** on the one hand,
and **greater span** on the other. Another way of putting this is that an
Integral Ethics attempts to honor and include the *most possible* perspectives (greater span), while giving proportionate weight to the *deepest* or
highest perspectives (greater depth).

Don't Be Partial: 4 Quadrants of Ethical Practice

There is another sense in which Integral Ethics encompasses all 4 quadrants. If your existence comprises these 4 basic dimensions of I, We, It,

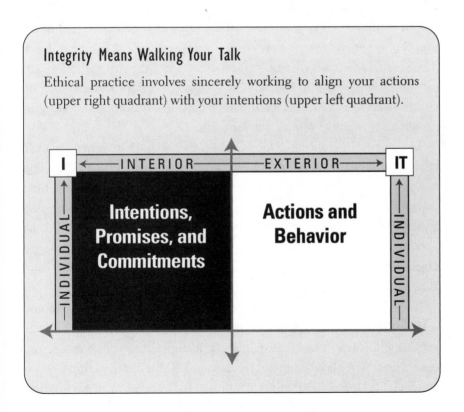

Integrity Means Walking Your Talk

Ethical practice involves sincerely working to align your actions
(upper right quadrant) with your intentions (upper left quadrant).

| **I** | ←——INTERIOR——— | ———EXTERIOR——→ | **IT** |

INDIVIDUAL

Intentions, Promises, and Commitments

Actions and Behavior

INDIVIDUAL

and Its, then it follows that your ethical practice can (and must) inhabit all 4 quadrants. Recall the different phenomena that arise in each of the 4 quadrants. How would you relate ethically to these different aspects of your being-in-the-world? What would an all-quadrant approach to ethics look like?

Upper-Left Quadrant, I

Your individual-interior or "I" space is the seat of your ethical **cognition**. Your interior level of development—or the number of perspectives you can hold in your awareness—will determine the range and depth of ethical choices you can make. The Upper-Left quadrant is also the domain of your ethical **conscience**, where you determine what you should uniquely *own* as yours—your responsibility, your fault, or your opportunity to make right. A key Upper-Left ethical practice is **self-reflection**, plumbing your own depths, examining your heart, and questioning yourself in the quest for moral clarity.

There are thoughts, intentions, and wishes in your Upper-Left quadrant that no one else may ever know. And yet, *you* must live with them. They are, in a manner of speaking, between you and Spirit in the 2nd person. But this also highlights the need for your ethical practice to include **shadow work**, as a means of removing emotional distortions and unwarranted assumptions from your judgments.

Finally, your Upper-Left quadrant is the domain of **intra-psychic** ethics. Simply put, this means, "How do you treat *yourself?*" Are you truthful with yourself? Do you abuse or neglect yourself? Do you hold yourself accountable? Are you *compassionate*, in both masculine and feminine modes as the situation requires, toward *yourself?*

Upper-Right Quadrant, It

What are your behaviors? What are their larger impacts?

If the body can be considered a temple, then how you treat this sacred vehicle is part of your Upper-Right ethical practice. This could include actions with respect to exercise, diet, appearance, the use of drugs, and even things like plastic surgery. But remember, there are multiple levels at which an Upper-Right ethics can function. Integral Ethics is not necessarily against using or modifying the body (including brain chemistry and genetics, as well as subtle and causal energy management) in unconventional ways. It asks us to discern between *pre*-conventional and *post*-conventional ethical expressions, which can sometimes be tricky because both are *un*-conventional.

As an extension of your bodily ethics, you might also consider how you treat *any* "it," whether a natural object, a cultural artifact, or a personal possession. Could there be, for example, an ethics to how you treat your laptop computer or your car? A book or a beautiful painting? Your relationship to these things might be merely instrumental, or it might be sentimentally charged. But there's a sense in which you have an ethical choice regarding how you treat the *things* in your life.

Behavior is the most eloquent and powerful expression of your ethics, reaching into all the other quadrants in practical, real-world terms.

Lower-Left Quadrant, We

The Lower-Left quadrant is where ethical practice is traditionally believed to reside, and it comes down to the question: "How should I treat *you?*" Through our ethical choices with respect to each other, we create a "We" space; and so we also ask: "How should we treat one another?" Lower-Left Integral Ethics is thus a practice of nurturing and evolving all the various "We" spaces we inhabit. Some of these "We" spaces of ethical practice include:

- Friendships
- Sexual relationships
- Marriage and family
- Work/school relationships
- Anyone we come in contact with (for example, the supermarket cashier)
- Animals (did you kick the cat?)
- Any *potential* "we"—national, global, species

Within all these "We" spaces of ethical concern there are various *levels* across which ethics is practiced. An *all levels* perspective changes the way in which you *communicate* your ethical care and concern within your various "We" spaces. Namely, you learn to speak in terms that the other can understand. A *mutual-Turquoise* friendship will have a very different ethical flavor than a *Turquoise-relating-to-Amber* family relationship (as you may have already experienced for yourself).

Lower-Right Ethics, Its

How do we care for the *systems* and *environment* on which our lives depend? This is the domain of Lower-Right quadrant ethics. It includes:

- The natural environment and ecosystems
- Technology infrastructure—transportation, Internet, etc.
- Home
- Government
- Schools
- Health system
- Economic system
- Business organization
- Justice system

Key questions here include, "How does my behavior affect the system?" and "How should we organize it?" (Where "it" refers to the system in question, a collection of "its.") Or from a vertically oriented perspective, we can ask, "What level of consciousness does this system reflect and support? Or, how can we make this system serve the greatest depth for the greatest span?"

The environmental movement's central concern is the earth system. So when we deal with questions of conservation, renewable energy, recycling, sustainability, land use, and so forth, these are Lower-Right ethical concerns. Civic responsibility, social activism, and political action engage both the Lower-Left and Lower-Right quadrants, often in the service of evolving our institutions.

On a more personal level, a Lower-Right ethical practice might be how you wish to organize, clean, and decorate your home. Just as your Upper-Right body can be a temple, and thus deserving of ethical regard, your Lower-Right living space could be considered another kind of temple.

The Art of Integral Ethics

In this section, we look at some of the more subjective aspects of Integral Ethics—how and why you might want to *creatively live* with an Integral ethical framework, on a day-to-day basis.

Three Reasons for Living Ethically

1. Feeling Good by Doing Good

Once we get ethics unstuck from lists of rigid rules, it is often equated with unselfish or altruistic behavior. But that too is a limited view. It presupposes a radical separation between self and other—a distinction that doesn't hold up at higher developmental levels. Of course, ethics can and often does show up as selflessness, but it can also be seen as the wisest form of *selfishness*.

Unethical behaviors create a much more complicated life. You have to remember your lies to keep them straight and otherwise avoid repercussions of your cheating and betrayal. Like a life of crime, it doesn't pay; it's a foolish way to live. An ancient spiritual insight says that one of the secrets of a happy life is to minimize your entanglements with negative karmas. Living ethically keeps your entanglements to a minimum, which keeps your consciousness clear and your subtle energy body healthy and open. You literally *feel* better.

Living ethically simultaneously benefits both you and everyone in your life. It enables you to live most happily, to bless others freely, and to minimize the inevitable unhappy entanglements that tend to accrue from unethically engaging the complications of life. You find yourself living in a field of goodwill, which is great for those who come into contact with you and also a very smart move.

Ethical behavior supports an intelligent, healthy, happy, fulfilled, productive, successful life. Ethics is not only how we can express our care and compassion for others—it's also a way to simplify our life and maintain a clear conscience. It's how we live with integrity, which makes us far more powerful and authoritative. It's how we earn respect—from others and ourselves.

2. Transforming to Higher Stages of Awareness

An ethical intention forces you to take the perspectives of others and thus grow in your own consciousness. Anytime you take another's perspective, not only do you better serve that person, but you also facilitate your own evolution. Transforming our consciousness in this way is one of the most important benefits of ethical living.

To review how this process of development works: At a certain developmental level, ethics takes the form of transcending chaotic selfish impulses and behaving according to moral laws. At this conventional (Amber) stage, morality means following strict rules that differentiate right from wrong. (Thank heaven for such rules! They make possible everything we call "civilized.")

But at a higher stage of development, our ethical framework starts to outgrow those perspectives, while still being capable of appreciating and including aspects of them. At this point, we start considering the underlying patterns of happiness and unhappiness that our speech and actions set in motion.

This leads to *post-conventional* ethical motives that embrace most conventionally moral behavior within a wider perspective, which is more capable of thinking in terms of paradoxes, shades of grey, contradictions, and competing values. It doesn't always conform to the old rules anymore (and sometimes creates the context for rebelling against them) and is therefore often misunderstood by both its proponents and critics.

But that's not the end of it. Ethics keeps evolving. Integral Ethics holds tremendous paradox, including caring passionately for the coexistence of all these (often battling) perspectives—while still unflinchingly facing and responding to the obligation to embody care and compassion through the specific, unavoidable hard choices of every individual life.

Ultimately, we go beyond merely avoiding doing harm to others. We start actively attempting to do good—through compassionate service and even a passionate personal mission.

3. Ethical Living Creates a Container for Awakening

Some openings into higher awareness confer a sense of mind-blowing freedom. Especially in a post-conventional ethical context, that can easily give rise to a subtle arrogance, the tacit sense that we are now operating beyond karma.* This is a huge error. Without a clear ethical practice, this subtle arrogance can easily lead to traumatic entanglements. We've all heard stories of apparently immoral behavior by supposedly enlightened spiritual teachers.

A classic stage on the Zen path is the experience of utter release from ordinary limitations—and it's wise to note that the *next higher* stage is sometimes called "falling from grace." Just because you've awakened from the "dream" of karmic existence, doesn't mean the dream goes away. The higher your stage of development, the harder it becomes to pretend that you're not connected to everything and everyone. Others may feel it too. You might even feel tremendously powerful and free. Ethical living prevents the dream (even as you awaken through it) from becoming a nightmare. When conventional self-protective or fear-based motives disappear, an ethical practice is what keeps us out of trouble.

On the positive side, ethics simplifies your relationship to the world of apparent others so that you're not distracted by petty conflicts all the time—and this makes it more likely that your awareness will open to the ever-present. Ethics in and of itself won't cause this awakening (you can no more attain the ever-present than you can your own nose!), but it can help you avoid doing the things that otherwise would *delay or prevent* it, and it can make you more capable of maintaining that nondual awareness once you realize it.

Take an Unflinching Look at the Costs of Unethical Behavior

Even though your ethical perspective evolves, there's a reliable measure for your moment-to-moment ethical practice—and it's always at hand. Like it or not, you are keenly aware of the difference between your actions that do and do not meet *your own internal ethical standards*.

---

*Here the word "karma" is used to mean what it meant traditionally. It refers to the law of cause and effect, which means that we tend to "reap what we sow," or that "what goes around comes around."

Awareness and Care

Awareness and care are two of the primary themes of Integral Life Practice. Awareness expresses Big Mind while care expresses Big Heart.

Integral Ethics:

- Involves sincerely bringing as much awareness and care as possible to the moment
- Shows up as behaviors animated sincerely by our greatest available awareness and care
- Serves to increase the awareness and care we and others will be able to bring to future moments

Thus, ethics is not just the cultivation of care and compassion. It is also the cultivation of *awareness*. I can only care for what is in my awareness. If my care is sincere, it asks for continual expansion of my awareness.

New awareness expands my circle of care and compassion. Care demands new awareness. Awareness grows, care grows, awareness grows, care grows. . . .

Do you inwardly wince, actually experiencing mental, emotional, or psychic pain, when you feel your unethical behavior? Do you glow with good feeling when contemplating your best behavior? An inner monitor makes us all aware of our ethical lapses, and our ethical exemplars—even in the muddy zones where we lack ethical clarity.

Our ethical lapses are closely associated with negative, unhappy, unskillful states of mind and emotion. We generally *behave* our worst when we inwardly *feel* the worst.

Not only do our ethical lapses occur when we're at our worst, but they also *set in motion a whole stream of effects and causes that tend to **keep** us at our worst*. Unethical actions often create and reinforce the same kinds of negative, unhappy, and unskillful states of mind and emotion that give rise to them.

Our most ethical behavior propagates positive, happy, skillful states of mind and emotion. Our most courageous and generous behavior happens when we're at our best, and it tends to set us up for future moments when we feel good and are able to act in accordance with our highest values.

We pay dearly for our ethical lapses. And wise ethical choices repay us handsomely.

- The *short-term* costs of unethical behavior are *unhappy, contracted, and unskillful states of mind and emotion.*
- The *long-term* costs of unethical behavior are worse—a *vicious cycle* of lies, self-contempt, and denial that erodes the foundations of our integrity and virtue.

When we do things we don't respect, or can't bear to openly confess, we automatically generate defenses to cope with our feelings. "Oh what a tangled web we weave . . ." In one way or another, we almost always hide our ethical lapses from others, and often even from ourselves. This robs us of free energy and binds our attention. And this gives rise to upset feelings that further sap our energy.

Deception has extremely high costs. It divides our psyche, undermines our self-esteem, compromises our core commitments, and just weighs us down. Self-deception has the highest costs. It results in psychological repression, driving aspects of our experience into the unconscious and thus building inaccessible layers of unconscious conflict within us. In other words , it *adds* to the shadow. This weakens our ability to show up with integrity, to make wholehearted choices and commitments, and to live most effectively and powerfully.

Both ethical and unethical behaviors usually become self-perpetuating patterns. Unethical behavior makes it harder to find our way back to wholeness and happiness. Ethical behavior not only makes us happier, it makes it easier for us to make good choices in the next moment.

Getting Off Easy

"Crunch!" went the fender as it crumpled behind me. "Oh no! I can't afford the extra insurance premiums, the embarrassment, the delay, the hassles . . . I glanced up, down, and around. No one had seen or heard what had happened! I quickly sped away.

Weeks passed. No phone calls from an aggrieved party. No fender-bender on my record. It seems I got away with it, doesn't it? I thought so at the time.

But 20-20 hindsight tells a different story.

For months I felt cunning, ashamed, less confidently able to own and inhabit my best instincts and highest aspirations. Inside, I felt like I was a sneaky, cheating rat. (I was!) I had placed my chips on getting away with things instead of being someone I'm proud to be.

And that choice continued to resonate for years. I had undermined my sense of integrity. I didn't feel I deserved or had a right to hold my head high and take a stand for what I saw to be noble or true. So I lived under a shadow from which I had to extricate myself, bit by bit, over years.

I paid a much higher, intangible price than the extra insurance premiums and the $500 deductible. Getting off easy can be extremely expensive.

What Integral Ethics Is Not

1. Conventional Ethics

We've already discussed the most common misconception—that ethics and morality are equated with conventional conformity or traditional social norms that hand down absolute distinctions between right and wrong.

Post-conventional and Integral ethics grow beyond these narrow definitions and see that ethical choices can be better discerned by one's *intentions*, rather than one's outward *behavior*.

This does not absolve us of responsibility for bad outcomes based on sloppy execution or for unintentional damage we may do to others. In fact, it provokes awareness and a sense of responsibility for the care and skill we bring to every aspect of what we do.

A deeper point: While criticizing the limitations of conventional ethical perspectives, people sometimes end up behaving irresponsibly in the name of a higher perspective. This is an example of the *pre/trans* (or *pre/post*) fallacy, where *pre*-conventional actions are mistaken for *post*-conventional ones, because they are both **non**-conventional. This is a common and baleful consequence of postmodern relativism. High postmodern insights can inadvertently open the way for regression into lower-level moral functioning.

Paradoxically, *Integral Ethics often reaffirms respect for conventional moral behaviors,* but for very different reasons. For example, because we value the importance of living in an orderly, lawful society, we might choose to obey the letter of the laws that we deem unnecessary. When driving, I might come to a full stop at a stop sign and signal my turn, even when no other cars are near the intersection. When we do this, it's not because we're bound by conventional ethics, but because we want to live in a society where everyone obeys certain rules. Such morality might look almost identical to conventional morality from the outside, but Integral Ethics is based on a deep, nuanced, and solidly post-conventional perspective.

2. Meek and Mild

The second common misconception is that high-level ethical or moral behavior necessarily means a total absence of (even healthy) aggression.

However, the ability to defend the boundaries of the self is a necessary stage in development and **a crucial developmental capacity**. Integral Ethics is developmentally informed and thus values the capacity for healthy defense of self-boundaries. Thus, there is a place for appropriate, skillful, healthy aggression in Integral ethical behavior.

There is no need to idealize care for others at the expense of care for self. Healthy care begins with care for self and extends in concentric circles to care for our family, friends, community, and world. We care for self *and* others, not others *instead of* self.

An individual who practices mature Integral Ethics must inhabit both masculine and feminine compassion when appropriate. Feminine compassion expresses itself as acceptance, care, nurturance, and sweetness. Masculine compassion expresses itself as discrimination, challenge, setting limits, and ruthless truth-telling—all motivated by love. We need to be able to mobilize both capacities in order to embody Integral Ethics.

3. Residual Guilt and Faux Ethical Lapses

A third common confusion comes in the form of false ethical conflicts. People sometimes think they must be experiencing an ethical conflict when they're actually just confused about contradictions between social messages and their own ethical instincts. This usually occurs while people are in the midst of outgrowing one set of moral and social structures and haven't yet fully inhabited their new perspectives.

For example, after thirty years of being a very sweet wife to her high-achieving husband, Judith was shocked to hear herself telling him "Go to hell!" over a minor inconsiderate act. "What's wrong with me?" she thought. "This is terrible behavior." She felt guilty, thinking she had behaved unethically. But she hadn't. Judith needed to show herself—and her husband—that she had outgrown the traditional submissive role she had been living out. Once she'd made some room for herself, she could animate kindness (or toughness) by choice, as an expression of a much freer way of being. Healthy self-love had burst a profane leak in the old code of behaviors.

Many people spend years sorting out residual feelings of guilt over intelligently realizing they can't necessarily tell the whole truth about all things to all people at lower developmental levels, in particular to authority figures like bosses, parents, or teachers, who aren't capable of accepting certain truths. There's a big difference between compassionately and openheartedly speaking as much truth as can be heard (when someone just can't yet hear and process it all in a balanced way) and its alternatives. On one hand, we might speak truths that are unkind, hurt others, or create separation. On the other hand, we can justify the withholding of information by conveniently assuming a posture of superiority and condescension that unnecessarily distances us from others. It can take great integrity and discrimination (and often years of learning and growth) to act skillfully on the basis of these distinctions.

When this kind of clarity is gained, such false ethical conflicts fall away. Nevertheless, these same situations may remain knotty practical problems of communication and perception, even ones that require new skills and awareness, and that require time to master with grace and ease. But they are not genuine *ethical* conflicts anymore.

Completing Your Karmas

Unethical behavior usually hurts somebody in particular or society at large. That damage leaves a legacy. Whether or not we actively feel guilty about a past misdeed, it almost always remains as a subtle loose end. It lingers as a festering or incomplete transaction with our world. It places limiting conditions on our integrity. It also shows up in the relationship with whomever we have hurt.

A useful word for this is "karma." We use it here not in its traditional sense (as we did on p. 271) and without intending all the often confused ideas that some people associate with this word. It's just a quick, economical word to refer to *the intangible burdens we unconsciously take on when we harm others*.

One ethical practice is to complete your incomplete karmas. You can confess and apologize. You can make financial restitution. You can ask for forgiveness. You can do favors or services to redress the imbalance you have created.

But some wrongs can't be directly or easily redressed. Sometimes those we've hurt have died. Or the consequences of our actions are beyond correcting. Or there are far too many karmas to correct them all individually.

We can do only so much to complete certain karmas. We can face them in a fully authentic way. We can allow ourselves to feel genuine remorse; we can grieve the losses that are too late to heal; we can repent sincerely. Real repentance is deeply sobering. It puts our feet on the ground and establishes us more firmly in our sincere ethical intentions as we go forward into the future.

In real repentance, we are no longer hiding from ourselves. Thus, something karmic has been completed, even when we haven't been able to address it directly with the people we've hurt. We complete our karmas as much as we can by showing up in life in a way that reflects our sincerity and highest intentions.

An operational definition for Integral Ethics in this context is, "Don't create new negative karmas and complete what you can of the old."

It's Not What You Did; It's What You Do Next

Many times, we become conscious of our impulses toward unethical behavior only after the fact. They dawn on us later, in moments of grim 20-20 hindsight. We see that we acted at variance with our ethical compass. We're caught like a deer in our own headlights, visible — at least to ourselves — as a lying, cheating, or otherwise dirty rat. It feels too late to be the person we aspired to be.

A wash of new impulses spills through us: "Will I get caught?" "Will others find out?" "What will they think?" "What can I do or say to make it better?" We feel ashamed. And we want to make the whole thing go away.

It's time to remember: *"It's not what you did; it's what you do next."*

This is a crucial moment of choice. It's the moment in which fake excuses, lies, and cover-ups often get set in motion, magnifying your bad karma. It's also your first best opportunity to nip that bad karma in the bud.

The big crime isn't merely the accident; it's also *leaving the scene of the accident.* It's not only the original scandal; it's *the cover-up.* It's not only what you did, but what you do next. Many of our worst ethical nightmares stem from the bad choices we make when we're already feeling bad about ourselves, and we don't want to face the consequences.

Seize the opportunity. Summon the courage to admit your mistake, to apologize or make reparations when appropriate, and to endure the embarrassment or costs of making things straight. Not easy. But the secret is this: *It's a bargain!* Concealing our misdeeds only heaps penalties and interest onto the painful price we want to avoid paying in the first place. It's smart to bite the bullet and move on with a lighter heart and a clearer mind. When you face your ethical lapse and take responsibility for it, you no longer have to conceal it, feel guilty, or feel less self-respect, thereby diminishing your free energy, attention, and personal power.

A key to authentic Integral Ethics is acceptance of your fallibility. When you commit to behaving ethically, in the back of your mind you know you're setting yourself up for a future moment when you'll discover you just blew it. That's 100 percent fine. In fact, it's the nature of practice itself.

Practice is like riding a bicycle. You can't guarantee that you'll never fall off the bicycle. After all, it's a long road, and you can't see what it will bring. You can only commit that if you fall, you'll waste as little time as possible dusting yourself off and getting back on the bicycle. You can rest assured that you can always do at least that.

Ethics and Your Relationship to Yourself

Abusive inner behavior toward oneself ranks high among the many psychological diseases of postmodern society. It's the case of the excessively harsh self-critic. Many individuals' inner parents are unkind, and their self-talk is peppered with expletives, hostility, insults, harsh negative judgments, and a lingering mood of suspicion. So your relationship to yourself is a rich arena for ethical practice, feminine compassion, and self-healing.

However, you also need to give yourself masculine compassion. Sometimes our negative self-talk is based on the very accurate perceptions of our conscience or of discriminative self-awareness. We've blown it! It's not just important to treat yourself compassionately; it's also crucial that you see yourself accurately and take responsibility for living up to your highest values and possibilities.

It can even be unethical to discard valid self-judgments, since they're our best guide to ethical growth and new self-responsibility. True ethical behavior in your relationship with yourself must draw on both masculine and feminine compassion in a continuously regulated balance.

Let's take a closer look at this crucial yin-yang dynamic.

Masculine Self-Compassion

Living consciously requires clear choices, limits, and boundaries. The river needs the riverbanks in order to flow to the sea. Without masculine self-compassion, practice can drift aimlessly.

Masculine self-compassion has two dimensions: **discernment**, or the unflinching courage to face unpleasant realities, and **discipline**, or the willingness to choose and enforce new behaviors and habits in place of old patterns that no longer serve.

Expressing your masculine self-compassion is a tremendous act of self-love. Through doing so, you earn more self-respect and empower yourself to show up in your life with more natural authority. This liberates tremendous energy and ability to focus — which goes right to your bottom line, enabling you to be the person you want to be in practice, work, and key relationships.

One of the core secrets of transformative practice is the enormous impact of intentionally intruding upon and interrupting your comfortable habits. To do so consistently is a secret of keeping your practice alive.

Feminine Self-Compassion

Masculine and feminine self-compassion can coexist quite well. Neither discernment nor discipline requires harsh judgments or a closed heart. You don't have to hate yourself to see your patterns and choose new ones. Feminine self-compassion actually greases the wheels of discipline, because it eases the tendency for parts of the self to get locked into unproductive resistance to each other.

The habit of negative self-talk doesn't change easily. Your first best step may be to soften and accept the inner abuser. An interior environment of self-acceptance and forgiveness has to begin somewhere.

Gradually, greeted with compassionate acceptance, the inner judgment and self-hatred will themselves begin to soften. You can't always change the self-talk, but you can relax in the midst of it and gently cultivate an inner atmosphere of acceptance and gratitude.

As you begin to treat yourself with more compassion and appreciation, it becomes natural and authentic to extend that compassion and appreciation to others.

The Ethics of Shadow Work

One of the kindest things you can do for the people closest to you is to become responsible for your psychological projections. When people are so preoccupied with past unresolved issues that they can't see us for who we are and relate to us openly in present time, we hate it!

And yet it is the nature of the human psyche that our most painful experiences are hidden in shadow. We are all prone to project our unresolved feelings onto important people in our lives—lovers, authority figures, mother and father figures, sibling substitutes, underlings—the list goes on and on.

When we do this, we indirectly and unconsciously discharge negative emotions and limiting images in the direction of those who trigger us.

We do the whole world a favor when we bring these tendencies into consciousness and start owning our projections. In the process, we make ourselves far more fun to work and play with (and, incidentally, improve the way others treat us in return).

Flying Under Altitude

The ethical importance of shadow work also holds for our "golden shadows"—the *higher* parts of us that we deny or repress. For example, if you're capable of making a highly nuanced, Turquoise discernment and taking action on its basis, but you're *flying under the radar*—because you don't want to get shot at—you might cop out and show up as if you were seeing things from a more socially acceptable, Green perspective. This kind of thing happens all the time, and important values get sacrificed whenever it occurs. Witness the many stultifying taboos—from anti-intellectualism to extreme political correctness—that people allow to proliferate unchecked and unquestioned.

For instance, "boomeritis," the unhealthy or "sour" side of Green, in its attempts to avoid marginalizing or subtly discriminating against anyone or anything, has often gone to the extreme of trying to shatter everyone's perceptual compasses, calling all developmental distinctions "elitist" and "patriarchal." While well-intentioned, this is a disaster, because it creates confusion about the reality—and verticality—of growth and maturation. In order not to fly under the radar, we must make necessary discernments and judgments of vertical depth.

Participating within a community of fellow Integral Life Practitioners will hold us accountable to our true capabilities and encourage us to straighten up and fly *at our highest authentic altitude*. An example of this is an exercise sometimes done during Quaker meetings—"Let the next thing out of your mouth be from your highest self." The injunction not to fly below altitude, not to function below our highest and best possibility, is a way to call upon this crucial aspect of vertical ethical practice.

Expanded Ethical Responsibility

As you embrace the disposition of 100 percent ethical responsibility, you'll begin to notice expanded perspectives.

For example, am I ethically responsible for the behavior of my spouse? Not entirely. But I have a responsibility to engage her, and I have some influence on her. I have some responsibility for the choices and behaviors we make as a couple. Similarly, I have some responsibility for the behavior of my children and of my pets.

Am I responsible for the behavior of the organization for which I work? For the institution I belong to? My community? My culture at large? My nation?

Clearly, I have less and less ability to personally determine the behavior of larger and larger groups. And yet, these groups have no locus of

responsibility other than their individual members. If I have no responsibility, then neither does anyone else. That doesn't fly. No way around it, we each do have some real and crucial responsibility.

In high stages of awakening, we are aware of our inseparability from the entire evolving Kosmos. Thus, as they awaken people often come to feel a profound sense of responsibility for the entire world. This is not grandiosity, but a passionate and serious commitment. Paradoxically, this does not call forth an overly heavy mood that suppresses humor, playfulness, and enjoyment, but rather one that inspires clear eyes, an open heart, and a straight spine. It's a commitment to facing your own hypocrisy—and growing beyond it. It shows up as a courageous willingness to creatively, seriously, and responsibly participate with others in shouldering your share of the hard work in this unfolding evolutionary adventure.

This is, of course, a profound koan (a Zen riddle, a question to be lived and learned from rather than glibly answered). Responsibility for our society and world is especially poignant because our human and natural world faces tremendous challenges, and because our institutions and societies play enormous roles in creating terrible suffering and destruction on a global scale. Together we face many challenges without obvious solutions.

How do we engage our responsibility for the groups and systems of which we are members? How do we exercise healthy care for ourselves while extending ethical, civic responsibility for our larger society and world? These are deep, difficult, and important questions.

As we mature, we grow in our capacity to engage these riddles. Our sense of responsibility for our world eventually becomes a healthy, powerful, and integrated commitment, entirely different from the naïve zeal of the idealistic revolutionary. Expressing an authentic sense of purpose, mission, and service to others and the world is a kind of heroism to which anyone can aspire. Such a balanced commitment is not just awake, but also grounded, sober, and stable. A sense of great urgency is held within a deeper patient acceptance. There is certainly great value in revolutionary idealism, but Integral Ethics *also* acknowledges the wisdom of reform, incremental changes, conservation, and practical idealism.

No Matter How Far You Travel, There's Always a Horizon

As we grow, our ethical practice evolves, and at each stage of growth, we can notice three ethical domains:

1. Ethical issues for which we are consistently responsible. (For example, most of us would never seriously considering committing murder.)
2. Ethical issues for which we are often but not always perfectly responsible. (This is the domain in which we are practicing and growing.)
3. More nuanced ethical responsibilities of which we're just becoming aware. (This might include shadow material and unintentional inconsiderate behavior, such as interrupting others, cutting into traffic, or indirectly communicating implicit negativity, for example.)

The key point is this: *everyone* **has an ethical practice with a growing edge**. A sincere practitioner is never morally complacent.

This is why the greatest saints' journals confess their selfish hearts and continual turning away from God. Meanwhile, the world in which all of us practice (including the highest saints) *keeps changing*, presenting us with new and more complex challenges.

The more deeply we understand ethical practice, the more humble we are, deeply aware of the endless layers of dynamic ethical challenge. Paradoxically, we also become simpler, lighter, and more self-accepting.

Since ethical dilemmas are unavoidable (not a sign of some terrible inner flaw in us), we paradoxically become more lighthearted about doing our best to swim with integrity in the murky waters of our wide and often rather weird world.

The Lightness of Integral Ethics

Conventional ethics involves restraining one's impulses and submitting to higher injunctions. It builds essential capacities that could be called "moral muscles." Early conventional ethics is mostly about obedience,

while more mature conventional ethics emphasizes responsibility to the values of the group to which you belong.

Early post-conventional ethics tends to focus on the virtues of choice, freedom, excellence, and independent judgment. Individuals with a post-conventional ethics aren't afraid to stand apart from the crowd and break free from oppressive moral constraints. More mature post-conventional ethics builds caring sensitivity for others, which can develop into a sense of stewardship and service.

Integral Ethics embodies the intelligence and capacities of *all* ethical levels. Its spirit is light and generous, not heavy or shadowed by guilt. Even though this section has focused on noticing the costs of ethical lapses and on expressing intelligent care in every moment, please don't relate to these instructions childishly, as if they were your inner parent's "shoulds."

Notice that Integral Ethics is an opportunity for happiness and freedom—an invitation to engage ethical practice in a spirit of caring curiosity, intelligence, and passionate aliveness. It is *not* a matter of recasting your entrenched sense of dutiful obedience into more expanded terms. Let your practice be ethical in the sense that it is heartfelt, caring, and generous, and let it remain informed by the fierce spirit that also chooses freedom and self-expression. *Be free* to care more and more fully. *Expand joyfully* into profound and ever-growing freedom and responsibility.

9

Living Your Life as Practice

Relationships, Work, Parenting, Creativity, and Other Additional Modules

The Flesh and Bones of ILP

If you haven't figured it out already, ILP is more than a nifty framework used to organize a bunch of scheduled exercises. It's not a glorified to-do list. (Check, check, check, done!) A living ILP involves a conscious orientation to the many waves, streams, and states of life as they flow through us moment by moment. It involves a willingness to learn from life—the ultimate classroom—and all the joyful and painful lessons it teaches.

So just because you show up for your yoga class and meditate doesn't mean you have completely fulfilled your ILP. Practice does not occur only on the meditation cushion, in the gym, or at the dojo. Even more essentially, it occurs in life's trenches. Practice is especially real and vital when we arrive late to the office, get into an argument with our lover, hear the baby crying again, or learn about a loved one's illness. Indeed, such tests and lessons, successes and failures, hirings and firings, love affairs and breakups, ecstasies and tragedies make up the guts of our lives and our practice.

A living practice involves accepting all of life's textures, blessings, and challenges as honored teachers. ILP invites you to view each life experience as a unique practice opportunity with a valuable lesson to bestow. Each new moment carries the karmic seeds of the previous moment while simultaneously bursting forth with its own creative signature never before witnessed. And as each instant transcends and includes what came before it—continuing some aspects of the whole past while bringing forth something new and alive—novel practice occasions spring into being. Every *now* is a new practice opportunity.

Practicing during the unscheduled and unpredictable twists of life requires a lucid intentionality and commitment to living consciously. ILP is the opposite of being on automatic pilot—mindlessly following inherited habits.

Between life's stimuli and our habitual responses exists *choice*. This means practice isn't an accident. It's chosen and re-chosen moment by moment and expressed through who we are, how we relate to others, and how we show up in the world.

Every area of life is a place to practice. And practice is particularly complex and dynamic when it involves relationships with *other people and systems*. These life areas are the focus of key additional modules of ILP, such as **Work, Intimate Relationships, Family, Finances, Friendships, Sex,** and **Service.** These are not the only additional modules; in fact, there are a virtually unlimited number.

The modules highlighted here are important and nearly universal. These modules are accessible dimensions of your own being-in-the-world, which can all be developed through practice. Everyone—regardless of their gender, race, creed, cultural background, geographical location, or sexual orientation—can participate in these fundamental areas of life. Yet the actual ways people engage and practice these modules will be radically diverse.

In general, the core modules of ILP focus on the top two quadrants—your individual growth and development. And in general, most of the additional modules of ILP focus on the bottom two quadrants—your growth and development as expressed in your social and relational life.*

---

*Although most of them involve relationships, some additional ILP modules address individual development. The Transmuting Emotions module (see chapter 4) and the Creativity module, for instance, are considered additional modules, but they are both usually practiced by individuals on their own.

The core modules are the core of practice. But life is the big game. We're tested most by our primary intimacies, our family life and parenting, our work, our creative expression, our finances, and in the rough-and-tumble of every other messy, relational area of life. All practice is a matter of bringing awareness and care to every moment of life, and no moment is unimportant.

Everybody's Got Their Stuff

Sustaining continual growth and change is not so easy. Almost all of us have adapted to unconscious patterns. Inborn tendencies interact with early life experiences, traumas, and relationship dynamics to lay down unique challenges for each individual. You may have dysfunctional behaviors, be identified with contracted sub-personalities, or locked into repetitive relationship cycles (as in the drama triangle of victim-persecutor-rescuer). Everybody's got their stuff.

Our stuff appears most clearly and painfully in our self-defeating patterns. People often leave a stuck marriage only to recreate the same

Figure 9.1

Individual and relational practices.

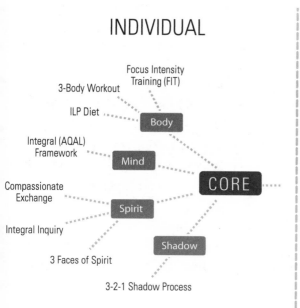
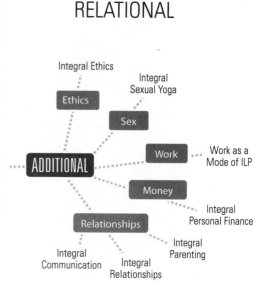

essential pattern with their next partner. At work, people often discover that their most limiting obstacles to effectiveness and success are their own unconscious beliefs, assumptions, and emotional patterns. Many people find it nearly impossible, even with decades of trying to act on good intentions, to free themselves from these limits.

Work and relationships are often the trickiest areas of practice, the acid test of maturity. These are the primary arenas through which people's patterns are mirrored, and in which their practice can show meaningful fruits — if they can really sustain enough presence, consciousness, and care, to supersede their habits and transform their work and relational lives.

Practice in all the core modules is still important, due to their synergistic impact on these other areas. Transforming your relationship to work, intimacy, family, money, or service, requires a full Integral practice.

It takes willingness to face your blind spots, unacknowledged feelings, and hidden drives (the Shadow module); to see clearly and make intelligent choices (the Mind module); to engage life with health, feeling, and an integrated body (the Body module); to be openhearted and awake to the ever-present Suchness of every moment (the Spirit module). It certainly requires a commitment to care for self, other, and Kosmos (the Ethics module).

But practicing these key modules in isolation is usually just the first step. All the capacities developed through practice in the core modules bear their most profound fruits when confronted with the untidy demands of everyday life. Thus, the Additional Modules are *very* important to most of us, even though they may not be universal. Some people choose a celibate, renunciate lifestyle, relinquishing conventional work and intimacies. But such choices are uncommon, and for most Integral Life Practitioners, several of the additional modules are as essential as the core modules.

Creating a life that works is important to almost everyone, whether or not they see it as a matter of practice. Integral Life Practice is a way to embrace the many tasks and goals that are crucial to a happy, functional life. The Integral disposition says yes to life on every level, which can

mean yes to relationships, family, work, and conventional success, affirming balance and ongoing growth.

But ILP frames it all as a continuous practice, rather than as an *ultimate* point. The ancient spiritual paths were founded on the insight that even the most excellent and blessed human lives are threatened by loss, sickness, old age, and death. They saw, quite deeply, that conventional fulfillment is fleeting. No matter how good your life can ever become, the moments of fulfillment will pass. This is a profound and enduring insight.

However, it doesn't necessarily follow (even though it was common in some of the ancient paths) that you should forsake certain kinds fulfillment altogether. Even though you will eventually die, health is still a very good idea in the meantime! It's possible to say yes to life *and* to awaken to that which transcends death. This inclusiveness reflects the Integral disposition. ILP helps you live an Integral life, saying yes to life while remaining aware that all fulfillments will eventually dissolve.

It's perfectly appropriate, within an Integral Life Practice, to commit wholeheartedly to goals for happiness and a successful career and relationship. In fact, it reflects a radical insight: there is no contradiction between life and death. There's not even a contradiction between trying to make life work and letting go into the inevitability of losing it all in the end. The Integral practitioner lives with these paradoxes.

So what about creating a life that works?

Effort, Surrender, Purpose, and Commitment

Creating a life that works requires effort. And yet too much effort can get in the way of practice. The most self-actualized lives often flow naturally and effortlessly.

As practice matures, you develop the intuitive skill it takes to live this paradox wisely—learning to bring effort and surrender appropriately to each moment of life. You'll get clear that when surrender is appropriate, it doesn't undermine commitment, leaving you to drift passively through your life. And when effort is appropriate it doesn't supplant or override your ability to open to larger forces, recognize what you can't control, or stay in touch with the present moment.

The natural evolutionary urge of the Kosmos arises in each of us as a drive toward self-actualization, awakening, and service. Every meaningful life has purpose. Some relate to ourselves—health, longevity, success, and happiness. And other aspects go beyond the self—an urge to make a contribution, to give our gifts, to serve our family, community, and world.

As we embrace our purpose, we can clarify a vision for ourselves—an intuitive picture of where our life and practice are taking us. That vision can become clear and specific, even to the point of being embodied in particular goals. When those objectives become clear, and we make a real commitment to realize them, tremendous power is unleashed. In chapter 10, we'll discuss practices for defining your life direction and clarifying your big picture as a part of the process of designing your ILP.

A Quick Tour of Some Additional Modules

Important additional modules include not just work and intimate relationships, but all the key areas we encounter in the school of life. Each of them is worth studying in depth. However, since every person's life is unique, there is a great deal of flexibility in what you might consider a true "module" of practice. Of course, we consider the 4 Core Modules, along with Integral Ethics, to be fundamental. But a life of practice can encompass *any* area in which you can cultivate your own development. Here are some suggested additional modules that could very easily be part of your Integral Life Practice:

Work
Work is a key area of practice since many of us spend more of our waking time working than in any other single activity. To be effective at work, most of us need to exercise *will*, or intention (a key area, even its own module of practice, to which we'll return later). The work module is an opportunity to incarnate grounded responsibility, mental and emotional self-management, functional effectiveness, time management, communication, interpersonal skills, and leadership ability. It is also a primary

opportunity to render service to others and to your community, and to fulfill and transmute your creative ambitions. It is also the arena in which to observe and cultivate your capacities and clarify your relationship to power, status, and personal identity. Practice in this module is usually multidimensional and continually evolving.

Money

No matter how successful (or unsuccessful!) you are in your work, managing your relationship to wealth and money is a distinct practice. It includes everything from balancing your checkbook to budgeting, from controlling your spending to setting goals for income and expenditures, from keeping usable records to making good investment decisions. Work is usually a necessary aspect of financial freedom, but financial management is the practice that usually matters most for security in old age and the opportunity to make creative use of money to serve others. Taking responsibility for a conscious relationship to money requires and builds important psycho-energetic capacities that can liberate one's creativity.

Time Management

Time management is a key aspect of the Work module for many people, but we make many important choices about how we use our time away from work as well. Time is your most precious and limited resource. Your relationship to time dictates your life's possibilities in countless ways. As your practice matures, your relationship with time can evolve, creating an efficient, free, and balanced rhythm of living, even while staying in touch with the timeless present.

Communication

Like time management, communication is an essential life skill. We all must learn to speak effectively to diverse individuals and groups, all of whom will hear what we say through any of a wide number of filters— different structures of awareness, values, identities, and morals. Effective communication requires listening and relationship skills. It will ultimately test you, exposing your weaknesses and drawing upon your strengths, thereby generating lessons and growth. Communication is a rich field of lifelong learning. And it makes the difference between an intimate relationship that stagnates and one that continually grows into deeper forms of loving.

Intimate Relationship

Many people's intimate relationships are their emotional home base, the dead center of fulfillment, frustration, insight, and growth. For everyone, it can be a central arena for learning and transformation. Intimacy and ecstasy are embodied here. Fears of abandonment and engulfment dance here, together with our primal needs for autonomy and communion. So it's a highly charged atmosphere. Throw in an array of hardwired differences and similarities that unite and divide men and women — and which show up in the play of masculine and feminine energies in relationships of any sexual orientation. It's a very spicy recipe!

To be a self-responsible individual, while living closely connected with a life partner and maintaining authentic love and mutual understanding, has never been easy. The accelerating pace of postmodern life has only made it more complicated. Traditional marriage and family patterns have been changing in fast-moving postmodern cultures, bringing unprecedented complexity into active, conscious, intimate relationships. The path of growth through committed relationship requires both partners to practice intensely, simultaneously, and in relation to each other, in the midst of many paradoxes. Even so, intimate relationships are among the richest and most transformational of life's opportunities. This profound yoga can be practiced in a wide variety of forms in traditional marriages, and in many new, non-traditional relationships as well.

Sexuality

Reproduction is vital to survival, so naturally our sexuality is one of the most powerful expressions of our primordial aliveness. We have an instinctual recognition of sexuality as the very psychoenergetic intensity out of which we were conceived and out of which our original human bonds were forged. It calls to us. Lived consciously, in all three bodies, sexuality can be profound, ecstatic, and transformative. It can be an occasion for the intimate exchange and circulation of life-energy. But it is always primarily an occasion for embodying intimacy, love, and care. Sexual yoga can draw from many practices, from ancient tantras to contemporary communication skills, and from passionate lovemaking to silent feeling-awareness, to celibate ardor for the Kosmic Beloved. Practiced consciously, sexuality can be a liberating and ecstatic practice.

Family and Parenting

Parental love is among life's most fulfilling experiences. But parenting is far from easy. Freud called it "the impossible profession," but it can just as accurately be called "the indispensable profession." Raising a conscious, loving, capable, and happy child is one of life's most important and challenging accomplishments. The task is huge: developing into a functional adult now requires much more than eighteen years, and parents' roles have expanded in other respects as postmodern life has become more complex. In the midst of cultural disruption, some traditional approaches to parenting are even more essential, while others are becoming inappropriate. Parents must provide their children's primary relationship and also create the structures that contain and shape their lives. This requires firm, age-appropriate, loving discipline as well as heartfelt authenticity. These are vital gifts, and to give them requires enormous commitment, courage, love, and discipline. It's a profound practice to keep showing up with as much awareness, care, and commitment as you can—even amidst all the chaos, delight, and heartbreak of launching one or more new lives. Practiced consciously, parenting develops great wisdom and compassion.

Community

We come to know aspects of ourselves only in group situations. We are social animals who learn through social feedback. We need to experience ourselves participating with others in communities of one kind or another—with classmates, friends, fellow practitioners, co-workers, and/or neighbors. We grow through our friendships, by receiving and giving. We grow through our relationships with other practitioners, in which we support others and are supported by a field of shared values and commitments. We also have responsibilities to our larger communities—local, national, and global. Some people fulfill this through community service of one kind or another; others engage in social responsibility or civic participation, including voting and politics, in order to express this responsibility to the larger community.

Service

Service with a glad heart is a direct way to tap into the energy that sustains life and uplifts the spirit. It is truly in giving that we receive most fully. One of the core secrets of happy living is the conscious practice of service with sincere intentionality. Everyone serves others, but not everyone approaches it in the spirit of service. And service can extend not just to other people but also to animals, plants, environments, systems, and to the whole natural world. As your devotional life becomes authentic and full, service is a way to bring that devotional spirit into action, using your whole body to enact your communion with the beloved Kosmos.

Nature

Communing with the natural world is key to many individuals' ILP. It may take the form of gardening, hiking, sailing, or doing physical service for nature by picking up trash or protecting endangered species. Wild plants and creatures can be profoundly healing and inspiring, and we can also enact our wholeness by taking care of them. Nature mysticism is an ancient and nearly universal expression of the Spirit module. Engaging the gross and subtle energies of natural environments, through all the senses, is just as central to the Body module.

Creativity

When people tap into "the muse," they make contact with a higher source of creative inspiration. Most dedicated artists pay their dues with long hours of perspiration too. Practicing an art requires discipline and surrender, and it can activate aspects of being that rarely surface in ordinary living. Opening to this creative flow is an inner yoga, one that shows up uniquely for each individual, whether their art is jazz improvisation, writing poetry, painting, dancing, singing, songwriting, acting, filmmaking, snowboarding, or graphic design. For many people, the practice of creativity is a key module, essential to their life practice. Creative expression can facilitate exceptional growth in one's whole human character and relationship to Spirit. For some individuals, practicing the cello is both central to their ILP and one of the deepest gifts they give to the world, independent of the notion of practice.

Will

The Work, Money, and even Relationship modules ask us to be capable of meeting our chosen goals and commitments. Almost all forms of practice imply a capacity to discipline ourselves. Underlying almost every human endeavor is the exercise of *intentionality*, or will. Your personal will can be approached as a module of its own. In fact, many well-known approaches to personal growth focus on the development of personal will, beginning with learning to discern priorities and make appropriate choices, maturing into making commitments, taking stands for what we wish to manifest in life, and ultimately becoming capable of magnetizing and enrolling others in our vision. This is not just a matter of having great "willpower," but of the *freedom* and *intelligence* of our willing. Full maturity means being able to exercise intention with extremely high effectiveness, but without undue stress or attachment to results. A highly developed will is usually essential to fulfilling one's life purpose.

The Affirmations practice presented later in this chapter is an excellent way to engage and cultivate your will. However, you'll also find that your *basic commitment to practice itself* will develop your power of intentionality in all other areas of life.

Using the Integral Framework in Daily Life

What makes ILP different from other approaches to practice is the Integral Framework. Practicing within an AQAL context—with your personal radar screen alert to the rich dimensions and perspectives present in every moment—enhances your lived experience. With a wider framework and consciousness you can literally let in more life, more reality. It's also true that an excessive focus on theory shrouds the actual territory it's attempting to illuminate. You can actually miss out on life, like a tourist with his head stuck in a map who forgets to look at the lush scenery all around him. Used wisely, however, the AQAL map illuminates life's evolving richness and depth so it can be experienced more fully.

You've already experienced how the multiple perspectives expressed by AQAL shed new light on familiar life areas such as Body, Mind, Spirit, and Shadow (the core ILP modules). Likewise, an Integral perspective offers unique contributions to the additional practice modules.

Integral theory does not tell you how to practice or how to live. Instead, it offers *new perspectives on practice and life, new possibilities, and new horizons.*

ILP strives for a balance between theory and practice, between the map and the territory. Having an Integral view clarifies the practice of parenting, sex, communication, leadership, and so on. Remember, the Integral Operating System works psychoactively. It changes you from the inside out and literally brings you to new vistas of experience.

Viewing Additional Modules through Five Integral Lenses

Each of the additional modules could be a book in itself (or several!). Our intention is not to cover each module in depth but rather to illustrate how the Integral Framework illuminates some of the additional modules, giving examples of how it can bring new perspectives to these important areas. Therefore, the rest of this chapter is organized using the AQAL elements: **quadrants, levels, lines, states,** and **types.**

Using the Quadrants

Taking more perspectives in any given area—from your relationship with your mother-in-law to your financial investments to your golf game—will deepen your practice in that area. A top athlete understands his sport inside and out, just as a successful businessperson gets to know his industry and customers from as many angles as possible. The reason is simple: the more perspectives you can hold, the more informed, intelligent, and appropriate choices you can make.

You can bet that a star basketball player picks up tons of phenomena that fly right over the heads of spectators. Behind a split second decision to shoot or pass lies considerations such as teammate chemistry, state of confidence, the opponent's defensive abilities, personal injuries, the coach's strategy, the score, the clock, and dozens of other factors, all seamlessly arising in the athlete's present moment awareness.

In the same way, so much goes into a yes or no response from a seasoned business executive who can rapidly discern subtle cues and indicators, connect the dots to a strategic plan and macro vision, and deliver a decisive answer. Leaders who push the edges of their discipline do so by taking perspectives with more depth and more span than most others. And they do it thanks to a lifetime of committed practice.

A good map can't prevent missteps, but it can reveal blind spots and help us maintain our footing when exploring new areas of life. Knowing where to look and what questions to ask are huge advantages.

The Work module shows up in all four quadrants. It is, after all, how you probably spend about one-third of your waking hours.

Choosing a job and career is one of your biggest life decisions. Discovering a right livelihood that serves you, others, and the world is often a hero's journey unto itself. Through work, you can express not only your character, but also at least part of your life's purpose. This is often a central thrust of practice, expressing a primal urge toward self-actualization and service.

You can bring a nuanced awareness to those investigations by using the quadrants as a multi-perspectival lens. The quadrant map won't explicitly tell you what career or job to pursue, but it will highlight the key, universal perspectives you can take toward any job or career. A quadrant mapping of some key questions you might ask about a job opportunity can be found in figure 9.2 on page 300.

A quick scan of the four quadrants can be used in virtually infinite ways. Here, it provides insight by zooming in on key dimensions that matter most without privileging or ignoring any. (The questions in figure 9.2 are just a small sampling of the many that might apply in each quadrant.)

If part of your Work practice includes working for a company approaching an Integral center of gravity or acting as an organizational change agent to transform your current company from within, then you can use the quadrants to designate the characteristics you're looking for in an Integral organization (see figure 9.3 on page 301).

Identifying your practice intentions in all 4 quadrants and seeing how they all relate and align (or tetra-mesh) with each other creates a powerful synergy for Integral Life Practice at work. Your work is consummated not just by what you do, but also by *whom you become* while accomplishing the tasks. The same applies to any ILP module.

Levels and Lines of Parenting

As you may recall, human beings grow through multiple *levels* along various *lines* of development. Nowhere is this more obvious than in the drama of a child growing up. Parents are blessed with the opportunity to participate in the most glaringly obvious and undeniable exemplar of the evolution of consciousness: the growth of a newborn infant into an adult.

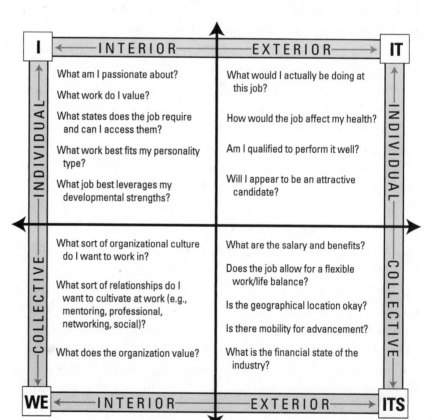

Figure 9.2
Job hunting in all 4 quadrants.

I ← INTERIOR — EXTERIOR → IT	
INDIVIDUAL What am I passionate about? What work do I value? What states does the job require and can I access them? What work best fits my personality type? What job best leverages my developmental strengths?	What would I actually be doing at this job? How would the job affect my health? Am I qualified to perform it well? Will I appear to be an attractive candidate? **INDIVIDUAL**
COLLECTIVE What sort of organizational culture do I want to work in? What sort of relationships do I want to cultivate at work (e.g., mentoring, professional, networking, social)? What does the organization value?	What are the salary and benefits? Does the job allow for a flexible work/life balance? Is the geographical location okay? Is there mobility for advancement? What is the financial state of the industry? **COLLECTIVE**
WE ← INTERIOR — EXTERIOR → ITS	

The entire history of consciousness evolution will be gradually reenacted through each little tyke. In just a handful of years, a newborn will develop through several major levels (or altitudes) of maturity from Beige to Amber and (hopefully) beyond.

Here's what makes parenting one of the ultimate Integral practices: every level of child development demands a corresponding level of parenting. The practice of Integral parenting is a whirling tango across the evolutionary dance floor in an attempt to keep in step with a sprouting human being.

In the Levels and Lines Story on page 302, Mark is at first unable to adapt his parenting to address Jamie at his developmental level. He has to learn how to translate his urge to communicate into terms Jamie can relate to. Many parent-child issues arise out of the developmental inflexibility of parents.

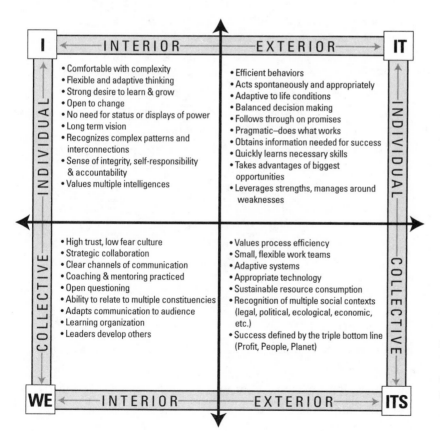

Figure 9.3

The 4 quadrants of an Integral organization.

A Levels and Lines Story

Susan was often saddened by her husband Mark's tendency to talk over their son Jamie's head. Mark loved his son, but he just couldn't help himself. He'd use simple words and make eye contact, but he just didn't get where Jamie was at. Again and again, he'd introduce abstract concepts. He'd lecture. And again and again, Jamie's eyes would glaze over.

Luckily, Susan's friend Meg was a developmental psychologist who pointed out that Jamie's awareness was at a stage of development that related best to myths and stories. With Meg's help, Susan and Mark considered other ways Mark could communicate the important life wisdom he so badly wanted to share with his son.

Together they found a story that communicated what Mark wanted to say. He told Jamie the story of the early 20th-century Olympian Glenn Cunningham.

As a young boy, injuries suffered in a terrible fire caused Glenn to lose several toes and all the feeling in his legs. The doctors told him he probably would never walk again. By trying hard and practicing often, he learned to wiggle his toes, and then his feet, and then to stand, and eventually to walk. He then even learned to run. As he ran and ran, he got faster and faster. He even began to compete in races. At first he didn't win. But he didn't let this discourage him from continuing to practice. After years, Glenn Cunningham, a former "cripple," became the world's fastest runner!

Jamie's eyes didn't glaze over this time. He loved the story. He asked his father to tell it again. And again! And gradually, he seemed to get the point. Mark noticed his goose bumps when he saw Jamie struggling to tie his shoes, failing again and again, refusing to give up, and eventually mastering his new skill.

Sometimes parents overestimate their child's capacities, as Mark did. But it's even more common for them to *under*estimate their child's capacities. In fact, it is a truism among child psychologists that parents tend, for the most part, to address their children at the developmental level at which the child was about a year previously! This is one way that many parents sow seeds of adolescent alienation.

Usually, a child's cognitive development advances ahead of his morals, values, and self-identity lines. This presents a valuable opportunity for parents and teachers to challenge children to think through specific situations and to discover for themselves their implications. Often this will help the child learn to bring his cognitive sophistication to bear in moral and interpersonal terms (where they have the most important impacts on others).

Understanding the unique psychograph of your child is important to Integral parenting. If, for example, you have a daughter with a high level of empathy, care, and emotional sensitivity, you can leverage that strength. You can invite her to participate in activities that allow her to express and cultivate the intelligence of her heart; for instance, offering peer tutoring at school or caring for a family pet. You can then encourage her to talk about her experiences or keep a diary, thus helping her connect mind and heart, and develop her intellectual self-understanding.

If your other daughter is a natural athlete who loves to dance, play volleyball, and ice skate, you can validate and appreciate her kinesthetic abilities by playing with her and accompanying her to sporting events. You can then suggest that she teach her skills to a younger sibling or a friend, thus helping her improve her communication skills, as well as learn to balance competitiveness with cooperation.

Skillful awareness of levels and lines implies meeting children where they're at while simultaneously creating conditions that help them develop to higher levels.

Discipline is an act of love. Children need clear rules, boundaries, and structures. And they'll sometimes test those limits and become upset if they're unable to exceed them. But over time, they'll be more disoriented and upset if they don't have clarity about their role and expectations. A skilled parent can set firm limits while remaining open to changing them when their children developmentally mature and the old approaches lose their effectiveness.

It is not easy to set limits for rebellious teenagers who are in the process of developing an autonomous self-sense. But they are much more willing to *co-design* agreements with their parents. At this stage parents often get the best results expressing their needs and being available to help without infringing on the teenager's responsibility for his or her choices and the consequences of those choices.

States of Practice

We experience remarkable states of body, mind, and spirit in the most special moments of our lives. But when our extraordinary states pass, they're gone. And the next moment will be different. If we try to cling to our exalted states, they wither in our hands. If, as William Blake put it, we "kiss the joy as it flies" we "live in eternity's sunrise." It doesn't work "to bind to oneself the joy." This is one of the core lessons to be learned about *states*.

States come and go all day every day. Changing emotions, stock market fluctuations, conversations, and the flu come and go, like the weather. Meditators experience various states of consciousness. Businesses pass through states of profits and losses. Artists enjoy states of creative inspiration and agonize through opaque periods of creative blockage. Lovers merge in mutual devotion and the next moment feel disconnected and hurt. States exist as the constant change and impermanence of phenomenal reality.

In a conscious sexual practice, couples may experience deep states of transcendental heart opening and mind expanding bliss. Yet one negative thought, one misplaced comment can snap a lover back into states of worry, fear, and regret. States can occur unpredictably and without warning. Someone walking through a forest, anxious and tense one moment, may experience a sudden oneness with his surroundings—an immediate and obvious identification with the ants, the birds, and the trees—in a transcendental state of nature mysticism.

Or, to give a more down-to-earth example, notice how your five physical senses can trigger

> He who binds to himself a joy
> Doth the winged life destroy
> But he who kisses the joy as it flies
> Lives in Eternity's sunrise.
> —William Blake, from *Songs of Innocence and Experience*

memories associated with vivid emotional states seemingly out of no-where: smelling the perfume of a former lover, hearing the harsh voice of an old boss, tasting the salty ocean, touching a dog's soft coat, seeing a deceased parent gazing up at you from an old photograph.

Finally, consider a parent's relationship with his or her young child. With an almost uncanny expertise, a young child can wear down the nerves of his parents to states of extreme vexation, frustration, and anger. Yet one well-timed smile or hug can melt a parent's heart and reopen the floodgate of love toward the child.

The practice of relating to states rides the paradox of effort and acceptance. Conscious living requires awareness and acceptance of all passing states. All states come, stay for a while, and then cease to be. Noticing ephemeral states and embracing the inevitable highs and lows of life's unstoppable currents is essential to mindful living.

Relatively speaking though, some states are more desirable than others. Politicians work toward a state of economic prosperity. Ecologists attempt to facilitate states of sustainability. Intimate partners in a conscious relationship seek deeper states of heart connection, mutual vulnerability, and care. Meditators may train to experience transpersonal, that is, subtle and causal, states.

An Integral Life Practice must include both *state acceptance* and *state training*. A leader practicing at work can learn from breakdowns: when the new hire turns out to be a flop, when the quarterly earnings don't meet expectations and the stock price gets slammed on Wall Street, or when a product defect requires a massive recall. With the insights gained from experiencing undesirable states, he can more effectively craft a business practice focused on a clear spirited mission, smart hiring, effective communication, strategic planning, and product quality.

In the same way, an artist can channel his suffering and past failings into a creative masterpiece. Artists know that creativity can't be forced. If it's not there, it's not there! Yet, in many cases, the simple act of accepting what *is* there unlocks the door to desired states. For example, mustering the courage to feel openly and deeply into anxiety or depression is often the most effective way to move beyond it. Similarly, many forms of meditation training access transpersonal states through the practice

Using States for Creativity

A creative practice births something new into being. Creative ideas, methods, technologies, interpretations, and aliveness transcend what came before them, while simultaneously growing out of and incorporating it all. (This is the nature of every evolutionary journey.) Great inventions don't magically pop out of thin air. As Isaac Newton famously said, "If I have seen further it is by standing on the shoulders of giants."

Innovators bring a new *perspective* to what already exists. They make *new connections*. The NASA scientist whose breakthrough led to the repair of the Hubble telescope mirrors made a creative association between high-tech space robotics and a German hotel showerhead. Who would have thought it? Practicing creativity involves seeing meaningful connections where others don't. Viewed from this perspective, the Integral Framework is a map for innovation.

The four-step practice outlined below can be used to enhance your creativity through state training and perspective taking—with an Integral twist.

1. Absorption: Learn as much as you can about the particular area where you'd like more creativity. Just dive in! You can do this through activities such as reading books, interviewing experts, or direct participation. You must befriend the giants before you can stand on their shoulders.

2. Incubation: Now drop what you've been absorbed in and change your context. If you've been at the office for twelve hours working on a complex problem—go home. If you've been reading a small library on a technical subject—watch a movie. If you've been consumed in relationships issues—travel somewhere by yourself. This context switch alone will alter your state of consciousness and activate different dimensions of your mind and brain.

Going further, touch into your gross, subtle, and causal bodies. Meditating, relaxing, sleeping, exercising, playing, and a variety of other practices put you in touch with different states and bodies and, hence, give you access to different perspectives. With the Integral

Operating System running in the background, surrendering old perspectives coupled with exposure to new perspectives sooner or later will generate the spark that sets your creative house on fire.

3. Illumination: Creative insights can come unexpectedly at any time. Creativity researchers commonly refer to the "3 Bs"—the bathroom, the bed, and the bus—all places where famous ideas have spontaneously emerged. All these places facilitate states other than normal waking consciousness, namely dream states and their corresponding alpha and theta brain-wave patterns. Late at night and early in the morning tend to be especially illuminating periods when you're in the *hypnagogic* state between waking and sleeping. The subtle dream state seems to free up inhibitions and make connections between seemingly dissimilar things.

When you're graced with a creative insight, be sure to write it down quickly and unfiltered. Carrying a small notepad and pen around at all times may be a good way to make sure you don't forget any creative ideas.

4. Evaluation: At this point you can use the AQAL Framework more explicitly to identify the exact nature of your creative associations. Analyze your insight from multiple perspectives (e.g., quadrants, levels, lines, states, types) until you understand how it works and fits into the larger picture.

Continue to critically assess your idea. Look for flaws that would not have occurred to you earlier in the creative process. Ask questions: Is the idea feasible? Is it useful? How can I further develop it? How can I successfully implement it?

of fully witnessing ordinary states. Loving what is can be the doorway into what can be.

Living Your Types

Types are *horizontal* differences, such as masculine and feminine or personality types like those described by the Enneagram, Myers-Briggs, and other such systems. Relationships are a rich area for exploring these differences. Take Tessa and Luke, for example. Every Sunday evening Tessa and Luke sit down together for their weekly check-in practice. By turns, they speak their truth of the moment. The sharing could cover everything from mundane highlights of the past week to interpersonal issues to emotional dynamics to questions about meaning, direction, and purpose. Even after four years of marriage, it's a mystery what will come out when they begin speaking.

While one person shares with full honestly and authenticity, the other's job is to listen with an open heart and mind. Well, at least that's the intention behind the practice. It doesn't always happen that way.

A pattern began to develop when Tessa would confront Luke about something and Luke would immediately become defensive and shoot back an elaborate and logical argument justifying why he acted as he did. When Tessa finally became aware of this dynamic, she mirrored Luke's defensiveness so he could clearly see it in himself. When he finally saw it and reflected on it, he recognized how this same defensiveness showed up in other areas of his life.

The next day, Luke created the affirmation, "I am open and vulnerable when confronted by someone I trust," and began to speak and affirm it every day.

In their next check in, Tessa communicated how hurt she felt when Luke broke a promise he had made to her. Luke opened his mouth in defense, then stopped abruptly. Beacons flashed and his affirmation, "I am open and vulnerable when confronted by someone I trust," streaked across his mind. Luke caught himself and chose to practice rather than react in his normal way. Dropping into his full being, he was able to take Tessa's perspective and empathically feel her hurt before even uttering a word. When Luke finally responded, he spoke from a different place. From there, the conversation flowed into a space of mutual recognition, understanding, and love.

Masculine and feminine types embody the most fundamental and simplest of typologies. Masculine and feminine elements are almost always manifesting in us simultaneously, reciprocally exchanged, in every moment and every practice.

A masculine orientation thrives in scheduled and structured practices: meditation every day at 6:00 a.m., weightlifting after work Mon-
day, Wednesday, and Friday at 5:30 p.m., and, in this case, relationship
check-in every Sunday evening. Masculine practice strengths include
discipline, focus, breaking through boundaries, confronting challenges
head on, staying on task, and taking action. Together, Tessa and Luke
use their masculine energy to stay true to their practice commitment
and show up together every Sunday evening to face the raw truth of their
lives and relationships.

Tessa drew from her masculine agency when she asserted herself and
confronted Luke. The sword of discrimination that cuts through confusion leaves the mark of masculine wisdom. Honest and direct feedback
that penetrates to truth is a form of masculine compassion. Likewise, lifting weights with focused intensity, concentrating with one-pointed focus,
managing time and getting things done, sticking to a new nutrition plan,
courageously facing one's shadow—all are masculine gifts used in a
living practice.

The spontaneous and flowing nature of the check-in embodies the
feminine aspect of the practice. Always open to the unexpected, the
feminine dances with life's practice moments and bathes in life's unscheduled jewels. The feminine tends to gravitate toward a more light,
playful, and humorous approach to practice—smiling and laughing her
way to enlightenment. A more feminine type follows the natural unfolding of her creative intuition, practicing through unanticipated conversations, nurturing relationships, and natural movements. Feminine energy
embodies the dynamic movement and the radiant mystery of a juicy
living practice.

Luke embodied the feminine side of practice when he opened to
Tessa's feedback. In that moment, he surrendered and allowed himself
to be vulnerable enough to receive her words, allowing them to pierce his
defenses and penetrate his psyche.

Typological systems with greater complexity than masculine/fem-
inine reveal more nuanced qualities. Some types tend to emphasize the
head, the heart, or the hara. Others are more introverted or extraverted,

or more intuitive or logical. Some emphasize avoiding errors, others avoid lost opportunities, while still others avoid rejection or engulfment. *Your practice style will differ depending on your type.*

The goal is not necessarily to strike a perfect balance among all possible types, but to leverage the gifts of your dominant orientation while keeping an eye out for ways to embody strengths of less dominant orientations. On the one hand, an extreme feminine type may struggle with sticking to a single practice for a set period of time, instead wanting to constantly change the practice or getting distracted by other things. On the other hand, an extreme masculine type may take his practice too seriously and allow it to get stale because he rigidly refuses to adapt to life's dynamic currents.

Finding ways to exercise capacities your type tends to exclude is often an important part of your ILP. It's important to outgrow our fixed patterns. Nevertheless, practices that match up with your personality type tend to have the greatest impact and usually are the most enjoyable.

The best managers, for instance, don't blindly follow the latest management trend. They forge a vital and unique style out of the natural gifts of their personality. They do it in a way that works for them, for their employees, and for the company. Great managers can have a wide range of personality types: sensing or intuitive, thinking or feeling, judging or perceiving, to use Myers-Briggs types as an example. Whether at work, with your child, or in the bedroom, the identical practice works better for some people more than others. Why? One of the key differences can be the naturalness and authenticity that are possible when your behavior is congruent with your typology.

Affirmations: A Power Tool for Actualizing Desired Changes

Affirmations are a powerful practice of directed intentionality. They can be used as a part of the Will module or to supercharge *any* core or additional module. Affirmations are useful when you are ready to make a real commitment to bring about a change in your life—whether it is a new behavior or a specific goal in your work or personal life. Speaking that intention is a way of aligning with the future you've committed to—resonating and affirming it.

The practice of using affirmations involves regularly repeating one or more statements of positive intentions. This can cultivate extraordinary changes if the practice is engaged with fierce intention, rigorous discrimination, and human maturity, but it can be an exercise in futility (and even silliness) if it is not.

Affirmations act as powerful attractors that work behind the scenes to call attention to life's unscheduled practice moments. When you repeat an affirmation, it flashes the message, "remember, remember, remember" whenever the relevant practice opportunity comes up.

For example, say you've decided to lose weight and have created an affirmation to reach your ideal weight of 150 pounds: "I weigh 150 pounds." An effective affirmation resonates with the different levels of your own psyche and begins to reprogram alternative voices and reoccurring thought loops that say, for example, "I will always be fat," or "I have no control over my eating habits." Repeating your affirmation every day will help you recognize nutrition practice moments and choose actions in alignment with your intentions—in this case, eating healthy foods and exercising. So when the restaurant server asks if you want the double chocolate fudge cake special, alarm beacons will sound and you will more likely choose and act from the reality of your future 150-pound identity.

An affirmation practice begins with a clear decision that a new reality will come to be. Engaged on that basis, it's a powerful tool for transformation. Essentially, you draw a line in the sand and declare, "This will be." By embodying that in an affirmation, and repeating it daily, you generate an alignment of all the levels of your being with your intention, and you keep broadcasting that resonance into your world. What once seemed painfully difficult (i.e., saying no to the cake) eventually becomes easy and natural (i.e., eating appropriately).

The practice involves finding a way to phrase an affirmation and relate to it, so that you're totally on board and you believe in what you are affirming. You must care about it; the affirmation must be something that you are invested in. Then, broadcast it from a place of real passion and speak it with certainty, more than just belief—a commitment of your whole being.

When you create an affirmation, it may be helpful to choose an area in life where you have difficulty recognizing practice opportunities. Then, explore this area of your life—whether it be friendships, sexuality, speech habits, addictive behavior, financial patterns, etc.—and form a vision of how this area could change to better align with your values and vision.

Now articulate this intention in words, working the phrasing over like you would a poem, getting the words exactly right, so you are really speaking what you have chosen to create. Once you have written the affirmation, the actual practice is to say it every day (or many times each day) consistently and repeatedly.

Affirmations can be used within an ILP to cultivate not just ordinary, but even extraordinary changes. In fact, some leading experts, including Michael Murphy, author of the authoritative volume *The Future of the Body*, believe they're among the most powerful tools for developing supernormal abilities.

Consider creating a few affirmations that powerfully address the areas of life where you're ready for real transformation. Then practice faithfully and notice how much more often you begin to wake up to some of life's unscheduled practice opportunities. You'll discover a powerful secret weapon for liberating the power of your intention. Affirmation practice works!

Guidelines for Affirmation Practice

1. **Always phrase affirmations in the present tense.** For example: "I am healthy." Avoid using future tense, for example: "I am going to be healthy" or "I will be healthy."

2. **Phrase them positively.** Always phrase affirmations positively. Negative statements will undermine your intended effect. For example, say, "I eat delicious, healthy food" rather than "I do not eat fast food."

3. **Make them short and specific.** This makes them easier to remember. If they are clear and specific, you can more easily visualize and feel them.

4. **State affirmations in the 1st person.** "I am" or "I do" or "My . . ." Some affirmations can be magnified by stating them three times, in 1st, then 2nd, then 3rd person. For example, "I trust myself." "You trust yourself." "Joe trusts himself."

5. **Make them *believable* (to you) by making them as close to the truth as possible.** They need to pass muster with the voices within you (like the "skeptic" or "editor"). Grandiose or unrealistic affirmations are not just silly, but ineffective.

6. **It's essential to *care* about your affirmations.** They depend on a strong **emotional** connection. It's important to make them real and inspiring to you.

7. **Repetition and persistence are essential.** Repetition imprints what is affirmed on all levels, increasing your comfort, belief, and congruence with what you are saying. Daily practice is important. Once you commit to an affirmation stick with it for at least three months.

8. **Act on your affirmations whenever you have the opportunity.** This has a huge impact on the subtle body, magnifying the power of affirmation practice.

9. **If affirmations are new to you, experiment with them gradually.** Find affirmations you can engage with minimal discomfort and reservations. Add others only when that feels natural and congruent. Let go also; it's appropriate for your affirmations to evolve over time.

Sample Affirmations
- I speak my truth with love.
- I honor my time commitments with grace and ease.
- I love myself unconditionally.
- I trust myself, and I trust Life.
- There is enough time for everything.
- My home and environment feed my soul.
- I attract abundance into my life.
- I keep my commitments to others and myself.

- I trust myself, my spouse, and our relationship.
- I surround myself with beauty and order.
- I attract blessings, luck, opportunities, appreciation, enjoyment, and delight.
- I choose what I eat to optimize my health, beauty, energy, and free attention.
- I take care of myself by getting sufficient rest and sleep.
- I happily focus my attention on my priorities and work efficiently.
- I forgive myself, my parents, and my patterns.
- I am a balanced powerhouse.
- I know what I want and I ask for it skillfully.
- I consult my 3 bodies as wise oracles for clarity on key decisions.
- I enjoy a profound empathy with others.
- I relax at will and am healthy in mind and body.
- I feel oneness with all existence.

Practicing Perfection

As we pointed out earlier in this chapter, all our efforts to make our lives work—which are the focus of many of the additional modules—are ultimately doomed. We suffer loss, get sick, age, and die. The good news is that everything and everyone (including you and all your "flaws") are *always already perfect*.

We don't *need* to practice to achieve perfection, we just need to wake up to the perfection that's already the case—coincident with our ordinary human difficulties, losses, mortality, and even the death of those we love. Nothing needs to be changed, achieved, found, or purified in order for this moment to be 100 percent full of radiant Suchness. And it's obvious—at least once we awaken to who we really are.

And yet, life kindly (and unkindly) requests us to grow and unfold and evolve. Which means practice is a good idea—in fact, indispensable. We hope this lends a sense of lightness and humor to the endeavor of Integral Life Practice.

This is the paradox of practice: Everything is always absolutely OK just exactly as it is, and as we are. And we are nonetheless called always to more goodness, truth, and beauty. Through Integral Life Practice, we rest as who we really are—while also aspiring to be who we know we can become.

Our essential health expresses how present we are to the Great Perfection. ILP can't help us manufacture the absolute self, but it can facilitate a profound *recognition* of something that is already present. It is like looking into a store window and seeing a hazy figure looking at you. You move your head around until you can see who it is, and with a sudden shock you realize that it is your own reflection in the window: you are witnessing your self.

Everything comes and goes, but the Witness is ever-present. The Witness cannot be attained, because it is ever-present. The Witness cannot be reached, because it is ever-present.

Notice: the clouds float by in your awareness, thoughts float by in your mind, feelings arise in the body, and you are the Witness of all of those. The Witness is already fully functioning, fully present, fully awake. The enlightened Self is 100 percent present in your very perception of this page. Enlightened Spirit is that which is reading these words right now: how much closer can you possibly get? Why go out and start looking for the Looker?

The great search for spiritual perfection is not just a waste of time; it is a colossal impossibility. This is because the enlightened Self is ever-present, as the Witness of this and every moment. You cannot cause something that is already here. In short, you do not *become* enlightened; you just wake up one morning and *confess* that you always already are, and that you have been playing the great game of hide-and-seek with your Self. And if that is the game you are playing, then certain activities—such as an ILP—can be engaged as part of the game, until you grow weary of the great search, admit the impossibility of becoming enlightened, and realize that you are already so, abiding then as the timeless Self that you have always been, smiling with the sudden shock that my Master is my Self, and I have been looking into the Kosmic window at my own reflection.

Absolute and relative, Self and self, perfection and evolution, stillness and practice. Paradox pervades a living practice. In this trans-logical practice space, we fully accept who we are *and* work hard to expand who we are. We savor the perfection of the present *and* listen to the evolutionary urge to grow.

All the core and additional modules of ILP—from Shadow to Relationships to Work—represent areas of *relative* development within the absolute context of ever-present awareness. Your essential health is your relationship with this fundamental paradox: all change occurs within the changeless; all transformation arises in stillness; all practices take place within perfection.

10

Navigating the Practice Life

Now that we've seen all the elements of Integral Life Practice, this chapter puts everything together. It's time for a practical, intimate, grounded conversation about what it actually takes to *live* an integrated life of practice.

How do you get started? How do you integrate ILP into your daily life? What does it feel like to live a life of practice? How do you keep practicing and growing in the midst of crises, distractions, and obstacles? What is the art of an ever-deepening practice?

Part I, **Designing Your ILP,** provides templates you can use to choose and keep track of your practices, in a way that takes into account the changes you might wish to make as your practice deepens and evolves.

Part II, **The Art of Integral Practice,** provides some down-to-earth insights—nuggets of wisdom and practical advice—to keep in mind as you journey forward on the practice path.

Part I: Designing Your ILP

Your Integral Life Practice *must* be personalized, because no one else has your life! The flexibility of ILP allows you to sculpt your practice into a customized form that's optimal for you.

We begin by guiding you through the design of an effective cross-training program that can become a sustainable *lifestyle*. The idea is to choose practices that you love *doing* and commit to a practice vision and way of living that you love *being*. But that's not the end of it—just as life never stands still, your Integral Life Practice can and should change over time—adapting and evolving with you.

The basic ILP injunction asks you to engage each of the 4 Core Modules (Shadow, Body, Mind, Spirit). To begin, choose at least one practice in each core module and exercise them concurrently, while living ethically. That's it for the short version! If you do this, you've got an ILP.

Many people, however, find a more structured design process to be extremely useful. The ILP design process below can help anyone get started with their ILP—regardless of previous practice experience, the number of modules included, or the amount of available practice time. The ILP design process can bring your practice vision to life.

1. Assess your current practices.
2. Identify what's missing.
3. Choose your practices.
4. Practice.
5. Be flexible.
6. Fine-tune continuously.
7. Get support.

Elizabeth and Jeremy
Two Examples of the ILP Design Process

We've created two fictional practitioners—Jeremy and Elizabeth—to give you examples of what it looks like to design an ILP. After getting a quick sense of their current life situations, follow along the seven design steps as Jeremy and Elizabeth customize their ILPs. Then you will be ready to design a unique Integral Life Practice for yourself.

About Jeremy

Jeremy is a 34-year-old entrepreneur who runs a small marketing firm and works fifty to sixty hours per week. His work requires him to understand the complexity of multiple perspectives and worldviews in order to communicate effectively. From the outside, Jeremy has a comfortable life: a stimulating job, a steady flow of clients, a suitable house, and a handful of good friends. He thought that this is what he wanted out of life, yet seemingly everything from his job to his relationships doesn't feel as satisfying as it once did. When he heard business expert Warren Bennis say, "Becoming a leader is the same as becoming a fully integrated human being," he began wondering what exactly this means. Jeremy would like to find more depth, meaning, and vitality in his life, but hardly has any extra time due to his busy schedule.

About Elizabeth

Elizabeth often feels overwhelmed by all the hats she wears: wife, mother, daughter, friend, volunteer, chauffeur, wage earner, care giver, chef, problem solver, and so on. She often feels frazzled and ineffective when doing so many things in a context of seeming chaos. Practice has been a part of her life for many years, although she has often struggled with how to fit it in and stay with it consistently. Faced with all her demands, she habitually hasn't taken much time to focus on herself and realizes that giving out her energy to others without giving back to herself is the likely culprit for her fatigue. Elizabeth desires more clarity, focus, and balance in her life—a sense of quiet in the center of the storm where she can address the tension between care of others and care of self. She's open and excited about bringing an ILP orientation to practices she's maintained for many years.

I. Assess Your Current Situation

You may *already* be doing an ILP, or at least major pieces of it! In this first step of your ILP design, scan your life to determine what practices you already have.

What are you already doing that could be considered a *practice*, an intentional activity that you repeat consciously and regularly for the purpose of health or growth? Identify what you already do for exercise, diet, study, meditation, and shadow work. What about work, relationships, sexuality, service, and money? This process will be much more meaningful if you list your practices in writing.

Now consider how your practices fit into an Integral context. Which current practices, if any, relate to the 4 Core Modules—Body, Mind,

Spirit, and Shadow? Which relate to the additional modules? Keep in mind that some practices, such as yoga and martial arts, apply to multiple modules.

Create at least five headings (Body, Mind, Spirit, Shadow, and Additional) on a sheet of paper and list the practices you're already doing underneath. Some sections will probably be fuller than others, and that's fine. You can use a practice design template or "ILP blueprint" for this purpose, like the sample on page 345. Or you can download one at www.Integral-Life-Practice.com.

If you don't have many current practices, don't worry. The ILP design process works no matter what your starting point is—beginner, advanced, or anywhere in between.

ILP Blueprint – Jeremy
Step 1: Assess the current situation.

BODY module

PRACTICES	DESCRIPTION	FREQUENCY
Weight training	Do light weight training when I get a chance.	1-2x/wk
Diet	Try to eat less junk food and drink less soda.	
Jogging	Take a jog in nature when possible.	1x/mo

SHADOW module

PRACTICES	DESCRIPTION	FREQUENCY
Nothing		

MIND module

PRACTICES	DESCRIPTION	FREQUENCY
Reading	Read marketing, personal growth, and philosophy books.	2x/wk

SPIRIT module

PRACTICES	DESCRIPTION	FREQUENCY
Meditation	Meditate for at least 30 minutes.	Tried once or twice; never stuck to it

ADDITIONAL modules

PRACTICES	DESCRIPTION	FREQUENCY
Work	Make a difference in the world through marketing sustainable products and services.	6x/wk
Relationship	Use online dating service and go out on dates.	2x/mo

2. Identify What's Missing

The next step is to locate any imbalances or gaps in your current practice. Gaps are important areas or modules you tend to neglect. Consider where you might need to take on new practices in order to have a truly *Integral* Life Practice.

Focus first on Body, Mind, Spirit, and Shadow, since these are the essential modules of ILP. Which of the 4 Core Modules have you been giving the least attention to? See pages 323 and 324 to learn how Jeremy and Elizabeth identify the gaps in their respective practices.

Jeremy has no problem meditating, but he tends to undervalue intense physical exercise. He could benefit from more structured strength

ILP Blueprint – Elizabeth
Step 1: Assess the current situation.

BODY module

PRACTICES	DESCRIPTION	FREQUENCY
Rock climbing	I love to go rock climbing with Rick (my husband).	2-3x/yr
Tennis	Play regularly in a league.	1-2x/wk
Yoga	Attend classes regularly.	1-2x/wk

SHADOW module

PRACTICES	DESCRIPTION	FREQUENCY
Psychological growth seminars	Deep personal work in 3-4 day seminars.	1-2x/yr

MIND module

PRACTICES	DESCRIPTION	FREQUENCY
Conversations	Have stimulating conversations with my husband and our friends.	1-2x/wk

SPIRIT module

PRACTICES	DESCRIPTION	FREQUENCY
Prayer	Attend evening prayer groups at my church.	2x/wk
Attend church	Fellowship, prayer, singing, and communion on Sunday mornings.	1x/wk

ADDITIONAL modules

PRACTICES	DESCRIPTION	FREQUENCY
Volunteer and service work	Very active in my church, especially in outreach. A major part of my social life.	2-3x/wk
Family time	Spend quality time together with Rick and the girls when we can.	

and aerobic training or from taking up a sport. In contrast, Elizabeth stays active, regularly engaging in rock climbing, tennis, and yoga. Spending time in silent contemplation would bring more balance to her practice. Make sure you're somehow practicing—at a minimum—with Body, Mind, Spirit, and Shadow.

As your practice deepens over time, this process of tailoring it can become more refined and nuanced. You may eventually customize your practice in a way that accounts for your unique strengths, weaknesses, and tendencies—your overall AQAL constellation, including your personality type, your psychograph (the levels of your various developmental lines), and your tendencies to gravitate toward certain quadrants over others. The most effective design for your practice is neither too tight nor too loose. You should be able to readily engage and enjoy your practices, but they should also challenge you. They should refresh and reorient your energy and attention, while also integrating seamlessly and pleasurably into your daily life.

Once these fundamental bases are covered, take a look at which additional modules may need attention. What's happening in your work and career, intimate relationships, sexuality, financial management, and family life? You might even look further into other areas, such as your relationship with the natural world, your close friendships and social life, and your home and work environments. Jeremy not only neglects shadow work, but he wishes he had a more active love life. Maybe there's a connection! Contemplate the patterns that show themselves; they may reveal opportunities for major transformation.

You can also use the 4 quadrants to evaluate your ILP's cross-training balance among the four fundamental dimensions of your being. Locate the dimensions that you are presently neglecting, and those you're overemphasizing.

Jeremy tends to pay too much attention to the I dimension; he can balance his self practices by sharing more energy with family, friends, and community (the We dimension) or by focusing more on the world (the It and Its dimensions). You might speculate that Elizabeth tends to get overly absorbed in the exterior world (Its) and sometimes loses herself when serving others (We). She identified gaps in cultivating inner awareness, self-reliance, and autonomy (I).

What's your pattern? This simple exercise can have revolutionary power to set a clear, integrating, and growth-promoting direction for your whole life.

This is also an opportunity to identify any current practice commitments that are vague, as well as the places where you're not facing the

ILP Blueprint – Jeremy
Step 2: Identify what's missing.

BODY module

PRACTICES	DESCRIPTION	FREQUENCY
Weight training	Do light weight training when I get a chance. **A more formalized and intense workout program would serve me**	1-2x/wk
Diet	Try to eat less junk food and drink less soda. No system. **Again, I want a more formal diet plan here that I can really stick with.**	
Jogging	Take a jog in nature when possible. **Something to touch into my subtle body while making connections with other people**	1x/mo

SHADOW module

PRACTICES	DESCRIPTION	FREQUENCY
Nothing	Add a practice here!	

MIND module

PRACTICES	DESCRIPTION	FREQUENCY
Reading	Read marketing, personal growth, and philosophy books. **I'd also like to learn more about Integral Theory and its implications.**	2x/wk

SPIRIT module

PRACTICES	DESCRIPTION	FREQUENCY
Meditation	Meditate for at least 30 minutes. **Maybe I could try just 5-10 minutes before heading out the door for work.**	4-5x/wk

ADDITIONAL modules

PRACTICES	DESCRIPTION	FREQUENCY
Work	Make a difference in the world through marketing sustainable products and services. **I feel isolated. What other people or organizations could I partner with to expand my business and circle of relations?**	6x/wk
Relationship	Use online dating service; go out on dates. **This online thing just isn't working. I want to find a woman who also desires a conscious relationship.**	2x/mo

facts of your life. What's necessary to make your ILP full and effective? Based on your assessment of your current situation, note the modules where you believe practice gaps exist and where you would like to add new practices or refine old ones in order to create a fuller, more balanced ILP.

ILP Blueprint – Elizabeth
Step 2: Identify what's missing.

BODY module

PRACTICES	DESCRIPTION	FREQUENCY
Rock climbing	I love to go rock climbing with Rick (my husband). I haven't done this in almost two years, so I shouldn't list it as a practice. However, I do want to plan a rock climbing trip in two months.	
Tennis	Play regularly in a league. I'd like to explore more of the inner game of tennis. Why do I get angry when I miss an easy shot?	1-2x/wk
Yoga	Attend classes regularly. What kind of yoga would activate my subtle body more?	1-2x/wk
Morning routine	I'd like a simple 5-10 minute routine I can do every day at home.	5-7x/wk

SHADOW module

PRACTICES	DESCRIPTION	FREQUENCY
Psychological growth seminars	Deep personal work in 3-4 day seminars. I think a daily practice that I can do on my own would complement the seminars.	1-2x/yr

MIND module

PRACTICES	DESCRIPTION	FREQUENCY
Conversations	Have stimulating conversations with my husband and our friends. I would like to learn more about Integral Theory and higher awareness, but I just don't learn best through reading books. Maybe there's another way?	

SPIRIT module

PRACTICES	DESCRIPTION	FREQUENCY
Prayer	Attend evening prayer groups at my church. I'd like to complement the groups with my own regular meditation practice.	2x/wk
Attend church	Fellowship, prayer, singing, and communion on Sunday mornings.	1x/wk

ADDITIONAL modules

PRACTICES	DESCRIPTION	FREQUENCY
Volunteer and service work	Very active in my church, especially in outreach. A major part of my social life.	2-3x/wk
Family time	I'd like to make sure to spend at least a short amount of quality time together every day, plus, once a week, to plan a more extended occasion.	
Sex	I'd really like to add a practice here!	

3. Choose Your Practices

Now you're ready to fill in the gaps by determining new practices to which you're willing to commit. You may also choose to delete or modify any of your current practices that have become stale and ineffective and no longer serve their original purpose. (You can see how this process worked for Jeremy and Elizabeth on pages 329 and 330.)

It may take some trial and error to find the right practice mix for you. Consider your uniqueness and your typology as you individualize your practice. Some of us are particularly open in one dimension of our being, for example in the head, the heart, or the hara, and particularly closed in another. For instance, we know one ILP practitioner whose heart and feelings are open and alive but who tends to be disconnected from his hara. He intentionally designed his ILP to include a particularly devotional, yet physically active form of hatha yoga. It powerfully engages his heart energy in a practice that is also gradually opening and strengthening his body and his kinesthetic intelligence.

When you're choosing your practices, remember: *more is not necessarily better.* The point is not to add practices upon practices until you get sick of practicing. Having too many practices can actually be *counter*productive.

That's why ILP takes a *modular* approach. It's also why we recommend the *Gold Star Practices,* which are a *distillation* and *condensation* of the finest practices anywhere. Even just one Gold Star Practice in each of the 4 Core Modules will cover the foundation requirements for an ILP.

Also remember that ILP is *scalable,* which means you are free to shorten or lengthen your practice sessions as needed. So time need not be an issue (or an excuse). You can engage your practice for as much or as little time as you have available—from a 1-Minute Module to a session that lasts for an hour or longer.

Here again, more is not necessarily better. In meditation practice, for example, it's far superior to commit to five minutes a day—and to actually follow through—than to commit to sixty minutes a day and skip it entirely. Your ILP will grow more quickly if you schedule short, manageable amounts of time, than if you over commit and give up in frustration when you can't meet your goals.

On days when you're pressed for time, the *1-Minute Modules* are a fantastic way to go. You'll find that even just touching in with a practice area gives rise to a sense of wholeness throughout your being. Being busy with *life* shouldn't stop you from having a *life practice*. Of course, if you're able to devote more time to practice, that's great too.

Take some time now to determine specific practices to add (or delete) from your ILP. Choose particular practices that fill the modular gaps you already identified in step 2. For instance, if you happen to neglect the Shadow module, then consider psychotherapy or a daily 3-2-1 process.

Though we've suggested numerous Gold Star Practices that we particularly recommend, the total universe of practices from which you can

Designing for Sustainability

Life is full of demands and distractions from practice. Most people don't feel like doing practices *every day*. There are always other important commitments, which sometimes need to take priority.

Take all your needs and commitments (including your resistance and reluctant sub-personalities!) into account when you design your ILP. Discover a compromise that accounts for all the various voices inside you and their competing commitments.

Often, this assessment will result in less ambitious practice commitments. Even if you think it would be a great thing to meditate for an hour each day, you should only make it a part of your ILP if you can reasonably stick with your commitment over time.

Account for the fact that certain key needs (such as financial survival and primary relationships) may sometimes need to take priority. Even so, protect your practice as a cornerstone of your lifestyle, one that supports every kind of health: horizontal, vertical, and essential (see page 21).

With all that in mind, craft an ILP design that *you can happily sustain over time*. You want a workable, lasting lifestyle, not an intensive program that will only last a few weeks or months.

choose is as boundless as human creativity. You may want to do your own research. Check out the Internet or your local bookstore. Or find out what kinds of teachers live in your area and what practices they offer.

Many people find that they cycle—as their lives cycle—between periods of more and less intense practice. People also cycle between different kinds of practice. So there is nothing fixed about these initial choices. Start in whatever way you sincerely feel works best for where you are right now. Stretch a little beyond your comfort zone, and yet remember that it's important to *love* your practices. Satisfaction from intentional, long-term practice comes from enjoying the process intrinsically, apart from believing that it will confer future benefits.

At this point, it can be extremely valuable to record the results of your design process on an ILP Blueprint (see page 345 for a blank template, or visit www.Integral-Life-Practice.com where you can find all the forms you need), which helps organize your practices and gives you the big picture, allowing you to see your entire ILP on one page.

Elizabeth's ILP Blueprint on page 330 is appropriate for a beginner. It is simple, easy, and short. Remember, the main benefit comes from doing these practices concurrently. Integral cross-training means that just a few minutes from each core module is more effective than an hour from only one. So start easy! It's worth repeating: **more is not necessarily better**. Also notice that the blueprint includes a space for the practice you want to work on next.

Jeremy's more advanced ILP Blueprint on page 329 is worth considering by those who have been practicing awhile and want to add more dimensions to their practice. This is obviously just one example from a limitless number of possible designs. Advanced practice doesn't necessarily mean doing more practices, but going deeper by refining your practices and how you relate to them. Many advanced practitioners settle in at four or five main practices. Others do many more. But the essential point is to keep it livable, which usually means fairly simple—at least one practice in each of the 4 Core Modules, plus additional practices as appropriate.

In addition to the name and a brief description of your practices, be sure to write down *how often* you are committing to doing the practice.

The frequency will vary with the practice. So on your ILP design blueprint, indicate the practices you commit to doing every day, in addition to those you will do less often, whether that's every other day, five times a week, or just once or twice weekly.

Later, you'll want to include more occasional activities—such as meditation retreats, seminars, strenuous runs, fasts, or purifying diets—that you might do monthly, quarterly, or annually. Not all practices are performed every day or even every week. It's wise to periodically **refresh and recalibrate yourself**. Here are some examples:

Meditation retreats. Days or weeks of intensive sitting meditation, usually with a teacher or guide, can create the setting for powerful breakthroughs and glimpses of higher states of awareness. Retreats can reenergize and add clarity to your daily practice. Although meditation retreats of two to seven days are most common, they can also be as brief as one day or as long as a year.

Intensive physical training. Sometimes a new level of focus, motivation, fitness, and metabolic function becomes possible during a period of intensive training (for example, preparing for a long run or a triathlon, or adopting a new sport or martial art). Just make sure not to *overdo* it; the benefits will be much greater if you can sustain your gains!

Personal growth seminars. When a seminar convenes a community of practice and becomes a crucible for deep transformational work, it can set in motion a new level of awareness and responsibility. It can also be an occasion for working with a skillful or awakened teacher and fellow practitioners from whom you can learn.

Camping, vacations, treks. Removing yourself from the numbing effects of your daily routine can do more than recharge your batteries. Deep rest, play, and time in nature can powerfully change your perspective, enabling you to make clear, free, conscious choices that would otherwise elude you.

Dietary cleansing or fasting. Many systems of holistic health and nutrition recommend periodic cleansing. Done correctly, this can rest and rejuvenate the whole body, especially the digestive system. It can also recalibrate the palate, reducing cravings for unhealthy and unneeded foods. Note: be cautious and make sure you're well informed; naïve engagement of extreme dietary regimes can actually *create* health problems.

Vision quests. Although the term "vision quest" comes from Native American traditions, the practice is universal. At certain times in their lives, many spiritual practitioners choose to go into the wilderness for days at a time to engage in prayer and fasting and ask for spiritual inspiration. This has been a feature in the lives of Jesus, Buddha, Muhammad,

ILP Blueprint – Jeremy
Step 3: Choose your practices.

BODY module

PRACTICES	DESCRIPTION	FREQUENCY
FIT	Focus Intensity Training 1-Minute Module at home.	3x/wk
	Focus Intensity Training 30-minute workout at the gym.	2x/wk
Integral Nutrition	Eliminate all low-quality foods. Restrict portions. End late-night snacks.	6x/wk
Jogging	Take at least a 20 minute jog in nature on Sunday mornings.	1x/wk
Qigong	Attend Saturday beginners class with a local teacher and practice on my own in between.	3x/wk

SHADOW module

PRACTICES	DESCRIPTION	FREQUENCY
Psychotherapy	Explore shadow issues with Dr. Kluever, a local psychotherapist I trust.	1x/wk

MIND module

PRACTICES	DESCRIPTION	FREQUENCY
Reading	Read marketing, personal growth, and philosophy books.	~ 2 hrs/wk
Integral Theory	Study the AQAL model through books and the Internet.	~ 2 hrs/wk

SPIRIT module

PRACTICES	DESCRIPTION	FREQUENCY
Meditation	At least 5 minutes of the 1-Minute Module of Integral Inquiry.	4-5x/wk
	At least one 20-minute extended sitting meditation session on weekends when possible.	

ADDITIONAL modules

PRACTICES	DESCRIPTION	FREQUENCY
Work	Attend relevant industry conferences and conventions and network with other sustainable (or even Integral) marketers.	3x/yr
Relationships	Use affirmations to clarify and strengthen my relationship intentions.	1 min in AM
	As a practice, take emotional risks and ask someone I like on a date.	2x/mo

Moses, St. Teresa of Ávila, and most mystics, saints, yogis, and sages throughout history. At certain moments in your practice life, a vision quest can be profoundly illuminating.

4. Practice!

When it comes down to it, ILP is about actually *practicing*. This involves discipline, persistence, patience, and often quite a bit of fun. The

ILP Blueprint – Elizabeth
Step 3: Choose your practices.

BODY module

PRACTICES	DESCRIPTION	FREQUENCY
Tennis	Play regularly in a league and practice focusing awareness on my head, heart, and hara.	1-2x/wk
Ashtanga yoga	Practice with Ashtanga teacher who focuses on all 3 bodies.	2x/wk
Integral Nutrition	Eat fresh, whole, natural foods only, and minimize simple carbs.	6x/wk

SHADOW module

PRACTICES	DESCRIPTION	FREQUENCY
Psychological growth seminars	Deep personal work in 3-4 day seminars.	1-2x/yr
3-2-1 Shadow Process	1-Minute Module in mornings and evenings.	4x/wk

MIND module

PRACTICES	DESCRIPTION	FREQUENCY
Conversations	Have stimulating conversations with my husband and/or friends.	2x/wk
Integral dialogues	Listen to audio dialogues with leading Integral thinkers.	1-2x/wk

SPIRIT module

PRACTICES	DESCRIPTION	FREQUENCY
Prayer	Attend evening prayer groups at my church.	2x/wk
3 Faces of Spirit Meditation	Practice this meditation for at least 10 minutes on the days I don't attend church activities.	3-4x/wk
Attend church	Fellowship, prayer, singing, and communion on Sunday mornings.	1x/wk

ADDITIONAL modules

PRACTICES	DESCRIPTION	FREQUENCY
Volunteer and service work	Very active in my church, especially in outreach. A major part of my social life.	2-3x/wk
Family time	At least 30 minutes of quality time together as a family.	6x/wk
	At least one major outing or happy family occasion besides church.	1x/wk
Sex	Experiment with simple conscious sexuality practices (from my new Tantra book) with my husband Rick.	1x/wk

secret of Integral Life Practice is actually doing the practices you set for yourself.

It isn't easy to begin something new and really stick with it. Commitment and self-discipline are generally required. It typically takes about ninety days to establish a new healthy habit. But once you've carved a new groove in your pattern of living, it's much easier to keep with it consistently. So it's especially important to stay in alignment with what you committed to do, and what you're actually doing, for the first three months.

To accomplish this, many people find it helpful to *track* their practices. Tracking is a way to keep yourself on track. It can help you stay with your initial practice commitments and can also re-energize practice after years or decades.

Practitioners use different methods to track their practices. Some people enjoy using templates such as the one on page 346. (See the following pages for sample tracking logs for Jeremy and Elizabeth.)

Others find that keeping a practice journal or log is helpful, especially at the beginning. You might also record your insights and ideas in a regular notebook. The point is to find a way to gently monitor whether you're keeping up with the practices you've committed to. Tracking your practices also serves to remind you of where you've been and where you're going.

If keeping track of your practices doesn't appeal to you, that's okay. For some people, it's just not their style. The most important thing is your practice itself. Jump in!

5. Be Flexible

Once you're in a groove of regularly practicing, you can be creative about your practice design. For example, we know experienced practitioners who create a lot of room for play and improvisation in their ILP without losing focus. One woman has committed herself to intense physical exercise at least thirty minutes *every day* and for at least ninety minutes at least three days a week. She can choose among running, biking, weight-training, dancing, and yoga, depending on her schedule and inclinations.

ILP Tracking Log – Jeremy
Step 4: Practice!

BODY module

PRACTICES	#	MON	TUES	WED	THURS	FRI	SAT	SUN	TOTAL
FIT - 1-Minute Module at home	3x/wk	Y		Y		Y			3
- 20-30 minutes at gym	2x/wk		Y				Y		2
Integral Nutrition	6x/wk			Y	Y	Y		Y	4
Jogging	1x/wk							Y	1
Qigong	3x/wk			Y			Y		2

SHADOW module

PRACTICES	#	MON	TUES	WED	THURS	FRI	SAT	SUN	TOTAL
Psychotherapy	1x/wk				Y				1

MIND module

PRACTICES	#	MON	TUES	WED	THURS	FRI	SAT	SUN	TOTAL
Reading	2x/wk		Y					Y	2
Study AQAL	2x/wk				Y		Y	Y	3

SPIRIT module

PRACTICES	#	MON	TUES	WED	THURS	FRI	SAT	SUN	TOTAL
Meditation - 5 minutes	4x/wk	Y	Y	Y		Y			4
- 20 minutes	1x/wk							Y	1

ADDITIONAL modules

PRACTICES	#	MON	TUES	WED	THURS	FRI	SAT	SUN	TOTAL
Work - Networking	1-2x/m		Y						1
Relationships - Affirmation	7x/wk	Y	Y	Y	Y	Y	Y	Y	7
- Ask for dates	2x/mo						Y		1

NOTES

Next week I want to practice Qigong more on my own so I don't forget what I learn in class. I also need to get rid of some unhealthy food still hanging out in my kitchen.

In addition, she does a ten-minute morning ritual much like the 3-Body Workout. This allows her to make flexible, spontaneous, and fun choices several times a week, which helps her stay motivated and enlivened.

Ultimately, your ILP, like your whole life, can be a living work of art. As in any art, the *form* is critical. Don't use creativity as an excuse for sloppiness, which undermines the intensity and free awareness of the practice life. But don't become a prisoner of rigid forms either. Create opportunities to improvise, play, and be inspired by what moves you in the moment.

6. Fine-Tune Continuously

Periodically, throughout a life of practice, it's necessary to *refresh* your practices—to **redesign your ILP**. Practice evolves! Updating your practice keeps it dynamic and alive. It's healthy and appropriate for your practice to shift as you pass into new stages and phases of your life. In fact, to reflect deeply and consciously on the form of your practice is *itself* a practice.

Setting a **timeline** for your commitments can help you do this. You may want to literally write out, "I will do my new strength training workout 3×/week until September 1, at which time I will make a new exercise commitment that sustains muscle strength." (Remember that practice commitments that last at least three months are usually most productive.)

Some practices (such as daily meditation) can remain stable for decades. Others (such as some seasonal outdoor sports and certain kinds of physical exercise) might change several times a year. As you grow into new phases and levels of life, your ILP needs to evolve with you so that it continues to nurture and challenge you.

7. Get Support

It can be a challenge to practice in a vacuum. Your practice commitments become more meaningful when they can't just slip away unnoticed. When you let someone else know whether or not you do your practices, a basic accountability occurs. This keeps you honest and injects a clarity and crispness that can enable your practice to gain real traction.

Updated 3-Month ILP Blueprint – Jeremy
Steps 5 and 6: Be flexible and fine-tune continuously.

BODY module

PRACTICES	DESCRIPTION	FREQUENCY
FIT	Focus Intensity Training 1-Minute Module. **This practice is so easy and quick. I'm going to add a second muscle group: one muscle from my upper body and one from my lower.**	3x/wk
	Focus Intensity Training 30-minute workout at the gym. **This is working well as is.**	2x/wk
Integral Nutrition	Eliminate all low-quality foods. Restrict portions. End late-night snacks. **I slip sometimes, but in general, I'm doing it. I need to remember to use my hand & fist to judge portion sizes.**	6x/wk
Jogging	Take at least a 20-minute jog in nature on Sunday mornings. **Sometimes I enjoy having my Sunday mornings free.**	2x/mo
Qigong	Attend **Thursday intermediate** class with a local teacher and practice on my own in between.	3x/wk

SHADOW module

PRACTICES	DESCRIPTION	FREQUENCY
Psychotherapy	Explore shadow issues with Dr. Kluever, a local psychotherapist I trust. **I'm really getting a lot from my therapy. I intend to see Dr. Kluever for at least three more months.**	1x/wk

MIND module

PRACTICES	DESCRIPTION	FREQUENCY
Reading	Read marketing, personal growth, and philosophy books.	~ 2 hrs/wk
Integral Theory	Study the AQAL model through books and the Internet.	~ 2 hrs/wk

SPIRIT module

PRACTICES	DESCRIPTION	FREQUENCY
Meditation	At least 5 minutes of the 1-Minute Module of Integral Inquiry.	4-5x/wk
	At least one 20-minute extended sitting meditation session on weekends when possible. **I am getting a lot from regular meditation and I'll want to rearrange my commitments so I can meditate for 20 minutes every day.**	

ADDITIONAL modules

PRACTICES	DESCRIPTION	FREQUENCY
Work	Attend relevant industry conferences and conventions and network with other sustainable (or even Integral) marketers.	3x/yr
Relationships	Use affirmations to clarify and strengthen my relationship intentions.	1 min in AM
	As a practice, take emotional risks and ask out someone I like. **I'm less shy, and coincidences seem to happen more frequently. I'm beginning to meet some amazing women. I really like Susan.**	2x/wk

Updated 3-Month ILP Blueprint – Elizabeth

Steps 5 and 6: Be flexible and fine-tune continuously.

BODY module

PRACTICES	DESCRIPTION	FREQUENCY
Tennis	Play regularly in a league and practice focusing awareness on my head, heart, and hara. *My game has improved significantly. Next season, I'll be ready to play in a more advanced league.*	1-2x/wk
Yoga	Practice with Ashtanga teacher who focuses on all 3 bodies. *Wow! This practice has helped ground me in my hectic life. I want to increase the frequency of my yoga practice, but just a little.*	3x/wk
Integral Nutrition	Eat fresh, whole, natural foods only, and minimize simple carbs. *It's hard for me to maintain this practice when I eat out. I think I will spread out my one "free" day to cover the few times a week I eat out.*	6x/wk

SHADOW module

PRACTICES	DESCRIPTION	FREQUENCY
Psychological growth seminars	Deep personal work in 3-4 day seminars.	1-2x/yr
3-2-1 Shadow Process	1-Minute Module in mornings and evenings. *What a powerful process! I can't believe how much I've grown by using the 3-2-1 Shadow Process on my dreams. Journaling about it has been important. I think I'd like to consider trying out psychotherapy.*	4x/wk

MIND module

PRACTICES	DESCRIPTION	FREQUENCY
Conversations	Have stimulating conversations with my husband and/or friends.	2x/wk
Integral dialogues	Listen to audio dialogues with leading Integral thinkers. *I'm really getting into this!*	2x/wk

SPIRIT module

PRACTICES	DESCRIPTION	FREQUENCY
Spiritual instruction	Attend evening prayer groups at my church. *1 night a week is enough. I've become overcommitted & need to cut back.*	1x/wk
3 Faces of Spirit Meditation	Practice this meditation for at least 10 minutes on the days I don't attend church activities. *This is working. I often meditate longer.*	3-4x/wk
Attend church	Fellowship, prayer, singing, and communion on Sunday mornings.	1x/wk

ADDITIONAL modules

PRACTICES	DESCRIPTION	FREQUENCY
Volunteer and service work	Participate and volunteer in church activities.	2-3x/wk
Family time	Continue to create quality time together daily and weekly.	
Sex	Experiment with simple conscious sexuality practices with Rick. *This has reawakened me as a woman. Sometimes we see each other with fresh eyes, as if it were the first time. After 12 years! So grateful.*	1x/wk

Do you already have someone who can be your practice buddy, or a few practicing friends willing to meet periodically? Do you have a teacher, coach, mentor, or therapist who will support you? Do you already belong to a church, practice community, or sangha that will support you? Can you join or organize an Integral Life Practice group? Can you buddy up with someone in another city and support each other by phone and email? Even if you are alone, you may be able to create an accountability structure by keeping a journal and tracking your practices.

Updated 3rd-Year ILP Blueprint – Elizabeth
Steps 5 and 6: Be flexible and fine-tune continuously.

BODY module

PRACTICES	DESCRIPTION	FREQUENCY
3-Body Workout	1-Minute Module in the morning for at least 10 minutes.	5x/wk
Tennis	Play my conscious inner game in an advanced league.	1x/wk
Ashtanga yoga	Continue to deepen my integration of gross and subtle bodies.	2x/wk
Yoga retreat	Attend week-long workshops.	2x/yr
Integral Nutrition	Involve all four quadrant perspectives in my eating choices.	6x/wk
Ecstatic dance	Integrate my awareness with spontaneous ecstatic movement.	1x/wk

SHADOW module

PRACTICES	DESCRIPTION	FREQUENCY
Psychological growth seminars	Deep personal work in 3-4 day seminars.	1-2x/yr
Somatic psychotherapy	Deepen my integration and free up my patterns and choices.	2x/mo
3-2-1 Shadow Process	Do the full process, very consciously at least once a month.	1x/mo

MIND module

PRACTICES	DESCRIPTION	FREQUENCY
Integral discussion group	Meet with local Integral thinkers (including Rick) to better understand an Integral perspective on life, practice, and politics.	1x/mo
Integral dialogues	Listen to recorded dialogues with leading Integral thinkers.	1-2x/wk

SPIRIT module

PRACTICES	DESCRIPTION	FREQUENCY
Prayer	Attend evening prayer groups at my church.	1x/wk
3 Faces of Spirit Meditation	Practice this meditation for at least 15 minutes on the days I don't attend church activities.	4-5x/wk
Attend church	Fellowship, prayer, singing, and communion on Sunday mornings.	1x/wk

ADDITIONAL modules

PRACTICES	DESCRIPTION	FREQUENCY
Volunteer and service work	Participate at church and work with church leaders to help the church keep growing.	1x/wk
Family time	Continue to create quality time together daily and weekly.	
Sex	Regular conscious sex practices with Rick.	3x/wk

If you maintain it, your Integral Life Practice will eventually transform from a series of special activities to a seamless aspect of your everyday life. A supportive community not only accelerates this transition, but also informs your ILP at every step. Group interaction helps avoid pitfalls such as ignoring the shadow, breaking commitments, getting caught in an inflated sense of progress, and robotically going through the motions. Many people find that their practice benefits from the visibility and accountability a group can provide. Not to mention the fact that it just feels good to practice in the company of others.

Updated 5ᵗʰ-Year ILP Blueprint – Jeremy
Steps 5 and 6: Be flexible and fine-tune continuously.

BODY module

PRACTICES	DESCRIPTION	FREQUENCY
FIT	Practice Focus Intensity Training after work for 45 minutes.	3x/wk
Diet	Continue to eat only quality food, control portions and snacking, and choose organic foods.	6x/wk
Swimming	Swim laps at the health club pool.	2x/wk
Qigong	Practice in the neighborhood park with a local group.	3x/wk
Walking in nature	State park near my house.	2x/mo

SHADOW module

PRACTICES	DESCRIPTION	FREQUENCY
Journaling	Write in personal journal.	3x/wk
Personal growth workshop	The last two years I've grown tremendously from this, so I'll go back.	1x/yr

MIND module

PRACTICES	DESCRIPTION	FREQUENCY
Writing	Continue to publish integrally informed articles in marketing journal.	
Integral Theory	Participate in online integral discussion forums.	2x/wk
Reading	Continue to read. Especially interested in developmental psychology.	

SPIRIT module

PRACTICES	DESCRIPTION	FREQUENCY
Meditation	Meditate at a local meditation center with a community of practitioners every Monday, Wednesday, and Friday morning in addition to my weekend practice.	5x/wk
Integral Inquiry	On the days I don't meet with my sangha.	2x/wk

ADDITIONAL modules

PRACTICES	DESCRIPTION	FREQUENCY
Finance	Research and invest in socially responsible companies.	
Work	Meet with mastermind group of local marketing professionals.	2x/mo
Relationships	Schedule special time with my fiancée Susan.	3x/wk
Service	Volunteer with local community hospice.	2 hrs/wk

On the other hand, don't let a lack of community become an obstacle. If you don't have others with whom to practice—or if you're more of a lone wolf—don't be discouraged. You can still practice ILP and reap huge benefits. Just follow all the other steps. Everything else is the same; no worries. If you later decide you want to connect with a community, you'll enter it more conscious, healthy, integrated, and responsible.

The best support system involves people who are willing to share their own experiences and listen to yours, people who can sustain you during breakdowns and invigorate you during plateaus. Practicing together forms the basis of an Integral culture—a culture that honors the greatest spectrum of human capacities.

Spend Time in Good Company

All ancient spiritual traditions encourage aspirants to spend time with strong, sincere practitioners, "the company of the Holy." This is valuable, in part, because we're all continuously transmitting our states to one another. Spending time in a field of clear practice intention yields a wealth of instructive information. We attune to that field of clarity and thereby speed our own growth.

In fact, spiritual awakenings have most often been transmitted through lineages that passed them down from one awakened person to another. This usually took place only after many years of close study and apprenticeship in a monastery or other community of intense practice.

Your practice can be empowered and quickened if you spend time with other practitioners. In countless ways, practitioners supply each other with examples and support. They share their lives with each other informally, and this naturally communicates the nitty-gritty details of how practice can be lived. Our friends' examples of courage, clarity, and compassion inspire us to our best.

Practice can also be impeded by hanging out with bad company. Sometimes you can gain ground by spending less time with a former friend who depletes your awareness and energy, subtly luring you into unproductive patterns. For many people, addictive relationships to TV, computers, food, alcohol, or other drugs function as bad company.

Human tendencies—whether they are helpful or unhelpful—develop most fully within cultures that encourage them. What tendencies are encouraged by the company you keep?

On Working with a Teacher

Of course, there's another way of getting support: you can find a coach or a teacher.

For many reasons (including the importance of your self-responsibility, autonomy, and choice) we assume you will be designing your own ILP. However, this has built-in limitations: it means your practice is designed by the very person who has the *least* insight into your blind spots—you! How can you get around this?

One way, quite seriously, can be to ask your friends and family. Although their perspectives may have their own limitations, they are in a position to see what you don't, and they can sometimes function as effective teachers, if given the chance. Based on your best assessment of their advice, you can redesign your practice to address your blind spots.

However, the primary way to transcend your own blind spots, the one used by all the ancient traditions, is to find a wise teacher who will accept you as a student. All humanity's great spiritual traditions originated with great spiritual realizers and have maintained their depth over time through *lineage* systems. Individuals acknowledged for their wisdom and spiritual maturity in turn acknowledge others. This is how the esoteric heart of the tradition stays alive. Remember—the entire spiritual wisdom of humanity originated with great awakened realizers and their disciples. A truly awakened teacher can be an immense source of guidance, wisdom, and spiritual transmission.

However, at times lineage systems preserve unnecessary baggage as well, which can subordinate demonstrated wisdom and efficacy to traditional authority. In addition, some lineage systems seem to contain no checks or balances, and thus some apparently highly developed teachers have abused their spiritual authority.

Thus, the way to find a reliable teacher is often neither easy nor obvious. Not surprisingly, a new teaching role has begun to emerge—that of an Integral Coach. Here, an experienced practitioner acts as a senior peer. Such a person supports practitioners without the students having to defer to another's authority. The Integral Coach's legitimacy derives from his or her depth, skill, professionalism, and conformity to ethical standards instead of from a presumed spiritual superiority and authority. And an Integral Coach can help you design (and follow through with) an ILP oriented toward multi-dimensional growth. Those who work with an Integral Coach still self-author their practice commitments, but they do so with the intimate assistance of a seasoned guide.

An Integral Coach is not necessarily an *alternative* to working with an extraordinary teacher in a traditional lineage. An aspirant involved in a traditional relationship to a spiritual teacher or guru can sometimes work simultaneously with an Integral Coach who honors the teacher and lineage.

Many options are available, each with strengths and weaknesses. At some point along the path, most serious practitioners find someone they respect with more knowledge and wisdom. Teachers, coaches, or mentors who know a particular practice territory can see your blind spots especially clearly. A wise and caring coach or teacher naturally creates accountability and will ground your practice in a wider perspective, coaxing you beyond your comfort zones. You may also benefit from the teacher's or coach's presence and awareness. But despite its advantages, working with a teacher is not inherently obligatory; some practitioners mature to a significant degree on their own.

Core Values, Vision, and Life Purpose

The *ground level* foundation of practice is your daily discipline. As Yogi Berra said, "When you come to a fork in the road, take it." In other words, the most important thing about practice is . . . doing it.

The *high level* foundation of practice is the why of practice — its *meaning*. This includes your purpose in practicing, how your practice expresses your values, and how practice helps you actualize your purpose and realize your personal vision. It can be powerful to clarify this high level foundation by articulating your values, vision, and purpose.

To enhance the depth of your relationship to your practices and to anchor their meaning, you can articulate your values, vision, and purpose as a part of your practice design process—perhaps even doing it first, even before choosing your practices. Doing so can clarify and anchor the intention behind every specific practice you choose and answer the "why" of any practice moment. But it's optional; don't let this keep you from getting right to action!

Your values are what enduringly matter most to you. They determine what you pay attention to and act on. Here are a few examples of values: humility, wellness, advancement, financial freedom, family, integrity, spirituality, fairness, winning, sensitivity, duty, relationships, adventure, service, fitness, empathy, morality, security, and openness.

One way to clarify and prioritize core values is to articulate them as guiding principles for living. One form they can take is an I statement:

- My marriage is the crucible in which I kindle passion, commitment, and aspirations. It is our sacred container of love.
- As a continuous learner, I expose myself to new situations that require me to stretch beyond my existing comfort zones.
- By focusing on integrity, alignment, and commitment, I hold myself to the fire of walking my talk.
- Recognizing the need for replenishment, I regularly "sharpen my saw" with contemplative practice and return to source.

As you clarify your core values and guiding principles, you'll see how your practice expresses them.

Your vision is a compelling picture of a desired future. It is what you want to create; a target to orient toward that reflects how you might like yourself and your circumstance to manifest in the time ahead. While it is good to be ambitious and aim high with your vision, make it realistic too. As the poet Rilke said, "The future enters long before it actually happens." Your vision is a way to link up with your desired future, bringing intention and awareness to your latent possibilities.

A compelling vision paints a clear picture of a future that is better than the present. It evokes an emotional response. It clarifies direction and focuses your attention. It motivates and inspires you.

When articulating your vision, it's sometimes helpful to speak in the present tense from a targeted date in the future. For example: "It is now January 15 (of the next year) and I am (where? doing what?)." Visions of varying lengths— six-month, one-year, two-year, and five-year—can also be appropriate. You may want to articulate specific vision statements for your personal and professional life and perhaps also for your practice.

Here is an example of a vision statement:

It is September 1 of next year, and I feel embraced by supportive and loving relationships with my wife, family, friends, and associates. I am trusted and respected as a leader in my field, and increasing happiness is flowing naturally from my service and relationships.

Your purpose is your reason for existence. What is your unique contribution? (Don't let the word "unique" become a burden. It is perfectly fine to have vision, values, and purpose statements that may sound like someone else's.)

You can clarify your purpose by asking yourself *why* again and again. "Why is it important that you exist?" "What is the gift that you bring?" "What are you moved to be and do?" As you keep asking, the answers may become both more abstract and more essential: what is your central reason for being and doing what you do? Here's one example of a life purpose statement:

In the service of global well-being, my purpose is to embody the discovery and celebration of ever-greater depths of awareness and humanity.

Clarifying your purpose may be a lifelong process of refinement. Even so, articulating it can be powerfully catalytic.

If you decide to write out a statement of purpose, accept that it is a deep process. Your first version will probably sound awkward. Revise, and come back later to feel into it and make further revisions. When it resonates as true and feels right, it can function to orient your life, vision, and practice.

In a final example, we meet Tim, an ambitious 24-year-old graduate student, who can't wait to get started on his ILP. Let's jump to step 3 and see what practices he chose.

As you can see from the blueprint below, Tim signed on for a very demanding practice. On the following page you can see how he modified it after three months of actual experience.

ILP Blueprint – Tim
Step 3: Choose your practices.

BODY module

PRACTICES	DESCRIPTION	FREQUENCY
3-Body Workout	Full 45 minutes every weekday morning.	5x/wk
Nutrition	Eat optimally and only buy organic, free trade foods.	every day
Microcosmic orbit	On the subway to my graduate classes.	4x/wk
Ultimate frisbee	Participate in league and compete in competitions.	3x/wk

SHADOW module

PRACTICES	DESCRIPTION	FREQUENCY
Journaling	Keep an audio journal.	7x/wk
3-2-1 Shadow Process	Practice the 3-2-1 Shadow Process for 15 minutes.	3x/wk
Men's group	Participate in a men's group on Wednesday evenings.	1x/wk

MIND module

PRACTICES	DESCRIPTION	FREQUENCY
Graduate school	Reading, studying, papers, tests, etc.	6x/wk
Sex, Ecology, Spirituality study group	Read a chapter each week and discuss with local group.	1x/wk
Policy research	Virtual internship with Washington D.C. think tank.	10 hrs/wk

SPIRIT module

PRACTICES	DESCRIPTION	FREQUENCY
Individual meditation	Integral Inquiry for 45 minutes each day.	7x/wk
Group meditation	Zazen with sangha at local Zen center in evenings.	3x/wk

ADDITIONAL modules

PRACTICES	DESCRIPTION	FREQUENCY
Finances	Reduce my credit card debt.	
Intimate relationship	Find one!	
Friendships	Explore ways to deepen my current friendships.	
Service	Assist in local senior center.	3hrs/wk

Updated 3-Month ILP Blueprint – Tim
Steps 5 and 6: Be flexible and fine-tune continuously.

BODY module

PRACTICES	DESCRIPTION	FREQUENCY
3-Body Workout	~~Full 45 minutes every weekday morning.~~ I only stuck with this for 3 days! Now I only do the 10-minute version, which seems to work.	5x/wk
Nutrition	~~Eat optimally and only buy organic, free trade foods.~~ It's working better to eliminate junk food, emphasize raw food, and strictly limit snacking. Also, one day a week, I eat whatever I want.	6x/wk
Microcosmic orbit	On the subway to my graduate classes. - This practice still works great (although I've missed my stop a few times).	4x/wk
Ultimate frisbee	~~Participate in league and compete in competitions.~~ I've cut back here and now only play informally with a co-ed group. Less stress.	1x/wk

SHADOW module

PRACTICES	DESCRIPTION	FREQUENCY
Journaling	Keep an audio journal. - Every day is too much. Now I record an entry when I feel especially drawn to doing so.	open
3-2-1 Shadow Process	Practice the 3-2-1 Shadow Process for 15 minutes.	3x/wk
Men's group	Participate in a men's group on Wednesday evenings. My men's group has been extremely valuable for me. This is definitely a practice I want to continue.	1x/wk

MIND module

PRACTICES	DESCRIPTION	FREQUENCY
Graduate school	Reading, studying, papers, tests, etc.	6x/wk
Integral applications	Now that my study group has concluded, I'm looking at how I can apply Integral theory to my graduate work.	
Policy research	Virtual internship with Washington D.C. think tank. - I had to cut back my hours here.	4 hrs/wk

SPIRIT module

PRACTICES	DESCRIPTION	FREQUENCY
Individual meditation	~~Integral Inquiry for 45 minutes each day.~~ - Too much! I just didn't have enough time to sustain this practice. Now I'm doing a 1-Minute Module for 5-10 minutes. This, I can do consistently.	7x/wk
Group meditation	Zazen with sangha at local Zen center in evenings. - I love this group, but had to cut my attendance down to once a week.	1x/wk

ADDITIONAL modules

PRACTICES	DESCRIPTION	FREQUENCY
Finances	~~Reduce my credit card debt.~~ - I couldn't save as much as I hoped, but living simply has helped me save money.	
Intimate relationship	~~Find one!~~ I'm dating Mary now, who I met while playing Ultimate Frisbee. We've only know each other for 2 months but I'm happy how the relationship is unfolding.	
Friendships	~~Explore ways to deepen my current friendships.~~ - By cutting back on my other practices, I've had more time to connect and share with friends.	
Service	Assist in local senior center. This was wonderful, but again, too much. I've cut down to 1x/month, which I'm enjoying.	3hrs/mo

ILP Blueprint

BODY module		
PRACTICES	DESCRIPTION	FREQUENCY

SHADOW module		
PRACTICES	DESCRIPTION	FREQUENCY

MIND module		
PRACTICES	DESCRIPTION	FREQUENCY

SPIRIT module		
PRACTICES	DESCRIPTION	FREQUENCY

ADDITIONAL modules		
PRACTICES	DESCRIPTION	FREQUENCY

ILP Weekly Tracking Log
Week of _____

BODY module

PRACTICES	#	MON	TUES	WED	THURS	FRI	SAT	SUN	TOTAL

SHADOW module

PRACTICES	#	MON	TUES	WED	THURS	FRI	SAT	SUN	TOTAL

MIND module

PRACTICES	#	MON	TUES	WED	THURS	FRI	SAT	SUN	TOTAL

SPIRIT module

PRACTICES	#	MON	TUES	WED	THURS	FRI	SAT	SUN	TOTAL

ADDITIONAL modules

PRACTICES	#	MON	TUES	WED	THURS	FRI	SAT	SUN	TOTAL

Part II: The Art of Integral Practice

As you establish yourself in a regular practice, the *art* of practice begins to become possible. At this point, the emphasis shifts from specific practices to the evolving quality of your life itself as an expression of practice. We discuss this in two sections: **Everyday Expanded Awareness** and **Practice Tips and Principles.**

Expanded awareness is not just something that happens while meditating. Through practice, expanded awareness begins to pervade everyday experience. Below we discuss how you can cooperate with that process and how the principles of practice embodied in the core modules begin to show up in the way you experience every moment of life.

After a short discussion of everyday expanded awareness, we have a heart-to-heart talk about the practice life, expressed as a series of principles and useful tips for living an ever-deepening life of practice. We'll take in a series of perspectives that point to some key themes and smart moves that will help you get a feel for the art and craft of navigating the practice life.

Everyday Expanded Awareness

As you practice regularly, the quality of your consciousness will begin to change. The fruits of practice sometimes show themselves as deep changes in your whole way of being alive.

This can simply be a matter of your practices informing your everyday awareness. Your meditative states can begin to bleed into your waking consciousness. Your "inner game" body practices (such as conscious breathing) can become second nature and carry over into ordinary activities. A more Integral perspective can begin to shift your whole sense of identity and the way you process experience and information.

Everyday expansion of awareness is always a possibility. You can always awaken to what your awareness previously excluded. Your heart can always continue to open. You can always notice how to feel and function and relate in new ways. You can always discover how to relax and arrive more and more completely in your unique, radiant humanity. You can always conduct the energy of life more fully. Ultimately, communion can become so full that you can begin to feel like you are consciously lived by the larger Kosmos.

The Body Module

The key practices of the inner game of the Body module begin to inform not only your body practices, but also every life moment:

- You breathe consciously, with heart feeling, and use your breath to regularly re-center.
- You ground yourself with strength and authority through the hara, or belly center.
- You commune with and feel into life through the heart center.
- You shine with radiant consciousness through the head center.
- You use your subtle energy practice to maintain healthy states of mind and body.
- You consciously conduct and circulate the energy of life down the front of the torso and up the spine.
- You can tolerate, enjoy, and use more and more intensity rather than reacting and throwing it off.
- You move your body throughout the day, in loving, practical service of self and others.

The Mind Module

Mind module practices build your natural capacity to take complex perspectives and your ability to make intelligent use of AQAL theory.

The essence of the Mind module in your everyday experience is *clear seeing* or *discriminative awareness*. This engages not just mental sharpness, but the integrated feeling-intelligence of your whole being. This is expressed in several general injunctions:

- You intend to be consciously present in every moment of your life.
- You intend always to see more clearly, to cut through confusion.

- You notice, value, account and care for all the fundamental dimensions of your life and reality, the I, We, It, and Its.
- You relate consciously to shifts in your states of consciousness (like falling asleep and waking up).
- You naturally enjoy the paradox of holding many different perspectives, even and especially when holding a strong opinion.
- You insightfully and compassionately appreciate the wide variety of personality types you encounter.
- You try to fly a little higher (at your highest available level or altitude), and help others to do the same.
- You appreciate that everyone's perspective is both true and partial, including your own.

The Shadow Module

The shadow is, by definition, what you *hide* from your own awareness. Thus, shadow practice begins with that simple insight: some of your inner world is invisible to you and wants to stay that way!

What is it like to live day to day with that knowledge, in the disposition of a practitioner?

- You begin to live with a gentle ongoing psychological inquiry into your hidden psychodynamics:
  - "Why am I so triggered by that store clerk's minor rudeness?"
  - "Why won't I forgive my spouse's laziness?" And so on.
- It involves humility, trust, curiosity, openness . . . and, ultimately, *humor.*
  - Since all people have this same sneaky hide-and-seek dynamic going on, there's no need to be ashamed!
- What is there for you to notice?
  - "I'm afraid." "I'm hiding from myself and others." "I'm projecting my feelings onto others." It goes on and on, and it usually isn't pretty.
- As shadow work matures, you relax into the discomfort of self-awareness.

- You eventually no longer feel the automatic need to defend yourself against unflattering perceptions.
- You may even begin to welcome the new freedom that uncomfortable new awareness makes possible.
- You realize that self-defense is ultimately even more painful than self-awareness.

The Spirit Module

The everyday practice of meditative awareness involves recognizing the spirit, or Suchness, of every moment and of everything in life. It is a matter of resting in awareness itself, of noticing that no matter what happens, it arises *in awareness*.

- You notice you can relax your tendency to focus exclusively on what is arising and changing.
  - More and more you can rest in awareness itself, which is always *right here*, spacious, uncontracted, and deeply content.
  - You are even aware that *you are this awareness.*
- You recognize that gratitude is your natural, appropriate response to life.
  - The everyday practice of devotion is living in the presence of Spirit, living as one who is intimate with Spirit.
  - Since Spirit appears as everything and everyone, this is the everyday practice of natural, omni-directional communion and loving—a prayerful life.
- You notice you can also *contemplate* whatever arises, recognizing it all as the embodiment of Suchness itself.
  - The natural world can be recognized in its full mystical beauty. So can the elegant abstractions of mathematics. So can the inane excesses of popular culture or the dullest concrete freeways and parking lots.
  - The everyday practice of contemplation involves recognizing it all, seeing through it, and appreciating both its emptiness and its luminosity.

The Ethics Module

Everyday ethics is a sincere private commitment to doing what it takes to grow into a life of full integrity: walking your talk in every area of your life.

Everyday ethics is also expressed in goodwill toward others. As you take care of yourself by living a life of practice, your ability to care for others is liberated and magnified.

The fruit of everyday ethics is humility and deep self-respect, a meaningful and lasting integrity that frees you from living in denial, self-division, and self-contempt.

Everyday ethics can show up in action in many ways:

- You bring your full awareness and care to every present moment, practicing an ethical *sensibility*, instead of ethical rules.
- You begin to look for appropriateness and integrity, instead of merely personal advantage.
- You meet the moral dilemmas of everyday living intending to protect and promote the greatest depth for the greatest span.
- You try not to create new karmas, and try to complete what you can of the old.
- You treat yourself with both masculine and feminine compassion, listening to the voice of conscience without beating yourself up.
- You pay attention to how you can expand the circles of your caring responsibility for yourself, others, and your world.

Practice Tips and Principles

Once you design your ILP, begin doing practices in each of the core modules regularly and engage the everyday practice of expanded awareness. What more could there be?

A lot. There is no paint-by-numbers path to full consciousness. Life, in all its mysterious, tricky richness, seems to insist on offering unique lessons to each individual. To keep growing and practicing, year after year, you must participate, consciously, creatively, and wisely, in countless unique moments of choice. How do you do this fruitfully? There is no formula, but some principles can be detected. Let's consider a few key ideas to keep in mind while navigating the practice life:

Always Practice Discernment

Practice doesn't progress by rote. It progresses intelligently, with understanding. When understanding is present, practice gains traction and moves ahead. Intelligent understanding is a moment-to-moment pratice, sometimes called "discrimination" or "discernment" or "clear seeing."

Daily life calls upon you, again and again, to assess outer situations, people, opportunities, and choices. You must also assess inner feelings, states, sensations, and perceptions. Discrimination is the process of using your highest intelligence to see clearly, to cut through confusion.

Without discernment, sloppiness and misperception are inevitable. At worst, you can fall into *binary thinking*: the tendency to see reality in simplistic yes/no, black/white categories that obscure its authentic complexity and nuance.

Noticing additional perspectives always sharpens the mind. AQAL theory arms you with a set of penetrating distinctions that can aid your practice of discernment. Noticing all quadrants of a person or situation enhances clarity of thought and action, as does sensitivity to various levels of awareness.

The moment-to-moment practice of discernment requires all of your faculties, intelligence, feeling, intuition, and even instinct. It is a living yoga of awareness, always cutting through to clarity, putting you into ever fuller and more nuanced contact with reality.

Take Responsibility

Take responsibility for aligning your choices to higher possibilities. This is the essence of practice.

It is possible to learn to take responsibility for your patterns of thought, emotion, behavior, and relating that express and reinforce *contracted states and patterns.* When you see that attitudes, beliefs, moods, behaviors, or even practical arrangements in your life are not supporting your growth into greater awareness, care, and service, you can look for better options, make new choices, and act on them. One of these choices might be to reevaluate your ILP and commit to deepening it in some way.

This process sometimes shines light in new places. You can see your patterns, and you can take responsibility for them. And sometimes you probably won't. At the beginning, and also throughout life, serious practitioners uncover a hidden deep layer of competing commitments. Individuals don't act in accord with what they believe they want to choose for a good reason: they are *also* committed to something *else*, such as comfort or numbness, or the habit of contraction itself.

In this process, awareness is served. We can see our competing commitments. We can see the results of our past choices. We can see where our current habits tend to lead us. When we're lucky, we find it possible to choose to open into awareness, aliveness, presence, care, and responsibility.

Free Your Energy and Attention

When we live unconsciously, we enact habit patterns that consume a great deal of our energy and attention. This includes patterns of thought, emotion, distraction, fidgeting, eating, talking, and watching or listening to media. These are some of the ways we deplete ourselves instead of conducting life force.

Integral Life Practice gradually builds up our inner muscles. By using these muscles, we can free up and make use of bound energy and attention, making them available for personal effectiveness, practice, and a happier life. This is **masculine compassion** for the self, the self-toughness necessary to choose growth and transformation. Key practice capacities include:

- An ability to tolerate discomfort—both the discomfort of unflattering self-awareness and the discomfort of interrupting unconscious patterns of thought and behavior.
- An interest in taking perspectives—both the perspectives of others and meta-perspectives on our own perspectives.

- An appetite for increased energy and awareness that's stronger than the addiction to habitual consoling behavior.
- An ability to interrupt your unconscious habits and reap a rich harvest of liberated energy and awareness.
- An openness to conducting more and more of the vast force of life, tolerating more and more intensity, instead of compulsively discharging that life force and throwing it off.

Don't Throw Off the Life Force

I'd never done a meditation retreat, and, not realizing what I was signing up for, I signed up for a strict, traditional five-day Zen meditation retreat. We chanted in Japanese. We sat in silence, walked in silence, cleaned the kitchen in silence, and ate in silence hour after hour, day after day.

My back hurt; my legs fell asleep; flies buzzed around me and landed on my neck. It drove me crazy. But anytime I moved or fidgeted, the teacher hit me hard with his stick.

I almost went out of my mind with fury and discomfort. I could not believe I had signed up for such punishment. I hated, positively wanted to kill the teacher. Several times I remember thinking, "If he so much as pauses beside me with that stick again, I'm going to break it over his head and jam the pieces down his throat!"

The dogged, drone-like Zen students around me just kept submitting to mistreatment. I despised them. But somehow, I didn't bolt. I stayed. I kept sitting.

I kept feeling like a volcano was going to erupt inside me. When I felt an almost overwhelming urge to move my body, and I didn't, I would sometimes feel a wave of intensity pass through me that almost made me levitate. I felt so intensely uncomfortable, it was almost like being in an altered state.

But since there was nothing else to do, I did what I'd been told to do. I just sat. I took a breath. I relaxed. I stayed awake in the present moment.

And my state kept changing. Sometimes I felt ecstatic and thought I was getting enlightened. Then I felt horrible again. Then I felt bored. Then I felt like I couldn't stand another minute.

After a few days, I still was feeling all these things, but I was also beginning to feel a sense of amusement as I witnessed it all unfold. I began to feel some love, in the midst of my hate, for the spartan routines of the zendo. It was all utterly ridiculous, empty, perfect, transparent.

By the last day of the retreat, I was full of energy. It felt like I was a thousand-watt bulb, radiating in all directions! And at the same time, I was perfectly still, calm, and clear. I was so deeply at peace, I wasn't perturbed by my own insanity.

I realized that all week, my energy had been concentrated by the forms of the practice. The reason I was so bright and clear was that I hadn't been throwing away energy constantly in my usual ways, by talking or eating or fidgeting. The strict traditional routines were like a brick oven with a tight door, whereas my usual way of living was like an open fire on a windy hilltop.

It was a huge gift, and a turning point. Ever since, when I've put that understanding into practice, it's always shown me the key to ratcheting up my commitment, clarity, and energy.

It's transformed the way I experience discomfort and intensity. They don't drive me crazy anymore. I recognize them as golden opportunities to give my practice an extra edge.

Be Your Own Best Friend

The practice life involves making a choice for your wholeness and health, including the realization of your untapped potential. Thus, it is deeply *self-friendly*, even when it takes on forms of renunciation. This attitude of self-care expresses **feminine compassion** toward the self.

- A natural enjoyment of awareness itself (not unlike the native drive to scale hills and enjoy vistas).

- A grateful affinity for the pleasure inherent in healthy, conscious, embodied human existence, with enjoyment uniting feeling, breath, and awareness.
- A strong inner commitment to lifelong health and growth (often deeply linked to a commitment to serve others).
- Self-forgiveness, the openhearted acceptance of limitations, foibles, and karmas, even as you surrender yourself fully into their healing and transformation.

Resisting Resistance?

Resistance hurts. When we suffer, what we suffer most is our way of *relating to* our experience, rather than the experience itself. We anticipate suffering and tense against experience, destroying our ability to be present. Some pain may be inevitable, but the internal experience of resisting the pain is even worse. But how do you stop?

Awareness is the key. A central and universal aspect of practice is *noticing* resistance—and relaxing into the present moment. Meeting the

Be Tough *and* Gentle with Yourself

Sometimes we need healthy masculine self-discipline, and sometimes we need to shed all armor and nurture ourselves. In some moments, both masculine and feminine compassion apply. We can accept ourselves exactly as we are—even while we cut, gently, into our trance, exercising freedom from unconscious tendencies.

Balancing both masculine and feminine qualities appropriately is not a static ideal, but a dynamic play. Life is a little like whitewater rafting. It presents intense extremes between turbulence and calm, and every shade of middle ground between. It's alive with flowing currents. The art is to stay attuned to the changing needs of each moment.

experience of resistance with genuine curiosity often yields insight into the futility of resisting. When you do this again and again, resistance begins to relax naturally on its own.

But we don't just resist painful experiences. We also resist growth, practice, and new awareness.

It's common to resist your own deepest realizations and commitments. After all, they challenge your habitual patterns. They call you to a higher, but initially more difficult, way of life.

The secret of working with resistance to growth is to choose the middle way. Our first knee-jerk response to our resistance may be to try to be good by bearing down harder and overriding that defiant (or even shameful) unwillingness to change. We resist our resistance. But this *hyper-masculine* strategy doesn't work in the long run. It exaggerates the inner split between "good" and "bad" impulses, driving the unwanted parts of us into shadow. Generally, this results in periods of shame-based but apparently virtuous practice, punctuated by periods of impulsive rebellion, disorientation, and abandonment of practice.

Another response—one based on resigning oneself to the futility of resisting resistance—is to just validate one's feelings and act according to one's strongest impulses in the moment. Since feelings by their nature change constantly, this *hyper-feminine* approach makes for constant drifting without real commitment. We don't feel ashamed and hypocritically divided, but we don't get the benefits of practice either.

So the two most typical responses to resistance are (1) to force our way through it or (2) to go with whatever feelings are present.

The middle way requires staying compassionately related to all our contradictory inclinations. It's important to stay connected to the sober commitment to a lifelong practice. But it's also best to forgive and befriend resistance. Relaxing internalized "shoulds" that create a split between "good" and "bad" parts of the self is both transformative and a great relief. The either/or mentality can yield to a both/and curiosity, making room for spacious awareness in which our integrated choices can unfold naturally. When trying to rigidly enforce good choices, we imagine that we can drag ourselves kicking and screaming to enlightenment. We cannot.

But we can greet our resistance to practice with openness and curiosity. Maybe it will tell us something we need to hear. Sometimes resistance signals unmet needs totally unrelated to our practice commitment. Resistance can be an opportunity for shadow work, greater self-knowledge, and forgiveness. It might be a signal that we need to have more fun or bring balance to our life in some other way. And in the midst of all such specific messages, meeting resistance with spacious awareness always offers a glimpse of the non-problematic and perfect nature of this and every moment of life.

Whatever its message, our resistance will only shout louder if ignored. Yes, it's best to keep practicing, even though we feel resistance. If we face and befriend our resistance, it will most quickly yield its gifts. Then, instead of being *in the way* of our highest intentions, our resistance will *show the way* to them.

Practice Feels Good. And Bad. Feel through It All. And Let Go into It All.

Can you navigate your way through the practice life by becoming sensitive to what opens or closes your head center, heart, and hara? Can you simply become aware of the state of your body-mind and thus discern what is healthy and unhealthy, growth-producing and growth-inhibiting?

It's a reasonable question. Bound energy and attention deadens us or *hurts*. As we grow, we become capable of new vistas of good feeling. We can also experience profound peace, freedom, and even bliss as we more frequently enter into higher and deeper states of awareness. Thus, as you practice and grow, you will feel increasingly free, spacious, and happy, right? Isn't that one of the main reasons we practice in the first place? Shouldn't you be able to tune in to that higher enjoyment and just "grow toward the light," so to speak? Shouldn't you just "follow your bliss"?

Well, yes and no.

Refined sensitivity to what feels best can (very enjoyably) guide and quicken growth into more sublime awareness and experience. So feeling intelligently into the quality of your experience is an essential skill, and moving toward higher pleasures can refine you. But it can result in shallow narcissism too. *Feeling through* what's arising is perhaps even more essential. Remember the importance of tolerating discomfort? Practice requires both capacities, eventually establishing a relationship to pleasure and pain that is both rich and free.

The two most vivid and extreme symbols of transcending pleasure and pain—the wild tantric using alcohol and sex and the ascetic on his bed of nails—are just the opposite faces of the same iconic coin. They are exaggerated symbols of an important reality: the most highly developed practitioners are *free* in the midst of experience—*any* experience. There's no need to test ourselves with extremes of pleasure or pain, but an essential result of practice is a similar paradoxical freedom in the midst of life's cycles of feeling good and bad. Thus, sometimes practice is all about feeling *through* our pleasure and pain, and beyond them.

But not always. The strategy of transcendence easily becomes a form of avoidance. In fact, it's crucial to be able to let go fully into life and pay close, undefended attention to the qualities of your felt experience. An advanced practitioner can *be with* experience, exactly as it is.

And yet that principle isn't *always* primary either.

Practice means staying awake and alive in the multidimensional paradoxical dynamic of life. Good and bad feelings wash through. There's no formula and no immunity. What's the highest, most conscious opportunity available to you in this moment? Is it paying attention to your experience or to the awareness in which it arises, or both? Summoning your best, or surrendering to the flow? Any of these are possible. True practice is to stay alive, conscious, and present: What is happening right now?

Practice draws upon the awareness that the highest good is not the opposite of the bad. *Suchness is*—always already. It includes and transcends all arising phenomena, good or bad. You are always already free in this moment. Nothing is missing. So you always have a completely fresh opportunity to be present, practice, and awaken.

Expect Both Good Days and Bad Days

Brightness and darkness don't stop alternating just because you practice sincerely. In fact, practice itself stirs up both! Because practice creates life changes, it disturbs the status quo of your previous existence. Any system will try to restore its previous balance. Thus, *practice inherently calls up resistance to practice*. Bad days are built into the practice life, unavoidable. And so are good days.

If you practice only on good days, your previous habit patterns will remain strong. Your bad days will keep coming as before. And when your good days come along, and you're ready to practice again, you'll be starting over again near square one.

Alternatively, if you honor your intention to practice during your bad days, your unconscious patterns will weaken. On your good days, choosing to practice will feel most fulfilling and sometimes produce high state experiences or even glimpses of perspectives characterizing higher stages of awareness. However, on your most ordinary days, when nothing seems to be happening, consistent practice is an investment in future openings, a way to make yourself prone to "lucky accidents."

Not only that—bad days give you a prime opportunity to see fast transformational results. Your life and realization reflect the whole mix of your awareness and behavior—in good moments, bad moments, and those in-between. If you do better when it's hardest, the averages will soar. Developing to a whole new level of consciousness may take time. But operating more consistently at your best requires only clarity, willingness, and consistency. That can happen very quickly—and without delay it will transform how others experience you and how you experience yourself. This is one of the key ways that people see big changes in the first weeks and months of taking up a life of practice.

Missing a practice here and there need not be made into a big deal. Forgiveness is a given, and so is a fresh start. You can always choose to practice in the next moment, without regrets or self-recrimination.

At the same time, it's not efficient to abandon your practice. It wastes precious time and alienates you from important resources. Plus, it reinforces your tendency to abandon practice, so it doesn't strengthen your resilience to deal well with future challenges.

Every moment in the up-and-down phasing of your practice life offers you a valuable leverage point. A secret in the game of practice is that practice builds momentum and efficiency. Just playing the game—and staying in it consistently—magnifies the effects of each ounce of intention and effort you put into your practice.

- Practicing on good days boosts your peak experiences.
- Practicing on bad days transforms your lows and brings up your overall level of functioning.
- Practicing patiently at the plateau (when not much seems to be happening) plants the seeds of your next breakthrough.
- Abandoning practice wastes time and reinforces the wrong impulses.
- Staying in the game is far easier and more efficient than going in and out.

Don't Waste Time Beating Yourself Up

In all practice, efficiency is key. If you learn your lessons and act on them, growth progresses quickly. If you don't, it won't.

Obstacles to efficiency include such things as struggle with oneself, neurotic self-preoccupation, non-acceptance of what's already happened, blame, guilt, and obsession with the stories of one's difficult life, or the stories of one's family, group, or nation. Time spent struggling with oneself, especially in the vicious recycling of negative thoughts, attitudes, and feelings, binds energy and attention and impedes growth. Some of these things may be inevitable and abruptly trying to cut them off will only complicate things, but they need not be prolonged.

Practice *by its nature* brings unskillful unconscious patterns into view. Waste as little time as possible regretting or justifying them. When you see that you've been blindly self-possessed, and that you've wasted valuable time and created suffering in others and yourself, and you feel disgusted and ashamed—that's great! You don't have to defend, remedy, or explain it. Appreciate and welcome this precious awareness. It brings the opportunity to make a new and different choice in the next moment. Focus on that. Practice is making good use of such unflattering self-awareness, again and again, not resisting it.

In some moments, this comes naturally. In others, it can be tremendously difficult. It's hard to violate and abandon your ingrained habits. It takes grit, while wallowing, to get up and refuse to become bogged down again. Even those who practice fiercely in many areas of life usually have blind spots where they can flounder.

It's important to know that in forgiving your past mistakes and focusing on free, right action, you are doing something important. You are changing your luck, creating a better future. You are taking responsibility for the one part of the universe for which no one else can.

The best way to relate to what you want to leave behind is not to engage it. Even so, you may get tripped up into opposing it. Drop it, if you can, in mid-sentence, *as soon as* you see it. You don't need to find a good stopping place.

In any moment when you notice that circumstances, within or without, have shaken your practice intention, attend quickly to the business at hand: right action. Right action means healthy, regenerative, compassionate, constructive, effective, efficient participation in life. It includes both subjectivity and behavior. Show up, make the best choices you can, and embody them as well as possible in your actions, thoughts, and feelings.

Without avoiding responsibility for past mistakes, accept that they cannot be changed. Choose to show up in life *in the next moment* as wisely, courageously, and fully as you can. No circumstance, no past mistake, can take away this opportunity. No matter how challenging a hand you were dealt, or how poorly you played it up until this moment, you can play your current cards intelligently and honorably—starting, always, right now.

Keep It Simple

The essence of efficient practice is simple: in the moment you notice unskillful, unhappy life patterns, **honor your intention to practice**. That's all. Accept and let go of the past; enter into the next moment as a practitioner. Use this moment to relax the tendency to contract, and engage in the next moment with intelligence, compassion, and courage.

This opportunity is available in any moment. It applies even if you have completely abandoned your practice for years on end. The best thing to do is to return to practicing. In the moment when you realize that you blew it, and that you'd really rather live a life of practice, it's best to *just do it*. You don't need to first grieve your errors, be forgiven, or figure out how to do better next time.

Unlearn Resentment

The attitude of resentment must have been pretty deeply ingrained, because I must have had to shift my attention a hundred times before it got any easier.

I remember the day I first got the message. I was working a summer job making lattes, espressos, and cappuccinos. I hated that job. But I had been reading about practice and the attitude of service, and it came to me in a jolt. I realized that I had a perfect circumstance for practice, even though it was in the midst of a job I hated.

So I just started interrupting my habitual inner dialog of complaint. Anytime I noticed myself becoming even subtly resentful, I just took a breath and relaxed my heart and belly, and brought some extra sincerity to serving people.

At first, it was really hard. I was underpaid and overworked and disrespected. A few of my co-workers were putting out as little as possible, happy for me to pick up the slack. Sometimes they were even unkind. I had a lot of good excuses for becoming resentful.

That was the great thing about the job. I was serving people all day long. Some of them were lovely. Some were pushy, rude, lazy, mean, or unhappy. Each one gave me a unique opportunity to practice, learn, and grow.

And even after I started practicing, for all my good intentions, I was still mostly resentful. I felt like I kept lifting a loaded barbell as I took a breath, smiled, and did my best to open my heart to the next person.

But I kept faking it, and after a while it wasn't so fake anymore. I felt like I kept leaving my unhappiness behind. Again and again, I chose something else. And I found that, even in something as simple and humble as serving coffees, it is inherently satisfying to serve others.

Really, all of life is service, if you think about it. I became a bit happier as I persisted. And after a few days, I began to feel really wonderful.

I actually came to love that job. And it was a turning point. I learned something that's never left me: it's not smart to wait for my mood to change; the big benefits come from cutting through my bad mood, through action, whenever I get the chance.

Great practitioners fiercely minimize wasted time. They might be besieged by demons of doubt or fear, but once they regain awareness of their option to choose practice, they act on it without delay. They minimize their suffering by accepting it fully and moving straight through. In some traditions it is said that this very capacity marks the difference between those whose practice requires many lifetimes and those who wake up in this life.

To the degree that this has not been your habit, don't worry. You can build it. To the extent that you have contradictory habits, it's fine. You can release them, piece by piece. If you learn to keep honoring your intention to practice, and if you act on that intention with stable commitment, you will speed your conscious evolution and save yourself years of unnecessary suffering. And whatever suffering is necessary will immediately be given more dignity and hope.

Integrate Your Practice

As practice matures, it becomes a more continuous, integrated flow. Though it may begin as a trickle, it will gradually gather more momentum and carve deeper pathways in the terrain of your being. A new level of functioning becomes possible, as your Body, Mind, Spirit, Shadow, and other practice modules more fully complement, inform, and amplify each other—all in the midst of living an ethical life, as best you can.

The individual modules and practices can be experienced as aspects of a single multi-dimensional awareness and commitment. And yet each practice has a distinct personality. In fact, very specific specialized practices (like martial arts, yoga, nature mysticism, child rearing, or meaningful work) can become especially transformative by being Integrally articulated throughout all modules. This points to the ineffable nature of the *art* of practice.

Practice and the Fast Pace of a Busy Life

Many of us live extremely busy lives, balancing multiple diverse responsibilities, relationships, roles, and recreations. Busy people often tend to say yes to positive options and to act on them. That's exactly how many busy people take on new practices. They pack another hour of commitments into their over-committed lives. This often works fine, because regular practice can dramatically upgrade both happiness and effectiveness. But practice does not have to add to your time pressure.

Even though hard work and high output are wonderful, each of us also needs rest. We all need life balance even though each of us has unique needs. Adding more and more good things to your life can overload you, turning many of them sour. As we practice, we grow in our sensitivity to our limits and to our life balance. We become more serious about gracefully managing our commitments. It is great to live an active, creative, and dynamic life, but not a frenetic, narrow, overcommitted one.

There's no one-size-fits-all prescription for dealing with our busy postmodern world. The fruits of diligent practice may lead you to simplify your ILP, to make more active use of the 1-Minute Modules, or to cut back on other commitments. However, you may also learn how to thrive on chaos, flowing more freely through the wild ride of life, being energized by the rough and tumble instead of bracing against it. ILP will naturally appear as a very calm way of life in some individuals, and it will show up as a high level of happy dynamism in others.

Whatever Your Age, Make Hay While the Sun Shines

You can emerge into a new identity, a new way of being in the world, at any age. But typically, it doesn't happen as often during the years in which people are first establishing their careers and families. Rapid evolution, including major reconfigurations of our identity, often takes place usually before people reach their mid-thirties and when they approach elderhood, usually not before their mid-forties. A key secret of practice is to "make hay while the sun shines." When doorways to growth open, a secret of practice is to seize the moment and step through the threshold.

Let Love Open the Door

Love—in its simplest and most profound mysteriousness—is the open secret of authentic practitioners—a remarkably powerful way to make your Integral practice *more* Integral.

When you love, your subtle body opens into its native radiance. Your natural happiness shines. Your head, heart, and hara relax and synchronize. You feel more connected to yourself, to others, to existence itself. You're alive to the present moment. Your breathing is full of pleasure and feeling. You're not afraid to face anything.

Love facilitates and integrates—and transcends—practice in all the key ILP modules. Any practice done with love is exponentially more powerful than one done out of mere obligation or self-seeking. You can meditate with love, do yoga with love, cook healthy meals with love—the attitude of love will infuse any activity with the scent of divinity.

Whom or what does one love? It could be anyone or anything. Ultimately, it's everything and everyone, and nothing, no one in particular. It's not really any "other," but rather Suchness itself. Your Beloved is visible everywhere to the eyes of the heart.

Such universal love is the most natural thing in the world, not something you have to force or *try* to do. It's something you are already doing—or yearning to do and be and live. It's the true identity of every object of desire, the essence of every natural pleasure. When you recognize the omnipresent Beloved, it's like falling in love, returning to your deepest love, dwelling in a love that is always already, even if it has sometimes been so covered over that it's been hard to see.

Love is a choice, as much as a feeling. Sometimes you act on that choice while feeling dry inside. Because love is such a deeply natural orientation for all people, real love usually eventually breaks through and replaces effortful attempts at loving.

But love doesn't always come easy. When your heart closes, it can seem impossible to open and love. Usually, the most effective first step is a small and simple one. Find something to appreciate. It can be as simple and basic as food, clothing, or shelter—or a practice. In every moment, even until death, you have much to appreciate. Just notice what's there. In fact, this is a powerful devotional practice: paying attention not to how you look but to how you see. Love can see the forms of Spirit that are always before your eyes. Appreciation softens and opens the closure of the heart.

Once that occurs, especially if you practice, appreciation can grow into *gratitude*. A tiny breeze of gratitude can blow open the wide doors of the heart.

Remember, love is thus an *inherent aspect of spiritual reality*. It's not squishy, ungrounded, or sappy; it's real. And the devotion that sprouts out of love is a natural, healthy, accurate, and *appropriate* response to the human condition.

Allow Paradox to Expand You

A core Integral skill is the capacity to hold paradox and thereby to discover new depth. Many profound paradoxes must be confronted in the process of any life of practice. These paradoxes are not riddles we must seek to answer, but koans with which we live, questions we contemplate and allow to instruct us.

Here are five deep paradoxes worth considering:

1. Seeking
   * Reality is always already completely present.
   * Nothing real can be sought or attained.
   * Therefore I dedicate myself to sincere practice.
2. Life and Death
   * I practice to enhance my health, happiness, and awareness in a mortal body-mind that will inevitably change and die.
   * Thus, in my heart I keep saying a quiet yes to my inevitable death.
   * And yet at the same time, my whole being keeps saying a loud yes! to life.
3. Serving Others
   * Ultimately, there is no such thing as an "other."
   * No separate beings exist to serve and liberate.

- Therefore, I dedicate myself to the well-being and liberation of all sentient beings.

4. Commitment / Surrender
   - I embrace an utterly serious commitment to effective practice and service.
   - I humorously relax and surrender all attachment to outcomes.

5. Bliss / Compassion
   - I practice inspired by One Taste or Suchness, limitless love, freedom, and bliss.
   - I practice inspired by One Taste—limitless compassion, the willingness to feel everything, including all the pain and suffering of the world.
   - There is only One Taste—amidst and as the endless play of pain and pleasure, ecstasy and agony.

Seasons and Phases in the Practice Life

Practice takes time. And over time, as you engage practice, certain phases often unfold organically. A series of different "seasons" will appear, quite possibly in a sequence very similar to what follows. Since the dynamics of spiritual growth are complex, combining several kinds of development and maturation, individual experience varies.

Amidst the variety, however, many of the opportunities, challenges, and changing "weather conditions" of the practice life described here will arrive for you, sooner or later, if you continue to walk the path over years and decades.

The Honeymoon

At first, and usually for a period of at least several years, practice involves the process of establishing a new orientation in life, breaking old habits, and establishing new and conscious routines. This requires fierce discipline, but it liberates a tremendous amount of energy and awareness.

This is not to say that the road always begins smoothly. It's different for everyone. And each new moment is unique. But even though there may be good and bad phases, internal struggles, and episodes of resistance or self-indulgence, you're working a juicy transition. If you keep returning to practice, you gradually see big changes. Your life and consciousness shift—they're uplifted, refined, and clarified.

These early years are often a very enjoyable (even if also quite demanding) phase of practice—an invigorating and revelatory period of new clarity and choice, and a time of establishing a healthy new lifestyle and enjoying a more conscious existence.

The Plateau and Falling from Grace

After a time, most practitioners hit a plateau. Everyday awareness will have expanded to a new level and stabilized. The regularity of daily practice will have become second nature. The sense of discovery and revelation recedes. One's awareness is greater than before, but not changing as rapidly as it used to. There's less of a sense of excitement.

This can be a dangerous phase. At this point some practitioners, unaware that they had become addicted to the experience of expansion, begin to feel like their practices aren't working anymore. So they falter in their discipline. A few skipped days don't seem to exact a very high price, so the missed days accumulate. People sometimes abandon important practices or begin seeking extreme experiences in order to regain the highs of their honeymoon phase.

The practice life can slip away for weeks, months, or years at a time. Sometimes practitioners even feel like they've "fallen from grace." But grace, which can be tough, is also endlessly forgiving. So even this is of course just another occasion for awareness and maturation. Even the most reactive episodes and time spent slacking off in despair become lessons that naturally fold back into the life of deepening awareness and growth.

After all, the practice life is never any further away than your next moment of waking up into greater awareness and care—or the next occasion of sitting in meditation, working out, or consciously spending time with a loved one.

For many years, most practitioners keep learning the wisdom of returning to the fundamentals. They keep discovering the false lure of thinking they were ready, prematurely, to graduate to a higher, freer relationship to practice and spirit. For the most part, when their discipline weakens, so does their practice. Then they go back to the basics and it strengthens again.

The secret of realization is to sustain dedication to regular practice during the plateaus, which can last for many years. Superficial motivations toward the pleasure and reassurance of high experiences give way to deeper motivations to participate more fully, consciously, and responsibly in the full spectrum of life's bittersweet and mysterious totality. Maturity develops by consistently renewing one's practice, diligently, especially when it's least "sexy."

The Fruits

And then, entirely independent of all seeking strategies, there are graceful openings. Meditation deepens and becomes blissful and profound in unexpected ways. New, free capacities bloom; elegant and generous new possibilities and options almost magically appear. Awareness effortlessly expands. Qualities of love and devotion come forth spontaneously in even the most ordinary moments of life. There even may be the "happy accidents" of kensho and satori—of mini-enlightenments and not-so-mini-enlightenments! When this happens, everything is suddenly different. We find ourselves in a freer relationship to practice after all. Life and the world are transformed entirely. Such fruits and blessings of practice, ironically, become tests and lessons that stimulate another kind of growth. There's a strong tendency to feel like we own our graceful openings. We worked hard and now we're seeing results. We're gratified. Proud. Identified. Attached. And, inevitably, full of it!

It is virtually impossible to avoid all spiritual materialism. So you get to learn the lesson that identifying with attainment blocks growth. Only re-applying yourself to practice, humbly and directly, works. Only practice makes you "lucky," prone to the happy accidents of insight and awakening. And so you grow.

Periodically, new awareness dawns in a way that illuminates something that was previously shaping your participation in life. Who and how your awareness showed up (*the subject*) in the previous stage becomes an *object* of awareness. This is a new *stage* of participation.

As practitioners mature, transitions organically unfold, opening up new awareness, depth, and options. From the interior, some of these transitions are gradual and mostly invisible, whereas others unfold more dramatically—sometimes in ways that seem similar to the classic hero's journey.

The Dark Night

At a certain point (generally after years of dedicated practice) your practice life may seem to fall apart. Even God may seem to have abandoned you. You may lose all motivation, no longer able to believe that practice is going to get you anywhere. Awareness of the underlying selfish motives for practice may become so acute that you despair of the whole enterprise. You may find yourself helplessly dropping out of the whole game of transformation. All your motives and efforts have begun to rot.

You may discover that something essential is actually *dying*. The awful aloneness and sense of limitation that you may have hoped to escape through practice has now engulfed you (often, when your life otherwise seems to be going quite well!). Despair is inescapable: your aspiration to infinity will never succeed. You are going through a kind of death, one you cannot escape.

Congratulations. This defeat is the doorway to profound freedom. It's no consolation to the one who is dying, of course. But on the other side of this death is a rebirth. Once your practice fails conclusively, you will discover that it has succeeded. Instead of expanding consciousness, it is now exploding it—popping the whole balloon!

In a lifetime of practice, there may be a number of deaths (and rebirths!). Consciousness survives them all, and practice is resurrected, transformed in the process. What would earlier have been the abandonment of practice is now a radical surrender beyond any consoling identity or effort. You've rotted, fallen, dropped from every pose and pretense into your irreducible humanity, undistracted and unconsoled. You can't do practice in the same way anymore; now it's as though practice is "doing" you.

Responsibility

As practice continues to deepen, it becomes increasingly obvious that your current internal weather conditions, whether they feel good or bad, will pass soon enough. You naturally find yourself paying attention more stably to the One Thing that never changes.

And you find yourself doing the one thing that's always appropriate: sincerely relaxing beyond unconscious tendencies and bringing care and awareness to your world and relations—in every moment of daily living. You've landed on the only ground from which you never fall—responsibility for awareness, care, and presence—for practice itself. In a way, you're in love and faithful. Such responsibility is indistinguishable from surrender. It is a stability that rests in a ground deeper than all holding on and letting go.

This phase of responsibility contains all the previous phases—honeymoon, plateau, falling from grace, fruits, dark night, and all—flowing together in a stability that's by no means a homogenous gray. On the basis of such stable and trustworthy responsibility, the fruits of practice may even gracefully deepen—perhaps becoming the liberating illuminations described in our ancient spiritual traditions. Eventually, when openings occur, you just enjoy them without attaching undue significance. It's like a change in the weather. Some days are overcast, other days are clear, but the sun is always shining. Consciousness will change, cycle, stabilize, expand, dissolve, and resurrect. Everything will be different, but just exactly as it always was.

> *First there is a mountain.*
> *Then there is no mountain.*
> *At last, there is only a mountain, just like there always already was, right from the beginning. And it couldn't be more obvious.*

The Unique Self

Right now—no matter what you're experiencing, thinking, feeling, hearing, and seeing—where is it all arising?

It is arising *in* the awareness you truly are—the Universal Self.

The core of the "I" is the silent, still Witness, unchanging and deathless. This "I of the I" is the most universal and essential dimension of who you are and of every individual identity.

The Truth of the Universal Self Is Not the Only Truth

The ultimate truth about identity coexists with another, relative, truth—the uniqueness of each person, place, thing, system, and moment in time.

Every body-mind is shaped by a unique confluence of historical, genetic, familial, social, cultural, psychological, and energetic circumstances. But our uniqueness is not just something that happens *to* us from without.

Any parent of multiple offspring will attest that each of their children is a unique individual, whose character was always individual and particular, not just shaped externally by accidents of birth order, injury, and the changing dynamics of the family's experience. Parents come to know and love unique individuals, who are first themselves, and not primarily or essentially extensions of their genes, parents, or family legacies.

Thus, you are not *only* pure Awareness. You are also a uniquely constituted and very particular refraction of universal light, a unique flavor of universal consciousness, a uniquely shaped embodiment of universal awareness and passionate life energy.

The Goal of Practice Is Not to Disappear

The most awakened saints and sages are not bland and homogenous beings. They are very much themselves, at home in their bodies and in their uniqueness. Their personality is a vehicle for their transparency to the impersonal. They inhabit a particular locus in space-time, and they accept that destiny. They are not ashamed of their uniqueness. They don't shrink from their responsibility to manifest the energy and consciousness that they are. In fact, they know they can only do so in a way that reflects the particular limits of their body-mind, personality, and history.

The transpersonal manifests most fully through the personal. Thus, to awaken to the transcendental, we do not have to put ourselves through a process of erasing our uniqueness.

In fact, it is quite the opposite. We do have to accept and forgive ourselves for being the unique, sometimes awkward, sometimes graceful, cartoon character that we each seem to be. We have to forgive our rough edges, past traumas, and neurotic patterns.

When self-acceptance is full and natural, our quirks distract us less, and the universal shines through, more brightly. Our uniqueness need not be viewed as a sign of the most constricted aspects of the self that are sometimes negatively associated with ego. Our uniqueness is just the way that ever-present is-ness chooses to manifest as us.

Free individuals may purify their limited patterns when appropriate, but they don't let themselves get hung up. They let the universal essence shine through their particularity and uniqueness, including the aspects that sometimes seem goofy, quirky, or weak. They accept themselves and thereby conduct the love, light, and consciousness of spirit *most fully*.

The most awake practitioners don't try to disappear. Instead, they let themselves be a uniquely flavored conduit for the universal conscious force of life.

Unfolding the Soul

Discovering, unfolding, and manifesting your uniqueness involves a profound journey into your personal unknown. This is the work of the **Soul module.**

Soul work is not equivalent to shadow work because it concerns an entirely different category of shadow—not into what was *repressed*, but into what is just barely *emergent*. It is not equivalent to the work of the Spirit module because it awakens downward into the personal and particular rather than waking up into Suchness.

Nonetheless soul work connects and integrates with both shadow and spirit. You may find your own process naturally integrating all these modules. Sometimes awakening into radical freedom cannot be separated from a simultaneous awakening into deep dimensions of your own unique embodied individuality. But being a person isn't easy. We resist it. So that's where soul work starts.

You Can Only Play the Cards You're Dealt

Life is sometimes compared to a game of cards. Each individual holds a unique hand. Our responsibility is to accept the cards we were dealt, and to play them as well as we can.

To do this we have to forgive the bad cards we hold. We may wish we held different cards, but if we have been given an alcoholic parent, acne, a family legacy of shame and non-communication, a squeaky voice, or a tendency toward being overweight, that's just what is.

We also may have been dealt a hand that contains especially difficult cards that affect large groups of people—being born into a persecuted minority group or during a time or place affected by war, disease, poverty, political or ethnic oppression, or environmental toxicity. These cards are hardly unique to our hand, and yet they can exert powerful shaping effects on our options. *Even then*, they affect each person's hand in a unique way. They also present complex challenges (and opportunities) for individual choice and creativity.

No matter what—*if we don't accept every card in our hand, we can't play our best.* We'll be compromised by guilt, resentment, or self-hatred. The deep game is not about being dealt a better hand, but about playing the cards we're dealt with as much intelligence, care, and creativity as we possibly can.

People born with handicaps sometimes face diminished possibilities with a courage and spirit and creativity that ennobles everyone who comes into contact with them. People born with beauty, privilege, wealth, and fame sometimes make poor use of all their advantages, diminishing themselves and those around them.

The first step is to forgive the cards in your hands. Open your heart to the quirky, noble, tragic, comic human idiosyncrasies of the character that shows up as you. Be willing to live the life you were given. As that acceptance takes root, you can wholeheartedly and authentically engage the unique—and perfect—opportunity of your birth.

We Keep Arriving in the World, Stage by Stage

As a child develops, his or her uniqueness unfolds. More and more of our uniqueness emerges as we grow from childhood through adolescence and into adulthood. The process continues in adulthood as we develop into higher stages of awareness.*

We are always more fully incarnating ourselves. We emerge both as the universal awareness or Self that we truly are and as the very particular unique self that we also really are. So we're always discovering new dimensions of who we are, and sometimes they're surprising.

At critical junctures, we have the opportunity to catch a particularly revealing glimpse of how our fuller self can next unfold. Then, we can more easily see and step into the noble and quirky role we were each uniquely born to play.

There Is Much More to You Than You Know

The process of fully inhabiting yourself takes in countless forms, both linear and nonlinear.

It can be valuable to take a direct, intentional, and intuitive look at who you are in the process of becoming and to make choices that support what's emerging. For example, if your leadership capacities seem ready to manifest, you can accept a promotion or apply for a new job.

It can also be profoundly catalytic to open to your unknown future through deeper psychic processes. Sometimes you catch a glimpse of

---

*This applies to both high state-stages (such as causal and nondual awakenings) and to high structure-stages (such as Indigo and Ultraviolet).

who you're becoming just through seeing what bubbles up through your deep subconscious in the form of synchronicities, dreams, images, and intuitive connections.

Often, this nonlinear aspect of practice and growth feels like a mystical journey. It is a big part of how life unfolds its greatest fulfillment and service to others. The voyage can be deeply gratifying and even joyous, and yet it is also long and demanding.

As we engage this journey, we find our unique way of belonging to our world. We come into possession of the unique gift we are able to give others. We recover a deeper sense of personal meaning. We get in touch with how we can contribute to life. We land more fully in our bodies and communities and world.

Such practice will eventually free up a vast amount of energy and attention. Arriving in yourself ever more fully is good, beautiful, and true. It catalyzes you to live your greatness and to fulfill your life's purpose. Service becomes self-actualization. As the Protestant theologian Frederick Buechner put it, you discover the place "where your deep gladness and the world's hunger meet."

The Courage to Be Born

Practice requires courage, because, like birth or death, it is a transformative ordeal. If we persist, it will eventually destroy us as it redefines our personal identity. Real evolution is both wonderful and terrible.

Although we long to discover and fulfill our life purpose, we are also afraid of finding what we're looking for. We don't want it to shake us up too much. We fear threats to our familiar and secure ways of relating to life. We probably already suspected the truth—that growing to fulfill our total potential would be harrowing.

Yet we have no choice if we don't want to be imprisoned in an identity that is too small for us. Eventually we must venture forth. We must leave what is familiar, sacrifice our sense of security, and endure a life-or-death journey. We must endure the cold seasons that temper and strengthen our souls, as well as the hot seasons that forge the alloy at our core.

Thus, crucial passages in this journey must be traveled alone, sometimes in extreme discomfort, with no assurance of safety. They require us to find new grit, endurance, commitment, and creativity. Though not fulfilling in a conventional way, the practice journey is real—and profoundly alive.

We are the ones who must set out on this journey, but it's one from which we can never return. If we're lucky, it will be completed by someone who transcends and includes all that we are, by someone greater than we are, and yet is utterly and authentically our very self. The journey can be completed only by the uncompromised human being we each have the unique potential to become.

To Find Your Calling, You Must Heed the Calls

Life will sometimes send you signals. Part of the growth process involves learning to notice them. If you keep finding yourself involved in the same dynamic at work or in relationship, it's wise to pay attention. You may be getting a call to learn deep and important lessons. Recurring dreams may hold hidden messages. Strange coincidences may point the way to unexpected doorways into important new terrain. Words or music that resonate particularly deeply and stay with you may be hints. These signposts may help you clarify a key choice or point to a dimension of your being that needs to come forward.

Sometimes the call confronts you more forcefully, requiring you to reevaluate the meaning and direction of your life. You may lose your job or relationship. Conversely, you may receive an important and unexpected job offer or another positive life-changing opportunity. Deaths or accidents can change the course of our lives. But so can a love affair or a sudden windfall.

Be Still and Listen

You can cultivate awareness as a practice by deliberately opening to the emerging unknown. This practice can include any and all the ways you come to know yourself. It begins with curiosity about the kind of illumination that can organically emerge from darkness. Methods for tapping into your soul's unknown range from depth psychotherapy to exploration of subtle experiences to creative artistic exploration to journaling.

It takes intelligent, intuitive discrimination to become alert to important clues bubbling up from your subconscious. At first, this new information might speak in a still, small voice. You may notice apparently irrational urgings that lead your life in totally unexpected new directions. Symbols may emerge from meditation or dreams that suggest a different kind of work, role, or identity through which to give your unique treasures to your community.

To Hear Your Call Brings Responsibility

All you can do is pay attention and be willing to heed the call when life speaks to you. But noticing life's signals also requires the discriminative intelligence to avoid falling into superstitious credulity that naively attributes significance too easily.

Nonetheless, if you pay attention, you will be shown where you need to go. Life may move you through a whole series of experiences, each of which progressively clarifies something new about who you are and what your unique contributions will be.

Some of these lessons can be brutal. Others are exquisitely graceful. Each unique instruction prepares you in a special way for what is to come. All your experiences play a part in shaping the unique form of your contribution to your community and Kosmos.

As your unique service becomes clear to you, you have no choice but to fulfill it. Eventually, it can seem as though all your moves are dictated by the needs of the world around you. You become free, but not free to do *what you want* (as if life were a smorgasbord and you were its hungry consumer). You become liberated to do *what you must* (as if you were a faithful servant, called into battle by a wise master).

Keep the Channel Open

There is a vitality, a life force, an energy, a quickening that is translated through you into action, and because there is only one of you in all of time, this expression is unique. And if you block it, it will never exist through any other medium, and it will be lost. The world will not have it. It is not your business to determine how good it is, or how valuable, or how it compares with other expressions. It is your business to keep it yours clearly and directly, to keep the channel open.

— Martha Graham as quoted by Agnes DeMille in *Martha: The Life and Work of Martha Graham* (New York: Random House, 1991).

With Practice, All Things Come. Uniquely.

It is said that grace and blessings are indistinguishable from good luck. And the more we practice, the luckier we get. We make our luck by continually bringing ourselves forward into the process of practice.

We make our luck by doing our practices each day. We make our luck by bringing awareness and care to every moment of our lives. We make our luck by listening to life and learning the lessons it provides.

As we persist in the life of practice, even in the midst of misfortunes and reversals, we lay the foundation for a more graceful existence.

As this happens, our lives flow more naturally, with less effort. More of us arrives here in this body, this life, this world. Our whole being comes together more fully, better able to participate in the events of life. We become able to give more of ourselves to others, and thus we receive more. More life flows from us, and it naturally follows that more life flows through us and into us as well.

As we surrender into our unique and particular expression, the universal energy and consciousness of life can embody itself through us more fully, with less obstruction.

As our unique self incarnates more completely, we find ourselves conducting the infinite and universal energy and consciousness of life in the way that only we can. Our unique voice makes its special contribution to the Kosmic symphony more purely, more loudly, more distinctly.

Uniquely Universal

What is the satisfaction of completing this journey? If so much of us gets burned off in the process, who is it that gets to enjoy becoming the unique you?

Who is it that gets the satisfaction of self-actualization, of incarnating your purpose, of giving your special gifts to the world? Who experiences the victory that comes with the fulfillment of a long ordeal of practice and emergence?

Who is it that wonders about these things? In whose awareness do these questions and ordeals and practices arise? In whose awareness is the duty done? In whose awareness is the humor enjoyed?

It is the same universal Suchness you were all along, from the beginning. In the fulfillment of your journey, you are liberated to be the
one you always already were—with nothing attained that wasn't the case
all along.

So why did you bother?

Looking back, it is all so obvious. It was clearly inevitable, and arbi-
trary. Looking back, there is only pure gratitude for every step you took.
Looking back, there is only freedom, utter freedom, to be the pure awareness you were all along.

Now you are finally free to be the Freedom you've been from the beginning. "Just this" is the ultimate reward that comes from inhabiting the
particular cartoon character you drew from this Kosmic deck of cards.

INDEX

Page numbers for definitions are in boldface.

ABOUT THE AUTHORS

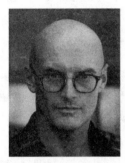

KEN WILBER, the developer of an integral "theory of everything" that embraces the truths of all the world's great psychological, scientific, philosophical, and spiritual traditions, is the author of over twenty books, including *No Boundary, Grace and Grit*, and *A Brief History of Everything*. He is the founder of Integral Institute, a think-tank for studying issues of science and society, with outreach through local and online communities such as Integral Naked, Integral Education Network, and Integral Spiritual Center. His personal website is www.kenwilber.com.

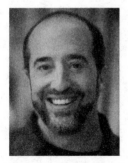

TERRY PATTEN has been walking the path for over thirty years. As a seminar leader, coach, theorist, and practitioner, he was a key member of the team that developed Integral Life Practice with Ken Wilber. Previously he was the founder and guiding spirit behind the consciousness technology catalog *Tools for Exploration*. The author of four books, Patten has guided hundreds of people in discovering and deepening their practice and in actualizing their higher potentials. He lives in San Rafael, California, where he works as a coach, consultant, writer, teacher, entrepreneur, and grassroots conservationist. His personal website is www.integralheart.com.

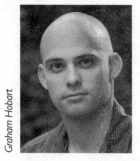

Graham Hobart

ADAM B. LEONARD is an educator, business consultant, author, entrepreneur, adventurer, and, of course, ILP practitioner. He was originally trained as a Foreign Service officer at Georgetown University and went on to pioneer the discipline of integral communication in graduate school. Adam specializes in applying the integral approach to individual, team, and organizational development. He has led ILP groups at several educational institutions. Adam co-authored the *Integral Life Practice Starter Kit* (Integral Institute, 2005) and *The Integral Operating System* (Sounds True, 2005), in addition to co-editing *The Simple Feeling of Being* (Shambhala, 2004). His personal website is www.adambleonard.com.

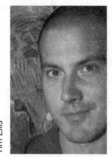

Tim Ellis

MARCO MORELLI is a freelance scholar, writer, and poet. He was a member of the start-up team that launched Integral Naked, along with many other groundbreaking projects at Integral Institute. He served as creative director for Ken Wilber's book *The Integral Vision* (Shambhala, 2007). His previous books include *Rubén's Orphans: Anthology of Contemporary Nicaraguan Poetry, Mirrors In Love,* and *The Joy of Nihilism & Other Poems.* His personal website and blog can be found at www.MADRUSH.cc.

For more information about Integral Life Practice, visit
www.Integral-Life-Practice.com.